EPILEPSY

ITS PHENOMENA IN MAN

UCLA FORUM IN MEDICAL SCIENCES

UCLA FORUM IN MEDICAL SCIENCES
NUMBER 17

EPILEPSY

ITS PHENOMENA IN MAN

Edited by

MARY A. B. BRAZIER

BRAIN RESEARCH INSTITUTE
UNIVERSITY OF CALIFORNIA
LOS ANGELES, CALIFORNIA

ACADEMIC PRESS New York and London 1973

A Subsidiary of Harcourt Brace Jovanovich, Publishers

ACADEMIC PRESS, INC.
111 Fifth Avenue, New York, New York 10003

United Kingdom Edition published by
ACADEMIC PRESS, INC. (LONDON) LTD.
24/28 Oval Road, London NW1

Library of Congress Cataloging in Publication Data
Main entry under title:

Epilepsy: its phenomena in man

(UCLA forum in medical sciences, v. 17)
        Six of the 16 papers were presented at the
Symposium on Electrophysiological Processes in the
Epilepsies, held during the alumni reunion of the
Brain Research Institute, University of California,
Los Angeles, in July 1972.
        Includes bibliographies.
        1.   Epilepsy—Congresses.   I.   Brazier, Mary
Agnes Burniston, Date   ed.   II.   Symposium on
Electrophysiological Processes in the Epilepsies,
University of California, Los Angeles, 1972.
III.   California. University. University at
Los Angeles. Brain Research Institute.   IV. Series.
RC373.E64   616.8′53   73-2060
ISBN 0–12–128650–9

PRINTED IN THE UNITED STATES OF AMERICA

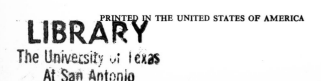

CONTENTS

* A participant in the Alumni Reunion of the Brain Research Institute, 1972.

* A participant in the Alumni Reunion of the Brain Research Institute, 1972.

CONTENTS

* A participant in the Alumni Reunion of the Brain Research Institute, 1972.

STRUCTURAL SUBSTRATES OF SEIZURE FOCI IN THE HUMAN
TEMPORAL LOBE

(A COMBINED ELECTROPHYSIOLOGICAL OPTICAL MICROSCOPIC AND
ULTRASTRUCTURAL STUDY)

W. Jann Brown

CONTRIBUTORS TO THIS VOLUME

C. Ajmone Marsan, National Institute of Neurological Diseases and Stroke, Building 10/4N262, National Institutes of Health, Bethesda, Maryland 20014

J. Bancaud, Hôpital Sainte Anne, 1 Rue Cabanis, Paris 14, France

Mary A. B. Brazier, Brain Research Institute, University of California, Los Angeles, California 90024

P. Buser, Laboratoire de Neurophysiologie, Université Paris VI, 4 Place Jussieu, 75230 CEDEX, 05, Paris, France

Paul H. Crandall, Brain Research Institute, University of California, Los Angeles, California 90024

O. D. Creutzfeldt, Max-Planck-Institut für biophysikalische Chemie, Karl-Friedrich-Bonhoeffer-Institut, D-3400 Göttingen-Nikolausberg, Postfach 968, Germany

David D. Daly, Department of Neurology, University of Texas, Southwestern Medical School, 5323 Harry Hines Blvd., Dallas, Texas 75235

L. Goldhammer, Department of Neurology, Georgetown University School of Medicine, Washington, D.C., 20007

W. Jann Brown, Department of Pathology, University of California School of Medicine, Los Angeles, California 90024

Robert Naquet,* Départment de Neurophysiologie Appliquée, Institut de Neurophysiologie et de Psychophysiologie, 13 Marseille 9, France

J. Kiffin Penry, National Institute of Neurological Diseases and Stroke, Building 36/5D10, National Institutes of Health, Bethesda, Maryland 20014

H. Petsche, Institut für Hirnforschung, Österreichische Akademie der Wissenschaften Schwarzspanierstr. 17, A 1090 Wien, Austria

Daniel A. Pollen, Massachusetts General Hospital, Boston, Massachusetts 02114

P. Rappelsberger, Institut für Hirnforschung, Österreichische Akademie der Wissenschaften, Schwarzspanierstr. 17, A 1090 Wien, Austria

Gian Franco Rossi, Istituto di Neurochirurgia, Universitá Cattolica del Sacro Cuore, Via della Pineta Sacchetti, 00168 Rome, Italy

Madge E. and Arnold B. Scheibel, Department of Anatomy, University of California School of Medicine, Los Angeles, California 90024

---

* Present address: Laboratoire de Physiologie Nerveuse, Centre National de la Recherche Scientifique, Groupe de Laboratoires de Gif, 91190 Gif-sur-Yvette, France.

JANICE R. STEVENS,   University of Oregon School of Medicine, 3181 S. W. Sam Jackson Blvd., Portland, Oregon 97201

J. TALAIRACH, Hôpital Sainte Anne, 1 Rue Cabanis, Paris 14, France

RICHARD D. WALTER,   Department of Neurology, University of California School of Medicine, Los Angeles, California 90024

PREFACE

In July 1972, the Brain Research Institute of the University of California, Los Angeles, held a reunion of its alumni. The scientific program of this reunion centered on eight symposia concerned with the various fields of neuroscience relevant to the work of the Institute. Among these was a symposium on Electrophysiological Processes in the Epilepsies. Of the six distinguished speakers in that symposium, five came from overseas, thus bringing an international overview to the problem of seizures, extending from basic neurophysiological mechanisms to the modern approaches to diagnosis and therapy.

In this volume, the papers given by the six alumni at the reunion have been joined by ten further manuscripts, contributed on invitation by workers in biomedical fields critical for the understanding of epileptogenesis. It has thus been possible to extend the frontiers of the subject to the wider field of the phenomena of epilepsy in man.

Mary A. B. Brazier

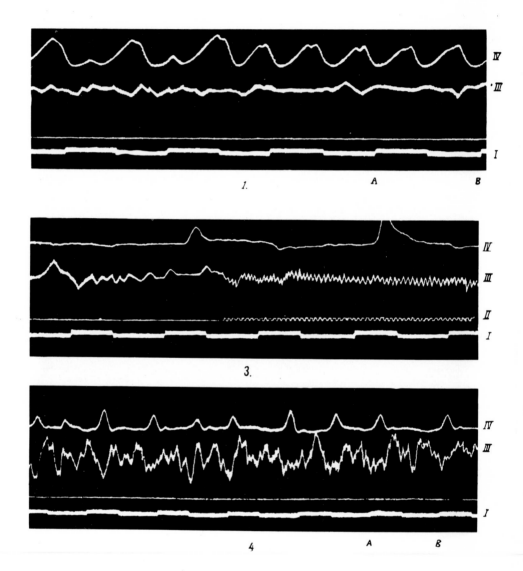

The first published photograph of the EEG changes in experimental epilepsy induced by electrical stimulation of the cortex in a dog. Top record: Line III = Spontaneous activity of the dog's cortex. Line IV = respiration. Line I = time marker. Middle and bottom records: Induction of an experimental seizure, the upper one showing stimulation and the lower one the resultant seizure activity. Line I = time marker (A to B = 1 second). Line II = stimulus signal. Line III = electrocorticogram. Line IV = respiration. All records read from right to left.

The frequency response of these nineteenth century instruments made them incapable of recording spikes; instead they recorded the disturbance caused by the seizure. (From Cybulski, N., and Jelenska-Macieszyna, Prady cynnosciowe kory mozgowej. *Bull. Int. Acad. Sci. Cracovie, Ser. B,* 1914:776–781.)

HISTORICAL INTRODUCTION: THE ROLE OF ELECTRICITY IN THE EXPLORATION AND ELUCIDATION OF THE EPILEPTIC SEIZURE

MARY A. B. BRAZIER

Brain Research Institute, University of California, Los Angeles, California

The role of electricity in the exploration of the epileptic nervous system emerged from two major and, at first, independent lines of observation and experiment. The fact that applied electricity could cause convulsions was at first accepted as being the same as any other traumatic insult to the brain—mechanical, thermal, or chemical. Such a view stemmed naturally from the influential Haller's (31, 39) concept of irritability based on experiments in which he pricked the brain and applied irritating fluids. These experiments led him to the erroneous conclusion that gray matter is insensitive to stimulation whereas white matter is the seat of sensation and the source of movement.

The realization that the applied electricity interacted with that of the cortical neurons had to wait for the discovery that the neurons were themselves the source of intrinsic currents.

In the earliest accounts, the electric stimulus is described as being applied within the brain rather than at its surface. In the mid-eighteenth century the Abbé Fontana (25) and Caldani (13, 14) (Galvani's predecessor in the chair of anatomy at Bologna) had convulsed their frogs by stimulation with frictional electricity. All these studies were carried out before evidence for the existence of "animal electricity" had made its controversial entry into physiology through the experiments of Galvani (27) and the attack on them by Volta (38). However, these rather indiscriminately applied stimulations of the brain continued and were soon applied to higher animals. Rolando (37), working in Sassari, extended the studies to pigs, goats, sheep, dogs, and also birds, reporting his findings in a text printed and illustrated by himself. But in the nineteenth century the goal was refined from the production of the disorganized, generalized muscle movements of the convulsion to an attempt to find brain areas that, on stimulation, provoked specific localized muscle contractions. This search continued in spite of the discouraging dicta of two very influential men: Magendie (36) who, because his own experiments had failed, pronounced the cortex inexcitable, and Flourens (24) who thought that success in the search for localization was more likely to follow from ablation experiments.

Yet why should these early workers have expected to find areas on the cortical surface that on stimulation evoked specific muscle or even limb movement? The neuron had not yet been identified as the unit of the nervous system and the pyramidal fibers were not yet known to be processes of cortical cells. Their hypotheses were extrapolations from the results of those who used ablation techniques, from the fantasies of phrenology in the first half of the nineteenth century, and from the startling claims of Bouillaud (8), of Aubertin (1) and of Broca (10) that there was a localized speech center in the human brain.

But meanwhile the search for localization of motor function persevered. Cabanis (12), the celebrated Idéologue in the Age of Enlightenment, had provoked convulsive movements in muscle groups that seemed to vary with the region of the brain he stimulated. But the crucial experiments were to come in 1870. As everyone knows, the pioneers were the two young doctors in Berlin, Fritsch and Hitzig (26), who demonstrated that certain regions of the cortex were excitable by electricity, as evidenced by elicited movements. Although Ferrier (20, 21) followed up and expanded their original findings in his classic book, "The Functions of the Brain" (22), acceptance of these concepts even then was far from general. An attack came from George Henry Lewes, whose name has almost faded from scientific memory; he was then a respected authority, and his "Physiology of Common Life" (31) was the best account of the nervous system available at the time.

Lewes, better remembered for his notorious liaison with George Eliot, wrote a pungent attack, both on Ferrier and on the original Fritsch–Hitzig concepts of functional localization (35). He deplored "the increasingly popular but thoroughly unphysiological conception of localisation." "We should marvel," he wrote, "to witness so many eminent investigators cheering each other on in the wild-goose chase of a function localised in a cerebral convolution." Just because stimulation of a cortical area evoked a movement that did not, in Lewes's opinion, prove it to be a motor center. "We do not," he wrote, "consider the centre of laughter to be located in the sole of the foot, because tickling the sole causes laughter." Lewes employed italics to emphasize his statement "*I do not think that Hitzig and Ferrier have proved the grey substance to be excitable.*"

He held that movements did not necessarily stem from involvement of cortical gray matter for the electricity could well be conducted through it without excitation until it reached the basal ganglia. This competing theory, suggested long before by Couty (18), was brought into prominence by Burdon Sanderson (11), the Jodrell Professor of Physiology at the University of London and a member of the Royal Society. He reached this conclusion from experiments in which he undercut the cortex with a sharp knife and then produced, by stimulation below the cortical layer, the same movements as he had evoked from the surface. This led him to direct stimulation of the basal ganglia and his method of approach is an interesting forerunner of modern stereotaxic methods. He wrote (11):

> In a brain hardened in alcohol, a needle plunged vertically, i.e. at right angles to the surface, from the active spot for retraction of the opposite ear, reaches the posterior part of the *corpus striatum* at a depth of from 10–12 millims. If a horizontal incision is made in the living brain, at this depth, and is met by two others, of which one is directed antero-posteriorly and the other transversely, and the part comprised within the incisions removed, a surface of brain is exposed in the deepest part of the wound which corresponds to the outer and upper part of the corpus striatum. If now the electrodes are applied to this surface, the movements . . . are produced in the same way as before, but more distinctly, the active spots are quite strictly localised . . .

If the cortex were not the originator of movements, then the alternative proposal was that they were secondary to sensation, and the direct effect of the stimulation was sensory rather than motor. The sensation was viewed as reaching the brain, where an "idea" then intervened and excited the basal ganglia to activate their motor function. This interpolation of an idea between sensation and motor output had in an earlier century differentiated the views of Glisson (29) from those of Haller (39) who omitted "psychic" perception between the irritation and the contraction. This hypothesis appealed to the Victorian mind because it provided a loophole for "free will" and a "voluntary movement." Stimulation evoked a sensation the result of which was that one willed to move a limb. This was much more acceptable than the thought of an automatic movement resulting from excitation of certain spots in the brain.

But the cortex was to come into prominence again through a major discovery—one which was eventually to be extremely important for the investigation of epilepsy (9). In the same year (1874) that Burdon Sanderson published his claims for the basal ganglia, Richard Caton, a young lecturer in physiology at the Royal Infirmary in Liverpool, applied to the British Medical Association for a grant to search for electrical signs in the brain of sensory impulses entering it from peripheral stimulation. He was given the grant and within a year had found what he was looking for—namely, a potential change when the animal received a stimulus such as a flash. But more important, as later years were to reveal, was his observation that his baseline was never still but always oscillated as long as the animal was alive. Actually this was the discovery of the electroencephalogram (EEG), published first in a brief note in the *British Medical Journal* in 1875 (15) and followed by a longer paper in 1877 (16).

Although demonstrated to the British Medical Association in London and reported at the Ninth International Medical Congress in Washington in 1887 (17) the discovery of the EEG went unnoticed by the clinical world in these two countries for 60 years. But not so in Russia or in Poland. Reinforced by the second and independent discovery of the EEG, 15 years later, by a Polish doctoral student, Adolf Beck (2), at the University of Jagiellonski in Kraków, and published as a thesis in 1891 (3), intensive work began in both countries, not only on evoked potential changes but also on the background on-going activity. Caton in 1877 had written that "the study of these currents may prove a means of throwing further light on the functions of the hemispheres." (16) And following the concept that these were "functional currents," the idea soon came that the dysfunctioning of the brain in epilepsy might be manifested in the form of EEG changes. The test of whether an epileptic attack was likely to be accompanied by abnormal EEG activity was first made in dogs by Kaufman (33) in St. Petersburg.

Pavel Yurevich Kaufman, the son of a doctor in Moscow, was born in 1877 and received his education at the Military Academy of Medicine in St. Petersburg, graduating in 1901. At this time the famous Bechterev held the chair of Nervous and Mental Diseases, and Pavlov that of Physiology, so that it was under these two great figures that Kaufman received his training. In 1904 he won his doctorate for his work in neurophysiology.

Kaufman decided to repeat the experiments of the early workers on the electrical activity of the brain with the advantage that 20 years' improvement in instrumentation could provide. By taking great care not to injure the brain, he was able to confirm that the "spontaneous" fluctuations were not currents of injury, as the skeptics claimed, but that the normal brain did, indeed, exhibit intrinsic electrical activity.

Kaufman initiated his own experiments after reading the works of all who came before him and, in fact, published a comprehensive review (33) of the EEG discoveries in the nineteenth century of Caton, Beck, Cybulski, Danilevsky, Fleischl von Marxow (23), and Gotch and Horsley (30). Unfortunately, however, this report, as well as the original papers reviewed, did not attract attention in the West, except for Berger who tried, mostly unsuccessfully, from 1905 to 1925 to repeat the experiments (7).

Kaufman was the first to express the concept that an epileptic attack would be accompanied by abnormal discharges and to test this postulate by examining the potentials of the brain during experimentally produced epilepsy. He stimulated the exposed cortex of dogs with an induction current and compared the discharges he found during the tonic and clonic phases. In his paper (33) he commented on the great difficulty he had in maintaining electrode contact during the seizure, and his inability to get as clear-cut a demonstration as he wished. Nevertheless, his contribution remains one of the landmarks in the basic development of what was later to become the electroencephalography of epilepsy.

Kaufman published his many experiments in very great detail, the most interesting in the context of this volume, are those on experimental epilepsy.

Many earlier investigators had provoked epileptic convulsions by chemical or electrical stimulation but had not attempted to record from the brain during the seizures. This was first attempted by Kaufman. His own description reads (in translation):

> How will the disorderly excitation which comes during an epileptic fit affect the electrical activity of the cortex? Indications of this are not found in the literature. In our experiments, epileptic fits were produced by irritating the cortex with an induction current, during which corresponding points on the opposite hemisphere were connected to the galvanometer.

Kaufman evidently knew that Beck and Cybulski were working along the same lines for he mentions that his results fully confirmed their findings and refuted the assumptions of Gotch and Horsley (30) who thought that the cortical potentials during fits were evoked responses, that is, responses evoked by afferent impulses from muscle contractions during the fit. By curarizing his dogs during the experiments, Kaufman ruled this out and demonstrated the abnormal electrogenesis of cortical neurons in epilepsy.

When World War I broke out with Germany, Kaufman left to serve with the army as a medical officer and the name Kaufman drops out of the scientific literature, for at this time he took the name of Rostovtsev and retained it to the end of his life.

At the end of the war he obtained an appointment at the University of Zakavkas, serving the region that used to include Armenia, Georgia, and Azerbaidzhan, and in 1925 he joined the department of physiology in the University that had been founded at Baku in the Caucasus. In 1930 this became part of the medical school under the Azerbaidzhan Medical Institute, and it was here that he spent the last 20 years of his life. He died in 1951 after achieving recognition as the leading physiologist of the Azerbaidzhan Soviet Republic.

At the time of his studies on experimental epilepsy, Kaufman had no camera so we have no illustrations of his records, but the work he had pioneered was taken up by the laboratory in Kraków from which Adolf Beck had, in 1890, received his doctorate for his treatise on the electrical activity of the brain and spinal cord. Beck had left Kraków in 1895 to take up a position at the University of L'vov but his old professor, Napoleon Cybulski, with another colleague, Jelenska-Macieszyna, continued the work and pursued the investigation of experimental epilepsy (19). They induced seizures by electrical stimulation of the cortex in dogs and monkeys and were on the whole more successful than Kaufman in overcoming the technical difficulties of interference by muscle potentials. After opening the skull under anesthesia (a mixture of equal parts of chloroform, ether, and alcohol), they then immobilized the animal in a plaster of Paris cast. (They have left a photograph of this rather unpleasing technique.) Their electrodes were nonpolarizable and placed directly on the pia.

The possession of a camera, however, enabled them to be the first to publish photographs of cortical potentials recorded during experimental epileptic seizures. They noted a great increase in both amplitude and frequency of the brain's potentials during these artificially induced seizures. The response characteristics of the galvanometers of that time were inadequate for recording spikes.

This first photograph that we have of the EEG in epileptic activity is shown in the frontispiece. The recordings are from a dog, respiration being registered on the channel marked IV, the EEG on III, a signal to mark the stimulus on II, and a time-marker on channel I. The recordings read from right to left. One of the EEG electrodes was on the occipital cortex, the other on the receiving area for the forepaw. They clearly pick up as artifact the stimulating current.

In describing their findings in experimentally produced epilepsy, Cybulski and Jelenska-Macieszyna wrote (19):

> The action currents of the cerebral cortex observed during an attack of artificially evoked Jacksonian epilepsy (Experiments I 16-IV-1913, II, 6-V-1913, III, 10-V-1913, plate 55, photograph No. 4) are distinguished chiefly by their intensity which is greater than in those occurring spontaneously or in the fluctuations in current recorded during stimulation. Their frequency also appears to be faster than that which can be observed in the same animals after stimulation of the extremities. The comparison represented in photographs Nos. 1 and 4 is noteworthy because these photographs which originated from the same animals (Experiment VII) and were prepared under identical conditions, very clearly present the difference between spontaneously occurring fluctuations in current, and those observed during an attack of Jacksonian epilepsy.

Photograph "No. 1" to which these authors refer is of the resting rhythm of a dog (the top record in the frontispiece). The EEG shows slow waves of low voltage in strong contrast to the activity in the seizure recording.

When electroencephalography moved from animal to man (4), its application to the study of clinical epilepsy was rather slow to develop. Only in 1931 (5) do we find Berger's first illustrations of the EEG in epilepsy, although, according to Jung (32), an entry in his journal in April 1929 notes that he had recorded from a man with "epileptic dementia." He never, however, gave much emphasis to EEG findings in epilepsy. The illustrations are not very contributory since clearly they are EEGs either of interictal or of postictal periods. It is not until 1933 (6) that Berger published an illustration that has been interpreted as a spike-and-wave discharge, recorded from a 15-year-old girl whose brief attack is described as an automatism. This lack of emphasis on epilepsy on the part of Berger may possibly be due to his approach to the whole subject of the currents of the brain as described by himself in a long review article (7) published 3 years before his death. In this he tells us that his interest was in "psychophysiology, the border area in which physiology and psychology come in touch with each other, the science which is to determine more accurately the connection between brain function and psychic processes; this was to be the area of my investigation."

Even before his attempts to record the EEG from man, and while he was still trying to repeat those on animals that had been demonstrated by so many workers, Berger's ruling interest was already focused on "psychic energy." Over the course of the 10 years following his appointment as Professor of Neurology and Psychiatry at the University of Jena, he was lecturing publicly on cerebral physiology and the search for a physiological basis for psychic phenomena. In 1921 he published a monograph on this subject. A great believer in telepathy, he constructed a hypothesis of wave propagation to explain it and devoted the last publication of his life, "Psyche," to an exposition of this theory.

Berger's goals in his electroencephalographic work were thus rather noticeably different from those of Kaufman in his development of experimental epilepsy, for the latter argued that abnormal neurons must be the common factor in epilepsy and in electrical discharges and was able to obtain evidence for this view.

However, in the 1930s interest in the role of the EEG in clinical epilepsy grew, sparked very largely by the classic paper of Gibbs, Davis, and Lennox published in 1935 (28).

From that date interest in this application of the EEG accelerated throughout the world, with the result that electroencephalography has become established as an important clinical test in the epilepsies. In due time, the argument of Kaufman that abnormal discharges indicate abnormal neurons, has led to the modern lines of research on the more intimate properties of neuronal tissue, both normal and abnormal, in terms of structure, of connections, and of electrical characteristics.

REFERENCES

1. Aubertin, E. (1825–1890), Considérations sur les localisations cérébrales et en particular sur le siege de la faculté du langage articulé. *Gaz. Heb. Med. Chir.*, 1863, **10**: 318, 348, 397, and 455.
2. Beck, A. (1863–1942), Die Bestimmung der Localisation der Gehirn-und Rückenmarkfunctionen vermittelst der electrischen Erscheinungen. *Centralbl. Physiol.*, 1890, **4**: 473–476.
3. Beck, A., Oznaczenie lokalizacyi u mozgu i rdzeniu za pomoca zjawisk elektry czynch. (Determination of localization in the brain and spinal cord by means of electrical phenomena.) Thesis, Univ. Jagiellonski, Kraków, 1891.
4. Berger, H. (1873–1941), Über das Elektrenkephalogramm des Menschen. *Arch. Psychiat. Nervenkr.*, 1929, **87**: 527–570.
5. Berger, H., Über das Elektrenkephalogramm des Menschen. *Arch. Psychiat. Nervenkr.*, 1931, **94**: 16–60.

6. Berger, H., Über das Elektrenkephalogramm des Menschen. *Arch. Psychiat. Nervenkr.*, 1933, **100**: 301–320.

7. Berger, H., Das Elektrenkephalogramm des Menschen. *Acta Nova Leopoldina*, 1938, **6**: 173–309.

8. Bouillaud, J. B. (1796–1881), *Traité clinique et physiologique de l'encéphalite ou inflammation du cerveau.* Baillière, Paris, 1825.

9. Brazier, M. A. B., *A History of the Electrical Activity of the Brain.* Pitman, London, 1961.

10. Broca, P. P. (1824–1880), Perte de parole, ramollissement chronique et destruction du lobe antérieur gauche du cerveau. *Bull. Soc. Anthropol. Paris*, 1861, **2**: 235–238.

11. Burdon Sanderson, J. S. (1828–1905), Note on the excitation of the surface of the cerebral hemispheres by induced currents. *Proc. R. Soc. Lond.*, 1874, **22**: 368–370.

12. Cabanis, P. J.-G. (1757–1808), *Rapports du physique et du moral de l'homme.* Bibliothèque Choisie, Paris, 1830.

13. Caldani, L. M. A. (1725–1813), Institutiones Physiologicae et Pathologicae. Luchtmans, Leyden, 1784.

14. Caldani, L. M. A., Letters to Haller. In: A. von Haller, *Mémoires sur les parties sensibles et irritables du corps animal*, 1760, **3**: 1–156 and 345–485.

15. Caton, R. (1842–1926), The electric currents of the brain. *Br. Med. J.*, 1875, **2**: 278.

16. Caton, R., Interim report on investigation of the electric currents of the brain. *Br. Med. J., Suppl.*, 1877, **1**, 62.

17. Caton, R., Researches on electrical phenomena of cerebral grey matter. *Trans. 9th Int. Med. Congr.*, 1887, **3**: 246–249.

18. Couty, L. C. (1854–1884), Sur la non-excitabilité de l'écorce grise du cerveau. *C. R. Acad. Sci. (Paris)*, 1879, **88**: 604–607.

19. Cybulski, N. (1854–1919), and Jelenska-Macieszyna, Prady cynnosciowe kory mozgowej (Action currents of the cerebral cortex). (In German.) *Bull. Int. Acad. Sci. Cracovie, Ser. B*, 1914: 776–781.

20. Ferrier, D. (1843–1928), The localisation of function in the brain. *Proc. R. Soc. Lond.*, 1874, **22**: 229–232.

21. Ferrier, D., Experiments on the brains of monkeys. *Phil. Trans.*, 1875, **165**: 433–488.

22. Ferrier, D., *The Functions of the Brain.* Smith, Elder & Co., London, 1876.

23. Fleischl von Marxow, E. (1846–1892), Mittheilung betreffend die Physiologie der Hirnrinde. *Centralbl. Physiol.*, 1890, **4**: 538.

24. Flourens, P. (1794–1867), *Recherches expérimentales sur les propriétés et les fonctions du système nerveux dans les animaux vertébrés.* Crévot, Paris, 1824.

25. Fontana, F. (1730–1805), Letter to Urbain Tosetti. In: A. von Haller, *Mémoires sur les parties sensibles et irritables du corps animal*, 1760, **3**: 159–243.

26. Fritsch, G. T. (1838–1927), and Hitzig, E. (1838–1907), Über die elektrische Erregbarkeit des Grosshirns. *Arch. Anat. Physiol. wiss. Med. Leipzig*, 1870, **37**: 300–333.

27. Galvani, L. (1737–1798), De viribus electricitatis in motu musculari. *Commentarius de Bonomensi Scientarium et Artium Instituto atque Academia Commentarii*, 1791, **7**: 363–418.
28. Gibbs, F. A., Davis, H., and Lennox, W. G., The electroencephalogram in epilepsy and in conditions of impaired consciousness. *Arch. Neurol. Psychiat.*, 1935, **34**: 1133–1148.
29. Glisson, F. (1597–1677), *Tractatus de ventriculo et intestinis.* Henry Brome, London, 1677.
30. Gotch, F. (1853–1913), and Horsley, V. A. H. (1857–1916), Über den Gebrauch der Elektricität für die Lokalisierung der Erregungsercheinungen im Centralnervensystem. *Centralbl. Physiol.*, 1891, **4**: 649–651.
31. Haller, A., De partibus corporis humani sensibilibus et irritabilis. *Comment. Soc. Req. Sci., Göttingen*, 1753, **2**: 114.
32. Jung, R., Hans Berger und die Entdeckung des EEG nach seinen Tagebüchern und Protokollen. In: *Jenenser EEG-Symposion* (R. Werner, Ed.). Verlag Volk u. Gesundheit, Berlin, 1963: 20–53.
33. Kaufman, P. Y. (1877–1951), Electrical phenomena in the cerebral cortex (in Russian). *Obroz. Psikhiat. Nevrol. Eksper. Psikhol. (St. Petersburg)*, 1912, **7–8**: 403–424 and 513–535.
34. Lewes, G. H. (1817–1878), *The Physiology of Common Life.* Blackwood, Edinburgh, 1859–1860.
35. Lewes, G. H., Book review of *The Functions of the Brain* by D. Ferrier. *Nature (Lond.)*, 1876, **25**: 73–74 and 93–95.
36. Magendie, F. (1783–1855), Des effets de l'Upas Tienté sur l'économie animale. *Bull. Soc. Philom. Paris*, 1809, **1**: 368–371.
37. Rolando, L. (1773–1831), *Saggio Sopra la Vera Struttura del Cervello dell'Uomo e degli Animali e Sopra le Funzioni del Sistema Nervoso.* Sassari, 1809.
38. Volta, A. (1745–1827), On electricity excited by the mere contact of conducting substances of different kinds. *Phil. Trans.*, 1800, **90**: 403–431.
39. Zinn, J. G., and Haller, A., *Mémoires sur les parties sensibles et irritables du corps animal.* D'Arnay, Lausanne, 1760.

SYNAPTIC ORGANIZATION OF THE CEREBRAL CORTEX AND ITS ROLE IN EPILEPSY

O. D. CREUTZFELDT

Max Planck Institute of Biophysical Chemistry, Göttingen, West Germany

The cerebral cortex is the most important structure for the manifestation of epileptic activity. Its threshold for the elicitation of seizure activity is much lower than that of subcortical structures, such as thalamic or lower brainstem nuclei. Clinical (motor and sensory) symptoms of seizure activity are predominantly of cortical origin. Even many "autonomous" symptoms may originate from cortical structures such as the temporo-basal cortex. The involvement of subcortical vegetative centers may be a consequence of the cortical seizure activity rather than a primary manifestation. The role of subcortical systems in the spread, synchronization, and termination of generalized seizures or in the triggering of cortical seizure activity is not denied, but it is as yet little understood. Different cortical areas may have different seizure thresholds, but the main threshold differences are those among the allocortex, the isocortex, and the cerebellum. The allocortex has the lowest threshold (30), whereas no self-sustained after-discharges can be brought about in the cerebellum.

Does the cerebral cortex have specific properties that make it capable of producing epileptic activity, especially self-sustained seizure activity? There are three main neuronal mechanisms which are discussed with respect to epilepsy (for further references, see 8, 28): (1) alterations of membrane properties; (2) increased synaptic excitatory responses; and (3) decreased synaptic inhibitory action. For the first mechanism, some experimental models have been found (such as the ouabain seizures and possibly penicillin seizures), but otherwise we have little proof of naturally occurring membrane disturbances which may play a role as basic disturbances leading to epilepsy. Of course, pathological membrane processes occur during seizure discharges of cortical neuron pools and are largely responsible for the sequence of events during a self-sustained after-discharge. In this paper we shall consider only the excitatory and (dis-)inhibitory hypothesis in the context of present knowledge of the functional organization of the cerebral cortex.

Neuronal Circuitry of the Cerebral Cortex

Although complex in its totality and not yet well understood in its function as a filter of sensory information and as an integrator of incoming and stored signals to produce coordinated motor output, the basic design of the cerebral cortex is rather simple. We can discriminate two fundamentally different types of cells, the pyramidal and the star cells (45, 48, 52). The former may send their axons out of the cortex as efferent fibers and (or) send recurrent collaterals back into the cortex. The star cells are supposed to distribute their axons only within the cortex itself. The fine structure of the cortex shows more-or-less clear distinctions in the different cytoarchitectural areas, but we do not know yet the functional significance of these cytoarchitectural differences. Nor do we know much about the significance of layering of the cortex. It seems that the cortical layers are more significant in higher animals such as primates, where—from the physiological and anatomical points of view—the upper three layers are clearly distinct from the lower three layers (11, 19, 27). But in the cortex of lower animals, such as the cat or the rabbit, neurons seem to be more homogeneously distributed across the whole cortex.

A functionally important principle of horizontal organization is the termination of afferent fibers. The specific thalamocortical afferents terminate mainly in the middle of the cortex (layers IIIb/IV) on dendrites of pyramidal cells and possibly also on star cells (19, 29). Other afferents terminate on more apical parts of the dendrites, for example, the "nonspecific" thalamocortical and the callosal afferents (22, 29). We still know very little about the termination of intracortical fibers. Some recurrent collaterals are supposed to terminate preferentially on basal dendrites of pyramidal cells (22), whereas others seem to run upward toward more superficial cortical layers (20).

The afferent synaptic input into pyramidal cells will, as a consequence, be quantitatively different depending on the depth, since the afferents terminate at different "strategic positions" relative to the axon hillock of the neurons—the presumed trigger zone for action potentials. Correspondingly, intracellular records of postsynaptic potentials will show differences in the forms and amplitudes of excitatory postsynaptic potentials (EPSPs) according to their origin (10a). In the cell of Figure 1, the steepest EPSPs are found after antidromic stimulation, that is, following activation of recurrent collaterals, whereas excitation of specific thalamocortical afferents causes flatter EPSPs and that of contralateral afferents still smoother EPSPs. Only if the contralateral cortex is stimulated so strongly that the terminals arriving at the stimulated side are also excited antidromically, are steep EPSPs recorded. Such records indicate that the electrotonic distance (which is a function of the membrane properties of the cell and of the actual distance of the synapse from the recording site, presumably the

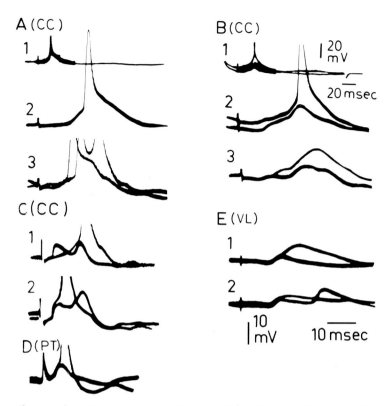

Figure 1. Shapes of excitatory postsynaptic potentials of a cortical neuron after stimulation of different afferent fiber systems. Cat, pentobarbital anesthesia, motor cortex. Intracellular recordings from a Betz cell. (A and B) Response after weak electrical stimulation of the corresponding point in the contralateral cortex (CC). Note the smooth and slow rise of the EPSP, indicating location of the excited synapses distant from the recording site (presumably the soma). (Calibration for recordings A and B at upper right.) (C) Supramaximal stimulus strength in the same contralateral location. Steep EPSPs are elicited, indicating location of the synapses close to the recording electrode. In this case, corticofugal transcallosal fibers were excited antidromically and the sharp EPSPs are presumably from intracortical recurrent collaterals. (D) Antidromic stimulation of the bulbar pyramidal tract (PT). The recorded cell has not been excited antidromically but a sharp EPSP, mediated via a recurrent collateral, is elicited. Its shape is comparable to that following strong contralateral stimulation (recording C). (E) EPSPs after weak electrical stimulation of nucleus ventrolateralis (VL) thalami. The rise time of these potentials is similar or shorter than that of the transcallosal volley (recordings A and B), indicating location of the synapses at similar electrotonic distances. (Calibration of recordings C, D, and E at lower right and at B1. [From Creutzfeldt *et al.* (10a).]

soma) is smallest for the EPSPs after antidromic recurrent excitation and largest after callosal excitation. This is in principal agreement with anatomical observations (22, 46). The effective functional distances of synapses of various origin from the soma will be different at different depths. In addition, it can be assumed that the number of synapses originating from one afferent fiber will vary considerably, ranging from *en passant* contacts with only one synapse to chains of synaptic contacts in a climbing fiber arrangement. Yet we know far too little about the fine anatomy of cortical neuronal synaptic contacts to be able to propose a good functional model of afferent synaptic organization. Identification of neurons from which records were taken and an exact correlation between electrophysiological and morphological measurements are necessary and will be an important task for the coming years.

An essential property of the cortical network is the existence of recurrent inhibition as well as excitation. Both can be demonstrated in the motor cortex by antidromic stimulation in the pyramidal tract. Such stimulation not only produces an antidromic action potential in Betz cells that send their axons down the pyramidal tract but also produces EPSPs in the same type or in other cells that do not send their axons down the pyramidal tract (43, 50). All neurons, however, show postsynaptic inhibition after antidromic stimulation (42, 43, 50).

Strong postsynaptic inhibition in the cerebral cortex is also found after direct electrical cortical stimulation (10, 15) and after stimulation of specific thalamocortical afferents (10, 15, 34). No differences in this basic functional behavior have yet been found in different cortical areas. The direct, primary afferent input to the cortical network is excitatory. After electrical ·stimulation of the specific afferents (optic tract or optic radiation), about 75% of the neurons in area 17 show a primary excitation (13, 24). The inhibition is of longer latency (54) indicating its transmission through recurrent collaterals and (or) inhibitory interneurons. Also anatomical findings suggest that afferent thalamocortical terminals are excitatory (19, 29).

The direct excitatory connection between afferent fibers and individual cortical cells appears to be very restricted. Recent findings in the primary visual cortex indicate that one cortical cell may receive its excitatory geniculocortical input from essentially only one or very few afferent fibers (9, 23; Creutzfeldt and co-workers, in preparation). A similar organization probably exists in the somatosensory projection areas also, as suggested by the high specificity of somatotopic and of receptor-type input to individual cortical neurons (as described by several authors).

The filter properties of the cortex, which are best analyzed in the visual areas with its orientation- and direction-selective neurons, are basically the result of the network properties of the cortex itself with its intrinsic inhibitory and excitatory connections, onto which the afferent input is multiply projected. This multiple projection has two aspects: (1) one thalamic relay neuron excites not only neurons at one cortical point but, through its branches, excites a relatively wide cortical area (up to a millimeter or so distant) (45, 48, 52); (2) neurons in one cortical cylinder are excited by different specific afferent fibers originating from different, although nearby points in the periphery (9, 26; Creutzfeldt and co-workers, in preparation), resulting in an overlapping, somewhat "fuzzy," multiple topographical representation. This input is then connected to a network of basically homogeneous intrinsic organization.

The connections between different cortical areas and the multiple projection of some sensory systems is another important aspect of the functional organization of the cortex. But this aspect will only be mentioned here.

Role of Disinhibition for Cortical Epileptic Phenomena

Let us now turn back to the question of this paper: What is the significance of such cortical synaptic organization for epilepsy? The presence of inhibitory mechanisms is not a unique feature of the cerebral cortex, for it is found in all thalamic relay nuclei (3, 18). Furthermore, it is found in practically all cerebral nuclei and can be considered a general wiring property of virtually all cerebral subsystems. A specific cortical feature, however, is the presence of recurrent excitation. This specific feature may, therefore, be of significance for the capability of the cerebral cortex to develop seizure activity.

It is still an open question whether disinhibition by itself is capable of rendering "epileptic" an otherwise normal neuronal system. The known convulsant substances, which produce more or less strong suppression of γ-aminobutyric acid (GABA) or glycine action (17), such as strychnine and Metrazol, can also produce abnormal convulsoid activity in single neurons (such as stretch receptors) or in peripheral ganglia of snails (6). It is probable, that, besides their inhibition-blocking action, they have a direct effect on membranes, leading to abnormal excitatory responses. Also ouabain acts directly on membrane mechanisms by interfering with the Na^+/K^+ pump in blocking the Na^+-dependent adenosine triphosphatase (ATPase) (4).

Nevertheless, we know several functional states of the central nervous system in which disinhibition is present but which do not lead to epileptic activity in otherwise normal brains. One example is that of flicker stimulation: single light flashes induce a mixture of excitation and inhibition in the neurons of the visual cortex (12) (Figure 2). This inhibition may be so strong that it completely suppresses the excitation of some neurons. During flicker stimulation at 7 to 15/second and above, however, the light-evoked inhibitory potentials disappear and only excitatory potentials are visible (33) (Figure 3). But neither in a normal animal nor in healthy humans does flicker stimulation induce seizure activity. Only if the central nervous system is rendered capable of developing such activity by the presence of other disturbances, is abortive or self-sustained seizure activity likely to develop during flicker stimulation. This is known from humans with photosensitive epilepsy as well as from the photosensitive *Papio papio* from Senegal (41).

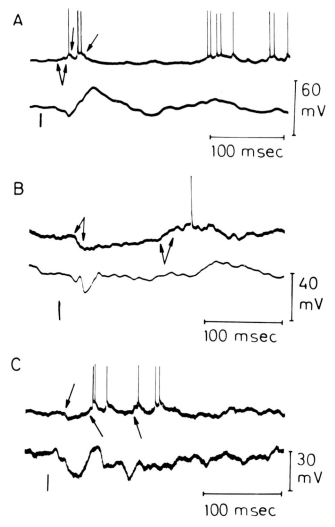

Figure 2. Postsynaptic potentials elicited in different neurons of the visual cortex by brief light flashes. Cat, pentobarbital anesthesia. Intracellular recordings in area 17. The vertical line on the left below each record indicates incidence of the flash. Downward arrows point to inhibitory postsynaptic potentials (IPSPs), upward arrows to excitatory postsynaptic potentials (EPSPs). Upper trace—intracellular record; lower trace—monopolar electroencephalogram record taken with an electrode near the cellular recording site. (A) A series of EPSPs and IPSPs is elicited by the flash. (B) The primary response is a large IPSP, whereas EPSPs are seen only as a secondary event. (C) A primary IPSP is followed soon by a series of EPSPs, which reach the firing threshold. [From Creutzfeldt et al. (12).]

Another well-known example of disinhibition is the augmenting response of the motor cortex, that is, the response to electrical 7–12/second stimulation of the specific thalamic projection nucleus (nucleus ventrolateralis). Single stimuli elicit a primary postsynaptic excitation, followed by a long-

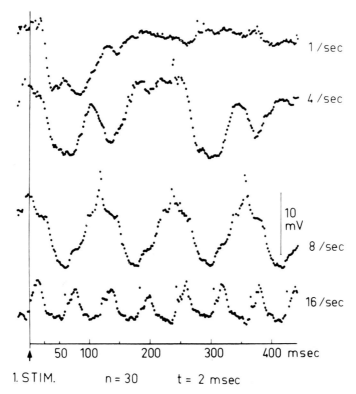

Figure 3. Disinhibition elicited in a neuron of the visual cortex by repetitive flashes at 16/second. Averaged records from an intracellular recording from an area 17 neuron. At the 1/second flash rate (top), only a short and small primary excitation is visible (small upward deflection), which is followed by a large inhibitory postsynaptic potential (IPSP) (downward deflection). Small excitations are superimposed on the IPSP. At 8/second, the amplitude of the IPSP is decreased. At 16/second, the IPSPs are no longer seen and broad excitatory postsynaptic potentials appear instead (unmasking). The arrow under the ordinate indicates the incidence of the first flash during the average sweep; n indicates the number of averaged sweeps, t = the bin width. [From Kuhnt and Creutzfeldt (33).]

lasting inhibitory postsynaptic potential (IPSP) (70–150 msec). But during 7–12/second stimulation, the IPSP disappears, unmasking a broad, large EPSP (40, 44). But here also, neither convulsive potentials nor seizure activity develop unless the cortex has been made "epileptic" by local application of strychnine or other substances (32).

The situation is different, however, if the cortex is stimulated directly with electrical stimuli above a frequency of 7 to 10/second. Single electrical stimuli to the cortical surface produce, like afferent stimulation, a primary excitation followed by long-lasting postsynaptic inhibition. But, as in the case of thalamic augmenting stimulation, the IPSPs disappear and the excitatory response becomes larger during a series of 7 to 10/second (or more) stimulations. In contrast to the stable membrane potential during afferent

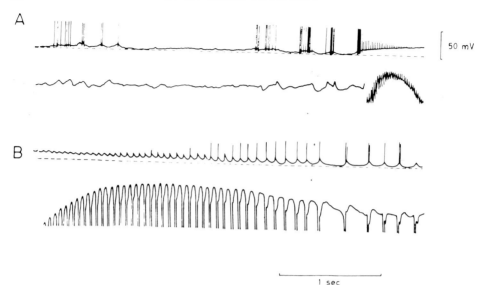

Figure 4. Intracellular (top) and electroencephalogram (EEG) record (bottom) before, during, and after a strong epicortical electrical stimulus series. Cat, pentobarbital anesthesia, sensorimotor cortex. (A) Intracellular record: the resting potential is indicated by a broken line. During the direct cortical stimulation (left, A) the membrane potential depolarizes and the action potentials disappear (inactivation of the spike generator). (B) Following the stimulus, the membrane potential shows oscillations while returning slowly to the base line. Action potentials appear only after recovery of the membrane potential. (EEG) Monopolar recording from the surface near the cellular recording site; negativity upward. Note the large surface-positive paroxysmal potentials (not fully shown) synchronous with the cellular oscillations during the self-sustained convulsive afterdischarge. [From Creutzfeldt *et al.* (16).]

excitation via physiological afferents, continued direct cortical stimulation leads to an increasing depolarization of the membrane potential beyond the threshold, resulting from direct excitation of the soma dendritic membrane by the electrical stimulus. If the membrane depolarization has reached a certain degree and if the stimulus series is then stopped, a self-sustained afterdischarge, that is, a focal seizure develops (Figure 4) (7, 16). This type of seizure may be considered as a "recovery discharge" (8) since, during the initial, oscillatory (tonic) and the later, periodic (clonic), synchronized cellular activities, the membrane potentials of the involved neurons recover from their "hyperdepolarization." Similar phenomena are also seen during pharmacologically or toxically induced seizures, but, under these conditions, the initial hyperdepolarization appears to be a consequence of repeated strong excitations due to the drug (1). These experimental findings indicate that disinhibition alone may not be sufficient to produce seizure activity and that, at least, some abnormal excitation is also needed.

Another example of this failure of disinhibition alone to produce self-sustained epileptic activity is that of chemically decreased inhibition. An increased blood ammonium level is known to result in spinal clonic activity (2), and an extremely high dosage by intravenous injection may even lead to generalized seizures (21a). It was recently discovered that such increased blood ammonium levels or even local electrophoretic application of NH_4^+ ions suppress IPSPs (36). This is not a complete extinction of IPSPs, but only a marked change of the "driving potential," that is, a decrease of the equilibrium potential of the IPSP (37). But at a dosage that significantly decreases the IPSP, seizures usually do not appear, although spinal myoclonus may be present. During pharmacologically induced seizures, cerebral ammonium levels are increased (51). Also during insulin-induced hypoglycemia, the blood ammonium level increases (53) and IPSPs decrease in amplitude (36). Cortical neurons show synchronized, grouped activity (38); but, as a rule, seizures do not appear. This finding also applies to human subjects: during insulin coma therapy, myoclonic jerks of essentially spinal origin are a frequent sign of deep hypoglycemia, but seizures are found only rarely and usually only in people who have a lowered seizure threshold and may have "latent epilepsy."

Visually Evoked Potentials in Patients with Epilepsy

In patients with epilepsy, we searched for possible characteristic changes in the visually evoked potential (VEP). An analysis of the neuronal basis of the VEP in animals had indicated that the different phases of the VEP can be correlated in a predictable way with neuronal activity patterns (12). The primary surface positivity is due to the initial geniculocortical excitation; waves I and III are simultaneous with the secondary excitation of one part of the cortical neurons and with the beginning of inhibitory responses in the majority of the cortical neurons (Figure 5). Waves IV and VI are clearly correlated to the large IPSP seen in most cortical neurons, regardless of whether or not they were primarily excited by the light stimulus. If a disturbance of inhibition were a primary cause in epilepsy, we would then expect a decrease of the amplitudes of waves IV and VI of the VEP. However, none of the components of the VEP was characteristically altered in epileptic patients. But the VEPs of the patient group as a whole showed larger interindividual variability than the control group (Figure 6a, b, c) (35). This increased variability was unsystematically distributed over all components: it could be due in one case to an increased amplitude of some components of the evoked potential, and in others to longer intervals between the different components. As a result, the mean potential calculated from all patient VEPs looked flatter and had a larger variability than the mean potential calculated from the control group. Also, the cross-correlation between the mean potential calculated from one control group was much lower for the epileptic patient group than for a second control group. Nevertheless, the total amplitude of VEPs from patients and

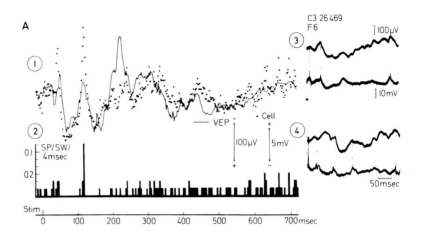

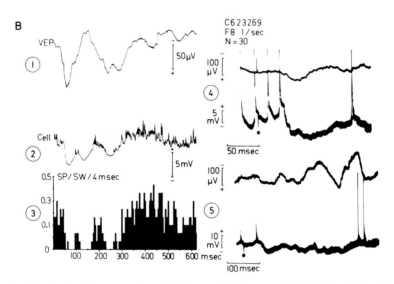

Figure 5. Correlation between the visually evoked potential (VEP) of the electroencephalogram (EEG) and those of single cortical cells. Cat, pentobarbital anesthesia, area 17/18. (A and B) Two different experiments. The EEG response was recorded against reference; negativity upward. Intracellular recordings (A3, A4, B4, and B5): original records show an early excitation followed by inhibition and secondary excitation in A, and primary inhibition in B (incidence of flash stimulus indicated by dot). EEG recordings (A1 and A2): continuous line is the averaged EEG response to 30 flashes; dotted line is the averaged intracellular response: PSTH of the cellular discharges in 2. (B1) Averaged EEG response; (B2) averaged cellular response, (B3) PSTH. The curves in experiment B are also averages from 30 stimuli. Incidence of flash at zero on abscissa. Bin width for PSTH, 4 msec. (Figure by courtesy of Dr. U. Kuhnt.)

control subjects did not differ significantly, nor was there a conspicuous absence of positive waves IV and VI. This indicates that, as a whole, a variation occurred in the time course of the sequence of potential components rather than in the amplitude. Only some patients with a markedly photogenic epilepsy may show considerably increased VEP, with both the positive and negative phases being amplified (21, 39). Recently, we have also investigated the photic driving response (8–18/second) of an epileptic and a control group. No significant difference in amplitude was found but there was a slightly larger variability in the patient group at the lower stimulus frequencies (8–11/second). The VEP changes were correlated to the background electroencephalogram (EEG) rather than to the type of epilepsy.

This analysis is in principal agreement with similar observations of other authors (5, 25, 39) and suggests that, except in the case of photogenic epilepsy, simple disturbances of synaptic transmission or inhibition cannot be revealed by the VEP method.

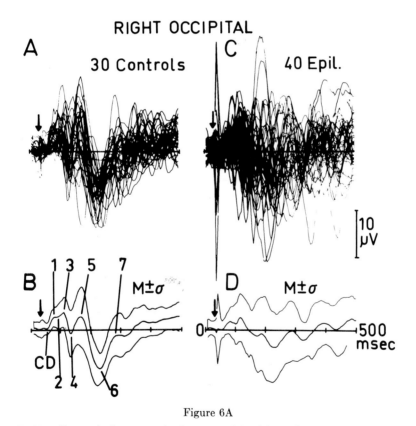

Figure 6A

Figure 6. Visually evoked potentials (VEPs) of healthy subjects (A, B) and patients with epilepsy (C, D). The averages from 100 responses were recorded from each individual and these curves were superimposed graphically (A and C). From each group of curves, the mean potential and the standard deviation were calculated (B and D). Note the larger variability of the VEPs recorded from patients with epilepsy in contrast to those from healthy control subjects. The numbers of individual wavelets (1–7) are indicated at the mean VEP from the occipital area. The VEPs were recorded against reference. [From Lücking *et al.* (35).]

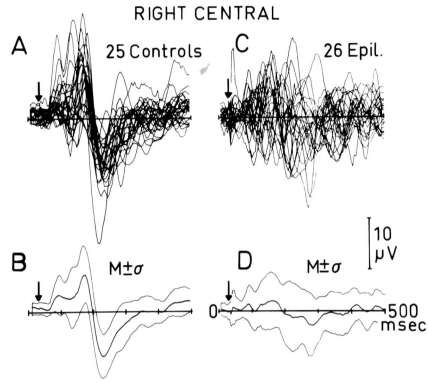

Figure 6B

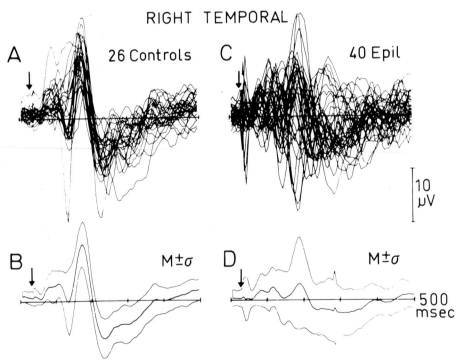

Figure 6C

CONCLUSION

The significance of subcortical structures in epilepsy has not been discussed in this paper, although subcortical nuclei may play a significant role for the development, spread, and possibly also the termination of actual seizure activity. But, since even the isolated cortex is capable of seizure activity (14, 47) and since final manifestation of epileptic activity is of cortical origin, cortical mechanisms must be considered as primary causes.

It appears that a lack of synaptic inhibition (disinhibition) is not sufficient to produce epileptic activity in the cortex. Disinhibition may, however, play an important role in epilepsy, as it may "unmask" abnormal excitatory phenomena and lower the threshold for elicitation of self-sustained seizures. Inhibition may also play a role in preventing the spread of focal epileptic activity to neighboring areas (31, 49). The mechanism of the basic excitatory disturbance in epilepsy, which has to be postulated, is not yet known, and may be of varying nature. The excitatory disturbances manifest themselves as hypersynchronous bursts of neuronal activity which lead to "sharp waves" in the EEG or to groups of such activities (dysrhythmia). If such hypersynchronous bursts appear too frequently, an abnormal depolarization of many neurons might develop within and around the "focus", possibly due to increased extracellular $[K^+]$. Such abnormal nerve cell depolarizations are the immediate cause of a self-sustained seizure.

The synaptic design of the cerebral cortex shows two characteristic features—recurrent inhibition and excitation. Recurrent inhibition is a feature common to practically all subsystems of the central nervous system, whereas recurrent excitation appears to be unique to the cortex (iso- as well as allocortex). It is therefore suggested that this specifically cortical organizational principle is relevant for the capability of the cortex to develop self-sustained epileptic activity.

If disinhibition plays an important role in the unmasking of basic epileptic excitatory disturbances, then investigation of the mechanisms of inhibition and disinhibition is important within the context of therapeutic measures to prevent seizures in patients with epilepsy. But in any search for the manifold primary causes of epilepsy, the study of abnormal excitatory mechanisms appears more important. Such abnormal excitatory mechanisms may involve postsynaptic excitation as well as excitatory phenomena of the neuronal membranes themselves. Any disturbance on the excitatory side may lead to cortical seizure activity, since the cortex is especially sensitive to hyperexcitation because of the excitatory connections between its neurons.

REFERENCES

1. Ajmone Marsan, C., Acute effects of topical epileptogenic agents. In: *Basic Mechanisms of the Epilepsies* (H. H. Jasper, A. A. Ward, and A. Pope, Eds.). Little, Brown, Boston, 1969: 299–319.

2. Ajmone Marsan, C., Fuortes, M. G. F., and Marossero, F., Influences of ammonium on the electrical activity of the brain and spinal cord. *Electroenceph. clin. Neurophysiol.*, 1949, **1**: 291–294.

3. Andersen, P., and Andersson, S. A., *Physiological Basis of the Alpha Rhythm.* Appleton, New York, 1968.

4. Carpenter, D. O., and Alving, B. O., A contribution of an electrogenic Na$^+$ pump to membrane potentials in aplysia neurones. *J. Gen. Physiol.*, 1968, **52**: 1–21.

5. Cernacek, J., and Cigánek, L., The cortical electroencephalographic response to light stimulation in epilepsy. *Epilepsia*, 1962, **3**: 303–314.

6. Chalazonitis, N., *C. R. Soc. Biol. (Paris)*, 1968, **162**: 1552.

7. Creutzfeldt, O. D., Neuronal mechanisms underlying the EEG. In: *Basic Mechanisms of the Epilepsies* (H. H. Jasper, A. A. Ward, and A. Pope, Eds.). Little, Brown, Boston, 1969: 397–410.

8. Creutzfeldt, O. D., Neurophysiologische Modelle der Epilepsie. *Nervenarzt*, 1972, **43**: 175–181.

9. Creutzfeldt, O. D., and Ito, M., Functional synaptic organization of primary visual cortex neurones in the cat. *Expl. Brain Res.*, 1968, **6**: 324–352.

10. Creutzfeldt, O. D., Lux, H. D., and Watanabe, S., Electrophysiology of cortical nerve cells. In: *The Thalamus* (D. P. Purpura and M. D. Yahr, Eds.). Columbia Univ. Press, New York, 1966: 209–235.

10a. Creutzfeldt, O. D., Maekawa, K., and Hösli, L., Forms of spontaneous and evoked postsynaptic potentials of cortical nerve cells. *Progr. Brain Res.*, 1969, **31**: 265–273.

11. Creutzfeldt, O. D., Pöppel, E., and Singer, W., Quantitativer Ansatz zur Analyse der funktionellen Organisation des visuellen Cortex (Untersuchungen an Primaten). 4. In: *Kybernetik Kongress* (O. J. Grüsser, Ed.). Springer-Verlag, Berlin and New York, 1971: 81–96.

12. Creutzfeldt, O. D., Rosina, A., Ito, M., and Probst, W., Visual evoked response of single cells and of the EEG in primary visual area of the cat. *J. Neurophysiol.*, 1969, **32**: 127–193.

13. Creutzfeldt, O. D., Spehlmann, R., and Lehmann, D., Veränderungen der Neuronaktivität des visuellen Cortex durch Reizung der Substantia reticularis mesencephali. In: *Neurophysiologie und Psychophysik des visuellen Systems* (R. Jung and H. Kornhüber, Eds.). Springer-Verlag, Berlin and New York, 1961: 351–363.

14. Creutzfeldt, O. D., and Stuck, C., Neurophysiologie und Morphologie der chronisch isolierten Cortex-insel der Katze. *Arch. Psychiat. Nervenkr.*, 1962, **203**: 708–731.

15. Creutzfeldt, O. D., Watanabe, S., and Lux, H. D., Relations between EEG-phenomena and potentials of single cortical cells. I. Evoked responses after thalamic and epicortical stimulation. *Electroenceph. clin. Neurophysiol.*, 1966, **20**: 1–8.

16. Creutzfeldt, O. D., Watanabe, S., and Lux, H. D., Relations between EEG-phenomena and potentials of single cortical cells. II. Spontaneous and convulsoid activity. *Electroenceph. clin. Neurophysiol.*, 1966, **20**: 19–37.

17. Curtis, D. R., Central synaptic transmitters. In: *Basic Mechanisms of the Epilepsies* (H. H. Jasper, A. A. Ward, and A. Pope, Eds.). Little, Brown, Boston, 1969: 105–129.

18. Fuster, J. M., Creutzfeldt, O. D., and Straschill, M., Intracellular recording of neuronal activity in the visual system. *Z. Vergl. Physiol.*, 1965, **49**: 605–622.

19. Garey, L. J., A light and electron microscopic study of the visual cortex of the cat and monkey. *Proc. R. Soc. Lond., Ser. B*, 1971, **179**: 21–40.

20. Garey, L. J., Fisken, R. A., and T. P. S. Powell, Patterns of degeneration after intrinsic lesions of the visual cortex (area 17) of the monkey. *Brain Res.* 1973, **53**: 208–213.

21. Gastaut, H., and Regis, H., Visually evoked potentials recorded transcranially in man. In: *Symposium on the Analysis of Central Nervous System and Cardiovascular Data using Computer Methods* (L. D. Proctor and W. R. Adey, Eds.). Natl. Acad. Sci., Washington, D.C., 1964: NASA, SP-72: 8–34.

21a. Gastaut, H., Seier, J., Mano, T., Santos, D., and Lyagoubi, S., Generalized epileptic seizures, induced by non-convulsant substances. *Epilepsia,* 1968, **9**: 317–327.

22. Globus, A., and Scheibel, A. B., Synaptic loci on visual cortical neurons. *Expl. Neurol.*, 1967, **18**: 116–131.

23. Gouras, P., Trichromatic mechanisms in single cortical neurones. *Science,* 1970, **168**: 489–492.

24. Grützner, A., Grüsser, O. J., and Baumgartner, G., Reaktionen einzelner Neurone des optischen Cortex der Katze nach elektrischen Einzelreizen des Nervus opticus. *Arch. Psychiat. Nervenkr.*, 1958, **197**: 377–404.

25. Halliday, A. M., The electrophysiological study of myoclonus in man. *Brain,* 1967, **90**: 241–284.

26. Hubel, D. H., and Wiesel, T. N., Receptive fields and functional architecture in two nonstriate visual areas (18 and 19) of the cat. *J. Neurophysiol.,* 1965, **28**: 229–289.

27. Hubel, D. H., and Wiesel, T. N., Receptive fields and functional architecture of monkey striate cortex. *J. Physiol. (Lond.)*, 1968, **195**: 215–243.

28. Jasper, H. H., Ward, A. A., and Pope, A. (Eds.), *Basic Mechanisms of the Epilepsies.* Little, Brown, Boston, 1969.

29. Jones, E. G., and Powell, T. P. S., An electron microscopic study of the pattern and mode of termination of afferent fibre pathways in the somatic sensory cortex of the cat. *Phil. Trans., Ser. B*, 1970, **257**: 45–62.

30. Jung, R., Hirnelektrische Untersuchungen über den Elektrokrampf. *Arch. Psychiat. Nervenkr.*, 1969, **183**: 206–244.

31. Jung, R., and Tönnies, J. F., Hirnelektrische Untersuchungen über Entstehung und Erhaltung von Krampfentladungen: die Vorgänge am Krampfort und die Bremsfähigkeit des Gehirns. *Arch. Psychiat. Nervenkr.*, 1950, **185**: 701–735.

32. Klee, M. R., and Offenloch, K., Post-synaptic potentials and spike patterns during augmenting responses in cat's motor cortex. *Science,* 1964, **143**: 488–489.

33. Kuhnt, U., and Creutzfeldt, O. D., Decreased post-synaptic inhibition in the visual cortex during flicker stimulation. *Electroenceph. clin. Neurophysiol.*, 1971, **30**: 79–82.

34. Li, C. L., Cortical intracellular synaptic potentials in response to thalamic stimulation. *J. Cell. Comp. Physiol.*, 1963, **61**: 165–179.

35. Lücking, C. H., Creutzfeldt, O. D., and Heinemann, U., Visual evoked potentials of patients with epilepsy and of a control group. *Electroenceph. clin. Neurophysiol.*, 1970, **29**: 557–566.

36. Lux, H. D., and Loracher, C., Post-synaptic disinhibition by ammonium. *Naturwissenschaften*, 1970, **9**: 456–457.

37. Lux, H. D., Loracher, C., and Neher, E., The action of ammonium on post-synaptic inhibition of cat spinal motoneurones. *Expl. Brain Res.*, 1970, **11**: 431–447.

38. Mergenhagen, D., Creutzfeldt, O. D., and Neuweiler, G., Beziehungen zwischen Aktivität corticaler Neurone und EEG-Wellen des motorischen Cortex der Katze bei Hypoglykämie. *Arch. Psychiat. Nervenkr.*, 1968, **211**: 43–62.

39. Morocutti, C., Sommer-Smith, J., and Creutzfeldt, O. D., Das visuelle Reaktionspotential bei normalen Versuchspersonen und charakteristische Veränderungen bei Epileptikern. *Arch. Psychiat. Nervenkr.*, 1966, **208**: 234–254.

40. Nacimiento, A. C., Lux, H. D., and Creutzfeldt, O. D., Post-synaptische Potentiale von Nervenzellen des motorischen Cortex nach elektrischer Reizung spezifischer und unspezifischer Thalamuskerne. *Pflügers Arch Ges. Physiol. Menschen Tiere*, 1964, **281**: 152–169.

41. Naquet, R., Photogenic seizures in the baboon. In: *Basic Mechanisms of the Epilepsies* (H. H. Jasper, A. A. Ward, and A. Pope, Eds.). Little, Brown, Boston, 1969: 565–573.

42. Phillips, C. G., Actions of antidromic pyramidal volleys on single Betz cells in the cat. *Q. J. Exp. Physiol.*, 1959, **44**: 1–25.

43. Phillips, C. G., Some properties of pyramidal tract neurones. In: *The Nature of Sleep* (G. E. W. Wolstenholme and M. O'Connor, Eds.). Churchill, London, 1961: 4–24.

44. Purpura, D. P., Shofer, R. J., and Musgrave, F. S., Cortical intracellular potentials during augmenting and recruiting responses. II. Patterns of synaptic activities in pyramidal and non-pyramidal tract neurons. *J. Neurophysiol.*, 1964, **27**: 133–151.

45. Ramón y Cajal, S., *Histologie du Système Nerveux de l'Homme et des Vertébrés*, Vol. 11. Reedited by CSIC, Instituto Ramón y Cajal, Madrid, 1952.

46. Scheibel, M. E., and Scheibel, A. B., On the nature of dendritic spines— report of a workshop. *Commun. Behav. Biol., Part A*, 1968, **1**: 231–265.

47. Sharpless, S. K., Isolated and deafferented neurons: Disuse supersensitivity. In: *Basic Mechanisms of the Epilepsies* (H. H. Jasper, A. A. Ward, and A. Pope, Eds.). Little, Brown, Boston, 1969: 329–348.

48. Sholl, D. A., *The Organisation of the Cerebral Cortex*. Methuen, London, 1956.

49. Spencer, W. A., and Kandel, E. R., Synaptic inhibition in seizures. In: *Basic Mechanisms of the Epilepsies* (H. H. Jasper, A. A. Ward, and A. Pope, Eds.). Little, Brown, Boston, Massachusetts, 1969: 515–603.

50. Stefanis, C., and Jasper, H. H., Intracellular microelectrode studies of antidromic responses in cortical pyramidal tract neurons. *J. Neurophysiol.,* 1964, **27**: 828–854.

51. Stone, W. E., Action of convulsants: Neurochemical aspects. In: *Basic Mechanisms of the Epilepsies* (H. H. Jasper, A. A. Ward, and A. Pope, Eds.). Little, Brown, Boston, 1969: 184–193.

52. Szentágothai, J., The anatomy of complex integrative units in the nervous system. In: *Results in Neuroanatomy, Neurochemistry, Neuropharmacology and Neurophysiology* (K. Lissak, Ed.). Akadémiai Kiadó, Budapest, 1967: 9–45.

53. Tews, J. K., Carter, S. H., and Stone, W. E., Chemical changes in brain during insulin hypoglycemia and recovery. *J. Neurochem.,* 1965, **12**: 679–693.

54. Watanabe, S., Konishi, M., and Creutzfeldt, O. D., Post-synaptic potentials in the cat's visual cortex following electrical stimulation of afferent pathways. *Expl. Brain Res.,* 1966, **1**: 272–283.

FOCAL EPILEPSY AND THE NEUROGLIAL IMPAIRMENT HYPOTHESIS*

DANIEL A. POLLEN

Massachusetts General Hospital, Boston, Massachusetts

For almost half a century the neuroglial scar (alone or as part of a meningo-cerebral cicatrix) has been recognized as the histopathological concomitant of the irritative source for those focal seizures which develop after anoxic or traumatic brain damage (2, 9). It would seem logical to look for a patho-physiological explanation of the irritative focus in terms of the structural, chemical, and physical changes that occur in the brain-damaged region. Such a search requires knowledge of normal brain function and of the de-rangements occurring as a damaged region of brain develops into an ex-citable focus.

Over the past 20 years there has been an extraordinary amount of electro-physiological work on the behavior of single neurons during drug-induced convulsive activity. These experimental models have been of interest in their own right, have led to an understanding of neurons subjected to in-tense synaptic bombardments, and have helped elucidate pathways for the propagation of seizures. However, I do not believe that these models, which by their very nature test the convulsive response of previously normal brain to some chemical agent—a *pharmacological* or *toxicological* problem—can help us much in our understanding of post-traumatic focal epilepsy, which is a *pathophysiological* problem.

For several years we had tried without success to formulate a model of impaired neural function in the focus (10). Our attention then shifted to a study of the normal function of neocortical neuroglial cells, of which protoplasmic astrocytes are the principal representative. Trachtenberg and I (15) studied the biophysical properties of these cells and found that they had high resting potentials (many values ranged from -70 to -92 mV), very short time constants ($\sim$385 μsec), and input resistances of 10.5 ± 4.9 MΩ. Orkand and co-workers (8) had suggested that neuroglial cells might serve as " 'spatial buffers' in the distribution of K^+ in the cleft system," and our data and calculations provided evidence that neocortical"

* Supported by U.S. Public Health Service Grant NB-14353.

neuroglial cells are ideally suited to buffer the immediate extracellular space at areas of synaptic contact against the increases in external potassium ion concentration that accompany postsynaptic and spike activity and to minimize the spread of potassium to other pre- and postsynaptic regions" (15). It is well known that local increases in K^+ concentration can set off seizures in otherwise normal brain (18) and that K^+ accumulates extracellularly during intense neural activity (1), and we, therefore, wondered whether an impairment in neuroglial function, especially with respect to extracellular K^+ homeostasis, might be a common factor in the development of the scar-related focal epilepsies (12).

Thus, based upon our work and a number of highly important findings already in the literature, we proposed a neuroglial impairment hypothesis for one factor in the development of focal epilepsy (12). Certainly a number of other factors must be of some importance and these have been discussed elsewhere (11, 12, 16).

Richardson and I (11) in combined histological and electrophysiological studies of physically induced glial scars and their border zones noted that an impairment of neuroglial function could come about in at least three ways: (1) by alteration of the normal neuronal–neuroglial anatomic relationship; (2) by either a primary metabolic defect or one secondary to vascular factors such that the neuroglial cell and its processes fail to maintain a very high internal K^+ concentration and restrict Na^+; and (3) by an inability of glial processes to distribute K^+ over required distances if process "space constants" were significantly reduced as a consequence of their slowly progressive packing with gliofibrils. Related aspects of the hypothesis are described elsewhere (12). We went on to study the glial scars developing 5–9 months after penetrating wounds or freeze lesions in the cat sensorimotor cortex (see Figure 1). The penetrating lesions were produced by inserting a blunt No. 18 gauge needle 2 mm into the cortex and dragging it through the brain until a trough of 3 to 4 mm had been made. No focal spiking was observed in the 5 animals with the penetrating wounds, and, on histological examination, the penetrating lesions were relatively circumscribed with narrow borders of fibrillary gliosis rather well separated from populations of normally appearing neurons.

However, focal spiking appeared in the scar border zones of most of the brains subjected to freeze lesions, and histopathological examination revealed rather wide zones of fibrillary gliosis, some regions of which contained many intact nerve cells (Figures 2 and 3). Thus, there is some evidence at the light microscopic level to support the first possibility, namely that the normal neuron–neuroglial relationship may be altered, and it would be tempting to interpret the difference in the excitability of the two types of glial scars as partly due to the presence of a relatively larger number of neuron cell bodies within a broader border zone of intense fibrillary gliosis in the freeze lesion series as compared with the sharp transition

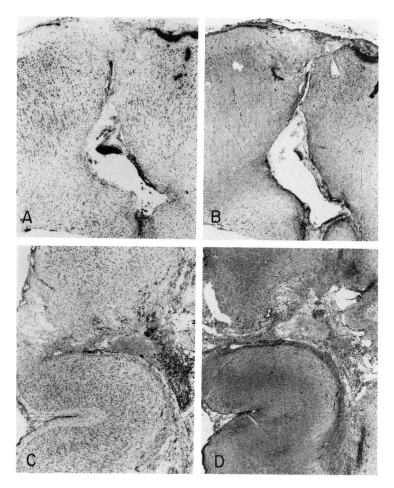

Figure 1. Penetrating lesions. (A) Surrounding the central destruction in the cerebral cortex is a narrow zone of incomplete damage with rapid transition into normal cortex. The most extensive cavitation is in the white matter. Cat No. 1; cresyl violet (CV); magnification ×27. (B) There is relatively little gliosis (dark-staining) surrounding the lesion. Cat No. 1; same area as in micrograph A; phosphotungstic acid hematoxylin (PTAH); magnification ×27. (C) Larger lesion than in cat No. 1, but damage to cortex is relatively circumscribed. Cat No. 9; CV, magnification ×27. (D) Relatively narrow zone of gliosis at the border of the lesion. Cat No. 9, same area as in micrograph C; PTAH; magnification ×27. [Reproduced by permission from Pollen and Richardson (11).]

zone in the penetrating wound series. Furthermore, at the electron-microscopic level, Wilder *et al.* (17) found normal neurons at the periphery of glial scars and noted that the extraneuronal neuroglial environment showed marked alterations.

With regard to the second postulate for impairment of neuroglial function, Tower (13) demonstrated that brain slices of scar tissue from epileptic patients, unlike slices of normal brain, fail to extrude Na^+ and take up K^+. Van Gelder *et al.* (3) have recently reported low concentrations of glutamic

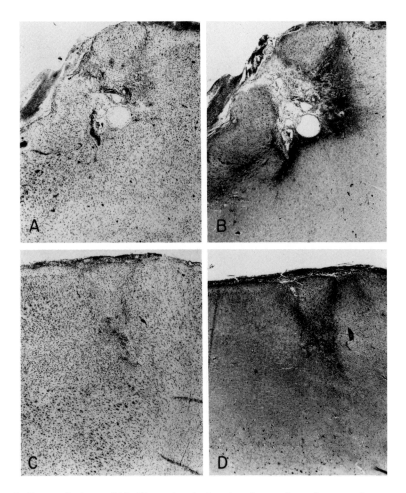

Figure 2. Freeze lesions. (A) Extensive lesion involves a broad zone of cortex, with deep cavitation. Cat No. 2; CV; magnification ×27. (B) The lesion is surrounded by wide gliotic regions which are situated in cortex. Cat No. 2; same area as in micrograph A; PTAH; magnification ×27. (C) Small lesion, but still affects cortex extensively. Cat No. 10; CV; magnification ×27. (D) The gliosis which is in the cortex is conspicuous. Cat No. 10; same area as in micrograph C; PTAH; magnification ×27. [Reproduced by permission from Pollen and Richardson (11).]

and aspartic acid in epileptogenic human brain, which suggested to them that there is an impaired energy metabolism in such tissue. Furthermore, there is evidence that in established scars, astrocytes show diminished quantities of glycogen and mitochondria (7).

With respect to the third postulate, it has been known that astrocytic processes in glial scars show an extraordinary increase in the number of glial fibrils (7) which, by taking up space inertly, could lead to marked increase in the internal resistivity and thereby decrease the space constant.

Thus there is some evidence consistent with three of the requirements of the hypothesis, but as yet there is no evidence sufficient to establish

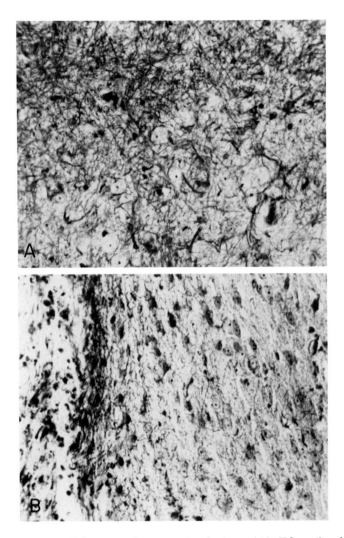

Figure 3. Comparison of freeze and penetrating lesions. (A) Edge of a freeze lesion with nerve cells surrounded by dense gliosis. Cat No. 2; PTAH; magnification ×400. (B) Edge of a penetrating lesion, with a narrow zone of dense gliosis near center of wound (left side of illustration), outside of which are many intact nerve cells and a few astrocytes and glial fibrils. Cat. No. 9; PTAH; magnification ×340. [Reproduced by permission from Pollen and Richardson (11).]

or disprove it. Tower (14) has recently amplified the neuroglial impairment hypothesis by suggesting that a second type of glutamic decarboxylase, which is present in glial cells and synthesizes γ-aminobutyric acid (GABA) from glutamic acid (6) and which is activated by Cl^-, may be important in releasing GABA upon neurons and thereby inhibiting them as excess K^+ and Cl^- enter the normal glial cell. Tower suggests that reactive astrocytes in gliotic areas may not respond to K^+ released from active neurons and, hence, hyperexcitability would persist.

Richardson and I (11) in fact attempted a direct intracellular microelectrode study to see if K^+ accumulated abnormally in the border zones of glial scars. We looked for changes in the hyperpolarizing undershoot of the action potential as an indicator of the extracellular concentration at various times after a first action potential had been set up. We encountered great technical problems, such as frequent microelectrode tip breakage, as we penetrated the scar zone. In one cell we found evidence of a probably abnormally slow removal of extracellular K^+, but the technical and sampling problems made the general study inconclusive. Furthermore, after completing the study we realized that our method could only test excitability in those regions where the spike undershoot was occurring; consequently, there has been as yet no test of excitability changes as a consequence of a K^+ buildup along presynaptic terminals or upon relatively distant dendrites. In view of the large "dendritic" potentials comprising the primary surface negative part of the electroencephalogram (EEG) spike, the input stage of the cell would seem to be the most likely place to look for the hypothesized abnormality to appear. Gutnick and Prince (5) recently noted that axons projecting into penicillin-induced cortical epileptic foci may be excited during spontaneous interictal epileptiform discharges, and they consider as one possibility that the increased axonal excitability may be related to large concomitant increases in extracellular K^+.

Grossman and Rosman (4) also carried out intracellular studies in glial scars resulting from freeze lesions and noted similar technical difficulties. They were particularly interested in determining the resting potential of neuroglial cells in the gliotic cortex. They found that "gliotic, epileptogenic cortex contains at least some inexcitable cells whose rates and amplitudes of depolarization following neuronal activity evoked by electrical stimulation were very similar to those of inexcitable cells in normal cortex." However, they noted that despite these findings "the present observations do not provide an adequate test of the hypothesis of local accumulation of K^+ in extracellular clefts in gliotic cortex . . ." because ". . . many inexcitable cells were found with low membrane potentials, and the activities of these cells may predominate in injured cortex."

The neuroglial impairment hypothesis still lacks critical testing. There is a lot of evidence, anatomical, chemical, and physiological, which is consistent with the hypothesis but which does not prove it. Testing the hypothesis has already provided a number of new problems, some technical in nature. Continued work along these lines is likely to offer a challenging and fruitful area for further research on focal epilepsy in the coming years.

REFERENCES

1. Fertizer, A. P., and Ranck, J. B., Jr., Potassium accumulation in interstitial space during epileptiform seizures. *Exp. Neurol.*, 1970, **26**: 571–585.

2. Foerster, O., and Penfield, W., Structural basis of traumatic epilepsy and results of radical operation. *Brain*, 1930, **53**: 99–119.
3. Gelder, N. M. van, Sherwin, A. L., and Rasmussen, T., Amino acid content of epileptogenic human brain: Focal versus surrounding regions. *Brain Res.*, 1972, **40**: 385–393.
4. Grossman, B. G., and Rosman, L. J., Intracellular potentials of inexcitable cells in epileptogenic cortex undergoing fibrillary gliosis after a local injury. *Brain Res.*, 1971, **28**: 181–201.
5. Gutnick, M. J., and Prince, D. A., Thalamo-cortical relay neurons: Antidromic invasion of spikes from a cortical epileptogenic focus. *Science*, 1972, **176**: 424–426.
6. Haber, B., Kuriyama, K., and Roberts, E., L-glutamic acid decarboxylase: A new type in glial cells and human brain gliomas. *Science*, 1970, **168**: 598–599.
7. Maxwell, D. S., and Kruger, L., The fine structure of astrocytes in the cerebral cortex and their response to focal injury produced by heavy ionizing particles. *J. Cell Biol.*, 1965, **25**: 141–157.
8. Orkand, B. K., Nicholls, J. G., and Kuffler, S. W., Effect of nerve impulses on the membrane potential of glial cells in the central nervous system of amphibia. *J. Neurophysiol.*, 1966, **29**: 788–806.
9. Penfield, W., Mechanism of cicatricial contraction in the brain. *Brain*, 1927, **50**: 499–517.
10. Pollen, D. A., and Lux, H. D., Intrinsic triggering mechanisms in focal paroxysmal discharges. *Epilepsia*, 1966, **7**: 16–22.
11. Pollen, D. A., and Richardson, E. P., Jr., Intracellular microelectrode studies at the border zone of glial scars developing after penetrating wounds and freezing lesions of the sensorimotor area of the cat. *Electroenceph. clin. Neurophysiol.*, 1972, **31**, Suppl.: 27–41.
12. Pollen, D. A., and Trachtenberg, M. C., Neuroglia: Gliosis and focal epilepsy. *Science*, 1970, **167**: 1252–1253.
13. Tower, D. B., Problems associated with studies of electrolyte metabolism in normal and epileptogenic cerebral cortex. *Epilepsia*, 1965, **6**: 183–197.
14. Tower, D. B., Fluids and electrolytes in the central nervous system: Factors affecting their distribution, with special reference to excitability and edema. *Electroenceph. clin. Neurophysiol.*, 1972, **31**, Suppl.: 43–57.
15. Trachtenberg, M. D., and Pollen, D. A., Neuroglia: Biophysical properties and physiologic function. *Science*, 1970, **167**: 1248–1252.
16. Ward, A. A., Mechanisms of neuronal hyperexcitability. *Electroenceph. clin. Neurophysiol.*, 1972, **31**, Suppl.: 75–86.
17. Wilder, B. J., Schimpff, B. D., and Collins, G. H., Ultrastructure study of the chronic experimental epileptic focus. *Epilepsia*, 1972, **13**: 341–355.
18. Zuckermann, E. C., and Glaser, G. H., Hippocampal epileptic activity induced by localized ventricular perfusion with high-potassium cerebrospinal fluid. *Exp. Neurol.*, 1968, **20**: 87–110.

CONTRIBUTION OF EXPERIMENTAL EPILEPSY TO UNDERSTANDING SOME PARTICULAR FORMS IN MAN

ROBERT NAQUET

Institut de Neurophysiologie et de Psychophysiologie, Centre National de la Recherche Scientifique, Marseille, France

In 1966 with the Killams (26) we discovered that a certain baboon from Senegal had photosensitive epilepsy. Because of this discovery, the *Papio papio* of Casamance has been considered since 1967, an animal model of great importance in the study of epilepsy (27).

At that time, as mentioned recently in the conclusion of a general review on the same subject (41):

> we embarked on a systematic study of this type of epilepsy including its electrical and clinical characteristics as well as the effect of certain cerebral lesions. We have looked for animals of the same genus, group, or species presenting the same symptomatology. Finally we have investigated pharmacological applications, both in the trial of anti-epileptic medication used or proposed in man and in improving the understanding of the neurochemical mechanisms of epilepsy. Experimentation is at a stage where the clinical data are no longer in doubt; with regard to the EEG data, certain points such as the exact origin of paroxysmal discharges and mechanism of photosensitivity still require clarification. The neuroanatomical investigation is just beginning and this model will allow the study of neuropathological events secondary to epileptic seizures (45). The entire field is still open for neurophysiological study, both of cell units and of preparations involving destruction of various cortical and subcortical regions; the possibility of a metabolic or neurochemical explanation is still only tentative. Breeding of animals with excessive and stable sensitivity, which has already been done for audiogenic epilepsy, may well provide answers to these various problems.

Since all the data concerning those various approaches to understanding photosensitive epilepsy have been analyzed in earlier works, it seems more interesting to present here only the more recent results, which we shall use in trying to understand certain clinical cases of photosensitive epilepsy, cases that are admittedly exceptional but whose interest lies in the very fact that they are extreme.

First of all we shall report the clinical data, then the new experimental data obtained from the photosensitive *Papio papio*, and in conclusion we shall discuss the deductions that one might make at the present state of our knowledge.

CLINICAL CASES

Initial Case

The first case was reported by Roger and his colleagues (46) and by Gastaut and Roger (22). This was the case of a 27-year-old man, Leo . . . Joseph:

an usher, free of previous pathological history, who came to consult one of us about a right hemifacial spasm which had appeared three years previously. At first this involved only an eyebrow tremor but later a complete blink; then the spasm spread to the whole of one side of the face. It was almost continuous with only rare periods of freedom. It was accentuated by strong sunlight, for which reason the subject wore dark glasses.

The patient complained of no other problem; however, detailed questioning revealed that very occasionally the right shoulder suddenly jerked upwards. Various treatments (genoscopolamine, barbiturates, diphenylhydantoin) had been found to be ineffective.

Examination revealed a characteristic hemifacial spasm beginning in the upper region of the face and then spreading to the whole hemiface. The jerks were rapid and quite soon became a tonic spasm with associated spasmodic generalized movements.

Careful exploration revealed, in addition to these right-sided jerks, some discrete intermittent jerks of the left labial commissure which were independent of the right-sided jerks. When the spasms had disappeared, neurological examination of the face and of the limbs appeared to be negative. However, when the facial movements were examined with extreme care it was possible to demonstrate a few discrete signs of right facial hypotonia.

Here, therefore, is a case of hemifacial spasm of the essential peripheral type. The only anomaly was the existence of rare jerks of the ipsilateral shoulder and of the contralateral face. This is not classical but one of us has emphasized for a long time how frequently a very searching interrogation and a thorough examination may reveal other abnormal movements unnoticed by the patient. As for the discrete facial hypotonia, this was found by Wartenberg (54) in almost all his patients.

The EEG showed a record with no continuous abnormality but characterized by brief paroxysms of bilaterally synchronous polyspikes and waves on absolutely normal background rhythms. The shape, distribution and chronology of these elements were absolutely identical to those generally observed in the myoclonic diencephalic epilepsies. The striking characteristic of these discharges was that they were not synchronous with the facial jerks; the latter were recorded perfectly well from the derivations using electrodes in the frontal pole and inferior frontal positions which picked up the muscle potentials from the orbicularis oculi and levator palpebrae superioris muscles. Hyperventilation made no appreciable difference to the resting record.

Photic stimulation did not apparently accentuate the occurrence of spontaneously visible discharges and did not evoke marked occipital following but its effect was most obvious on the rate of facial jerks. Each flash, in effect, provoked a single jerk whereas rhythmically repeated flashes caused rhythmic jerks which fused into a true tonic spasm when the frequency of flash presentation became sufficiently high.

Because of the similarity between this EEG and that of certain myoclonic epilepsies we performed an intravenous injection of trimethadione. The effect was spectacular: the effectiveness of photic stimulation started to decline after 15 sec. and disappeared completely after 30 sec. At the same time the clonus and spontaneous spasm disappeared and did not reappear until several hours after the injection.

After discussing the pathogenesis of this autonomic hemifacial spasm and the EEG characteristics of the myoclonus, Roger and his colleagues (46) concluded that in their case it seemed possible:

> to confirm that the hemifacial spasms cannot be differentiated from a myoclonic epilepsy of unilateral facial manifestation. The clinical picture of individual clonic movements grouped in a rhythmic or arhythmic fashion or fused in a spasm is highly typical of myoclonic activity. The EEG appearance is characteristic. The clinical picture in our case fits the classical type of hemifacial spasm called peripheral or autonomic. From a single case we cannot presume to classify this as facial myoclonic epilepsy.

In 1954, Gastaut and Roger (22) referring to the same case commented:

> we wished to show that facial epileptic jerks are not necessarily always related to focal cortical epilepsy but may derive from a diencephalic epilepsy and sometimes mimic, in their clinical expression, peripheral facial hemispasm.

The publication of this case inspired numerous discussions at the French Society of Neurology where Krebs (29) commented:

> the facial jerks of the patient had none of the characteristics of the contractions of peripheral facial hemispasm. This case does not show the dimpled chin, nor the concave nose, nor the paradoxical combination of elevation of the internal part of the eyebrow under the action of the frontal muscle and lowering of the eyelid under the effect of the orbicularis oculi.

Furthermore, he noted that Babinski (1):

> by analyzing these deforming and systematically unilateral contractions had demonstrated that they were marked by the particular feature of being identical to those produced by electrical stimulation of the branches of the facial nerve. He concluded that the facial hemispasm, having such intrinsic characteristics, could not be caused by anything but a direct disturbance of the facial nerve or of its nucleus, and that it was rational to refer to this particular form of facial hemispasm as peripheral.

Discussion of the case stopped at this point, leaving open the question whether this was facial myoclonic photosensitive epilepsy simulating a post-paralytic spasm, as Roger's group (46) held, or myoclonic epilepsy having little connection with facial spasm as Krebs (29) thought, or of some other etiology. This being an exceptional case, no solution was reached at that time.

Two Patients

The following two patients are twins (BON . . . , Giselle and BON . . . , Chantal) aged 14 in 1972, whom we have been following since 1970 and both of whom present the combination of a neurological syndrome suggesting spinocerebellar degeneration, aniridia, and epilepsy of the generalized type (12). We shall not discuss the neurological symptoms or the classification of this syndrome both of which are outside the scope of our subject, but we shall report only the electroencephalographic (EEG) data and those supplied by the study of visually evoked potentials (VEP), which seem to us the most significant for comparison with experiments on *Papio papio*.

In the resting EEG, either with the eyes open or closed, both twins showed discharges of generalized spikes and waves (see Figures 1 and 2). Photic stimulation increased the likelihood of their appearance for many stimulation frequencies, both with eyes closed and open. These discharges were sometimes accompanied by generalized myoclonus (Figures 3 and 4).

To study the VEP, photic stimulation was delivered by an Alvar Vareclat Tr stroboscope in the form of flashes, either isolated or paired at various intervals (30, 40, 60, 100, and 200 msec) at a frequency of 1 cycle/1.6 seconds. Later on, the VEPs were processed using an Intertechnique Didac 800 averager. Fifty responses were averaged; the cycles of excitability were studied using the classic method which consists of subtracting the conditional response (R1) from the response to paired stimuli; one thus obtains the single test response (R2): $(R1 + R2) - R1 = R2$. The value of the ratio R1/R2 represents the cortical excitability for a given stimulus interval.

Visually evoked potentials of large amplitude (as much as 300 μV) were seen from all derivations (Figure 5). In both twins the potentials were greater in amplitude over the right than over the left hemisphere.

In these two patients the occipital and inion-vertex responses corresponded to the classic data at least as regards their morphology; however, they were of much greater amplitude [particularly in the case of the late

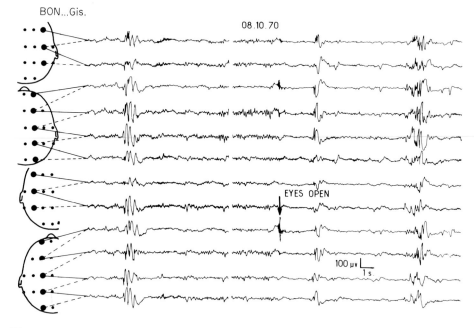

Figure 1. Resting record from BON . . . Gis. with eyes closed at left and open at right. Paroxysmal discharges occur in both conditions.

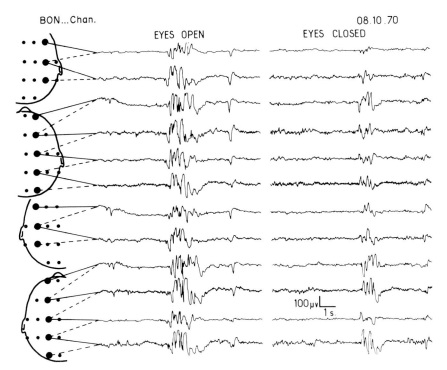

Figure 2. Resting record from BON . . . Chan. with eyes open and closed. Paroxysmal discharges occur in both conditions but are of larger amplitude with the eyes open.

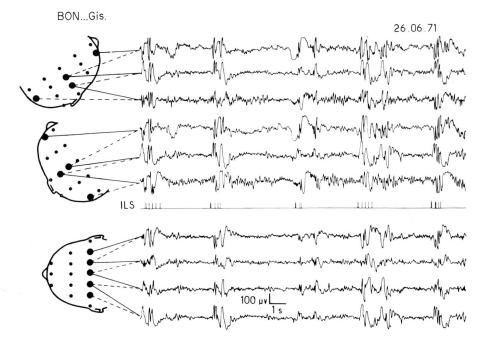

Figure 3. Effect of photic stimulation at various frequencies in BON . . . Gis. Paroxysmal features occur for various frequencies even for low ones. ILS—intermittent light stimulus.

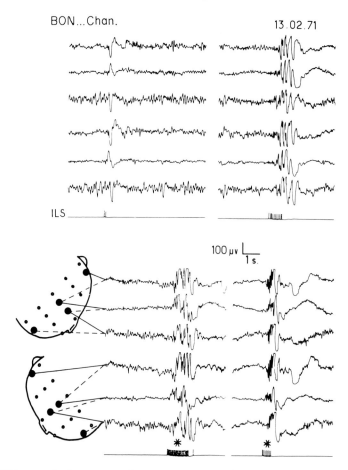

Figure 4. Effects of photic stimulation at various frequencies in BON . . . Chan. Paroxysmal features appear for many stimulation frequencies but polyspike-and-wave discharges, accompanied by myoclonus (star), occur only in response to frequencies close to 15 cps. ILS—intermittent light stimulus.

waves numbered V and VI according to the terminology of Gastaut and Regis (21); for example, even as high as 200–250 μV for wave VI]. The latencies of the late waves were shorter than in normal subjects (100 msec as against 130 msec for wave V, and 170 msec against 200 msec for wave VI). During the same stimulation sequence the occipital responses showed a certain variability in amplitude, probably connected to the level of alertness. No change suggesting habituation appeared during recording.

The most characteristic feature of the frontorolandic responses was the constancy of their occurrence (Figure 5). In amplitude they were often larger than 250 μV and sometimes were even greater than the occipital response of which they presented all the constant components (waves II–VI); these various waves occurred about 20 msec after their occipital equivalents. It is interesting to note that the large amplitude of waves II, III, and IV often gave these responses the appearance of true spikes and

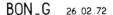

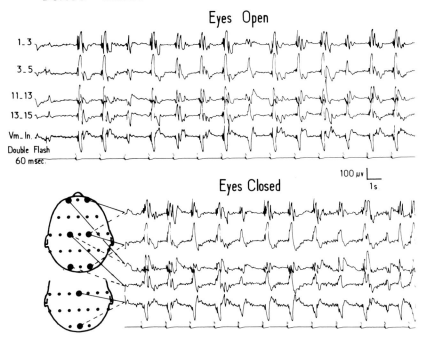

Figure 5. A series of evoked potentials obtained from BON . . . Gis. with eyes open and closed, using paired light flashes separated by 60 msec and delivered at a rate of 1/second. Each double flash triggers paroxysmal features which are bilaterally synchronous and symmetrical, often resembling spikes-and-waves. Vm-In—mid-vertex inion.

waves. The variability of the frontorolandic responses was parallel with that seen in the occipital region; in particular, eye-closing increased the amplitude and the stability of these responses.

In the occipital region the test response (R2) showed no important differences in morphology compared with the conditional response R1; however, the latencies of the various components were longer (from 10 to 20 msec), particularly for the R2 obtained for a stimulus interval of 30 to 40 msec; conversely, for an interval of 100 msec, the latencies of waves IV and V of R2 were found to be shorter by 10 msec. For intervals of 200 msec the latencies were equal. Study of the excitability cycles showed that the absolute refractory period was very short since R2 was already present for an interval of 30 msec. Starting at that interval, the late waves, V and VI, of R2 showed a facilitation which could reach 600% with the subject's eyes closed (Figures 6 and 7).

Facilitation of wave VI in these subjects was seen with stimulus intervals up to 200 msec. For the earlier waves this was not greater than 200% and disappeared after a 100-msec interval. It should be noted that this facilitation was seen even when the subject's eyes were open but in that case it was limited to the later waves, to intervals of 60 and 100 msec and was never greater than 350%; for the 200-msec interval, on the contrary, inhibition of the response was seen. From the inion-vertex derivation the only difference from the results just described was that the maximal excitability (600%) was seen for wave V and for the 40-msec interval (Figures 6 and 7).

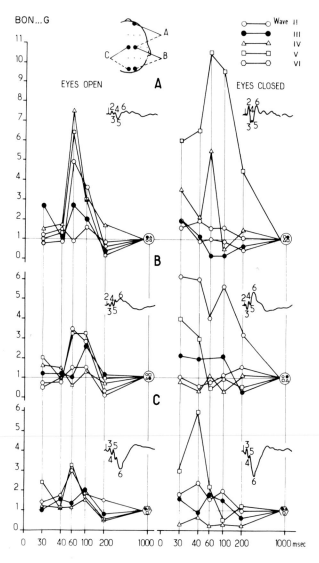

Figure 6. Comparison of excitability cycles of waves II, III, IV, V, and VI recorded from three different derivations (A, B, C) using bipolar linkages in BON . . . Gis. (Average of fifty evoked potentials recorded with eyes open or closed.) Abscissa: log scale; stimulus interval between 2 flashes. Ordinate: the ratio of amplitude R2/R1. There is considerable facilitation for waves IV, V, and VI when the eyes are closed, occurring in all derivations but particularly in the anterior region where it mainly affects wave V.

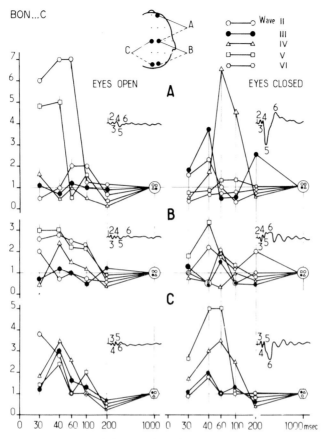

Figure 7. Comparison of excitability cycles of waves II, III, IV, V, and VI recorded from three different derivations (A, B, C) using bipolar linkages in BON . . . Chan. (Average of fifty evoked potentials recorded with eyes open or closed.) Abscissa: log scale; stimulus intervals between two flashes. Ordinate: the ratio of amplitude R2/R1. There is significant facilitation in both anterior regions with the eyes open or closed: with eyes open this involves waves V and VI; with eyes closed mainly wave IV.

In the frontorolandic region the findings for latency and absolute refractory period were identical to those described for the occipital region. Both twins presented very marked facilitation of waves IV and V, particularly for the 30–100 msec intervals, which reached 550 and 1100%, respectively at the 60-msec interval; for all the late components, a more or less pronounced facilitation was still present at the 200-msec interval. Consequently, the enormous amplitude of waves III, IV, V, and VI gave the appearance of a true spike or polyspike-and-wave. This facilitation was still great with the eyes open but did not exceed 750% (Figures 6 and 7). During the recording it was not unusual for single or paired flashes to trigger one for one paroxysmal evoked potentials such as have just been described, with a myoclonic jerk.

Dimov and our group (12) concluded that the twins present paroxysmal visually evoked responses and a long-lasting hyperexcitability involving the cortical regions explored. These results partially confirm those obtained by Morocutti and co-workers (37) and by Lücking and co-workers (32) in photosensitive epileptics, the differences which they found in their patients concerning largely the occipital VEPs.

It should be emphasized that the refractory period is shorter than that generally described in the normal subject (6, 20). Dimov and co-workers (12) commented:

> Since we had found nothing in the literature on normal subjects with which to make a comparison we carried out the same study on a normal subject and found that the visual evoked responses in the frontal region showed, at 30 msec, an absolute refractory period for waves II and VI and a relative one for waves III, IV and V: we were able to confirm in the same subject the existence of facilitation (200%) at 40, 60 and 100 msec for waves II, IV and V whereas at 200 msec there was inhibition of all components [see Figure 8]. In the frontal region in both twins there thus existed excessive hyperexcitability affecting most markedly the late waves of the response which is therefore made to look like a spike or polyspike-and-wave.

These results resemble those obtained by Bergamasco after Metrazol administration (5).

The eyes being open caused little change in this hyperexcitability, which may be related to the aniridia of both subjects. This possibility is backed

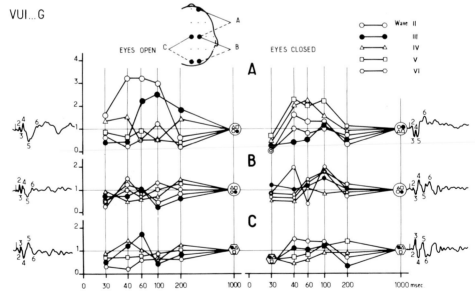

Figure 8. Comparison of excitability cycles of waves II, III, IV, V, and VI recorded from three different derivations (A, B, C) using bipolar linkages in a normal subject. (Average of fifty evoked potentials recorded with eyes open and closed.) Abscissa: log scale; stimulus intervals between two flashes. Ordinate: the ratio of amplitude R2/R1.

up by the absence of habituation which is a familiar observation in cases of aniridia (7). It is possible that the aniridia is instrumental in this photo-sensitivity which is greater than that usually found even in subjects present-ing excessive photosensitivity.

All these data were similar in both twins; it should, however, be pointed out that one was more photosensitive than the other in that the frontal responses were more paroxysmal and the hyperexcitability clearer in Giselle than in Chantal.

New Experimental Data from the Photosensitive *Papio papio*

Some of the experimental data are concerned with the study of various physical parameters that influence photosensitive epilepsy in *Papio papio;* other data involve the combined effects of facial nerve resection and discon-nection of the insertion* of the periocular musculature.

Effects of Variation of Various Physical Parameters

This study was performed by Serbanescu and our group (48) on two *Papio papio*—one very photosensitive, the other much less so. In order to describe the average reactivity of the intermittent light stimulation (ILS) three indices were chosen: the mean intensity of the paroxysmal discharge (I), the mean latency of the discharges (L), and the ratio of the number of effective stimulations to total number of stimuli (E).

When the animals were stimulated with varying wavelengths, it ap-peared that the most effective in revealing photosensitivity of both animals were the colors blue–green and dark green ($\lambda = 487$ and 538 nm); increase in the values of I and E, and decrease of L were seen simultaneously; the colors green ($\lambda = 544$ nm) and red ($\lambda = 676$ nm) were ineffective.

In the same way the paroxysmal discharges triggered by ILS were more intense, more frequent, and of shorter latency when the distance between the light source and the animal was decreased or when the surface area of the source was increased.

The effects of varying pupil diameter and of opening versus closing the eyes were also analyzed. It was found that increasing the pupil diameter increased the intensity of paroxysmal discharges in both animals, but more so in the more photosensitive animal than in the other. Closing the eyes also increased the response intensity but only when the pupils were dilated with homatropine.

In discussing pupil diameter, Serbanescu *et al.* (48) comment:

> the results as a whole show that increase in pupil diameter has a strong effect on level of photosensitivity, which it increases. It seems therefore that the size of the retinal receiving area is instrumental in the genesis of photosensitive paroxysms, as other authors have already suggested (8, 23, 30); Fernandez-

* In this article, for simplicity, we speak of *disconnection.* In fact, we disconnected the muscles from the sclera and resected the muscle bodies for several millimeters.

Guardiola and coworkers (16) suggested that the iris has a specific power to modify retinal excitability. But we observed that pupil dilatation increased intensity of paroxysmal discharges more in the animal which was the more photosensitive; that is, under our experimental conditions and with the two animals we used, the size of the pupil was much more important in the more photosensitive animal than in the other one. Could this, perhaps, be explained by a functional structural anomaly of the retina similar to the vestibular and cochlear anomalies described in the mouse with audiogenic seizures (4, 11)? It is not yet possible to answer this question.

Effects of Facial Nerve Resection and of Disconnection of the Periocular Musculature

From the work of Poncet (44) and of Naquet and our group (38) we know that rhythmic painless periocular stimulation combined with ILS is likely to facilitate the appearance of eyelid clonus and spread of clonus to the face and whole body. On the other hand (40), curarization of the animal reduces the size of the paroxysmal EEG discharges triggered by ILS. These discharges may, however, persist even though less intense, in the very photosensitive animal. Curarization may produce this effect either by suppressing the possibility for clonic signs to appear or because of the constant emotional stress which accompanies it. With the Killams (27) we demonstrated that "all disturbing influences in the laboratory during the test session markedly attenuated the response or blocked it entirely. These included excessive noise, light and general traffic."

Naquet and Menini (42) have shown that periocular anesthesia with 0.5% procaine blocks the clonic jerks elicited by ILS, but the paroxysmal EEG discharges persist. Saline injected in the same region affects neither the clinical nor EEG signs elicited by ILS. More concentrated doses of procaine block the electrical discharges as well, but it is impossible to be certain that the decrease in photosensitivity is not a consequence of a general effect of this agent (38).

In view of these results we thought it would be interesting to block this feedback mechanism, if it exists, by chronically immobilizing the eyes and eyelids.

First of all we resected the intraparotid part of the facial nerve on both sides for more than 1 cm (9). During the days immediately after the operation the animal kept its eyes open and no longer closed them when flicker was presented in front of it. In the absence of eyelid clonus, certain very photosensitive animals show clonus of the lower jaw, the head and the whole body, while the eyes remain half-open. In other animals the usual organization of the seizure disappears and a few isolated clonic movements of the body may occur with a latency usually rather long in relation to the paroxysmal EEG discharges (38, 41).

Results of this type of operation are by no means easy to interpret for the following reasons.

a. In the weeks immediately following the operation the animal rapidly became able to close its eyes spontaneously and also, because of the integrity of innervation of the levator palpebrae superioris, maintained the ability to make a certain number of movements of the eyelids.

b. Eye movements persisted because the nerves and muscles that control the eyes themselves were not affected. It seemed essential for the next phase to be surgical operation on these muscles. The surgical technique for this has been described by Dimov with our group (13).

c. Between the second and third month after the facial nerve operation a postparalytic facial spasm appeared.

We wish to comment first on the interaction between facial spasm and photosensitive epilepsy and then on operating on the periocular musculature and the effects on VEP and photosensitivity.

POSTPARALYTIC FACIAL SPASM AND PHOTOSENSITIVE EPILEPSY (9, 12)

The 6 *Papio papio* used in this study showed various degrees of photosensitivity, according to the classification of Killam and co-workers (28); 1 was not photosensitive, 4 were +3, and the remaining 1 demonstrated afterdischarges manifested by a generalized seizure after the end of ILS. Two of the +3 baboons were utilized as controls and were not operated.

Two to three months after the surgery, a postparalytic peripheral spasm appeared. Clinically, this spasm consisted of muscular twitches in various facial areas, mainly in the region where the superficial musculature is innervated by the inferior facial and particularly at the level of the triangular of the lips. These fragmentary myoclonic jerks may appear spontaneously or may be induced by various tactile, auditory, or photic stimuli. The latency of the average muscular response is 25 msec on electrical stimulation of the eyebrow arches. The latency of the average facial myoclonus to light varied little within the same animal, whether it involved the orbicular muscle of the eyelids, the triangularis of the lips or the platysma of the neck. But there may be individual variations ranging from 50 to 70 msec.* Analysis of successive single responses for a given muscle showed a large variability in latency (Figure 9). In one of the photosensitive animals, without any confirmed relationship between the two, the response was double: the first response appeared with a latency of 40 msec followed by a second one of 69 msec (Figure 10).

Regardless of the degree of photosensitivity, following repetitive stimulation, there is a rapid habituation to auditory and tactile stimuli but not to visual stimulations. For these latter, ILS may induce regular myoclonus up to 25 cps (Figure 11).

* Feger and colleagues (15) observed that upon photic stimulation in the cat, the latency of the blink reflex recorded at the level of the orbicular branch of the facial nerve is 35 msec; in man, Rushworth (47) found a latency of 50 to 60 msec for the blink reflex, and Marteret (33) a latency of 30 to 45 msec for an electrographic activity of the orbicular muscle.

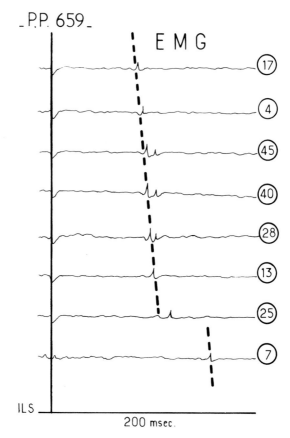

Figure 9. Different latencies for a given muscle [electromyogram (EMG) of triangularis of the lips] of unit responses to light flashes at 1 cps. *Papio papio* 659 is a nonphotosensitive animal. Top to bottom: shortest to longest latencies. Number in circle represents the number of flashes already given. ILS—intermittent light stimulus.

The appearance of facial spasm does not alter the degree of photosensitivity in a nonphotosensitive animal, and for higher frequencies, myoclonic responses cannot be obtained between 15 and 30 cps. In photosensitive animals, when ILS induces a paroxysmal activity in the frontal regions with or without slow waves which can induce polyspikes or polyspikes and waves, the myoclonic jerks reappear in the facial region where they previously occurred spontaneously. These are present at the same frequency as the paroxysmal discharges that they induced by ILS. During this activity, the correlation between the cortical discharges and the peripheral myoclonus is as follows: (*a*) the occipitally evoked potentials appear with a latency of 15 to 20 msec; (*b*) the frontal spike with a latency of 20 to 30 msec; the myoclonus follows the frontal response; it is reinforced as the amplitude of the frontal spike-type response is increased; it is decreased in amplitude or blocked during slow wave activity. The facial myoclonus always appears 10–12 msec after the spike recorded at the level

P.P. 671

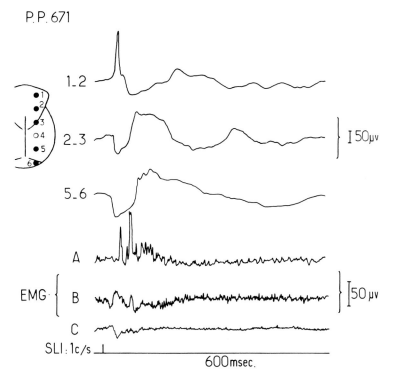

Figure 10. Relationship between paroxysmal visually evoked potentials recorded from the frontorolandic region (1-2, 2-3) and myoclonic jerks induced by flashes at 1 cps ILS = 1 cps) in a very photosensitive animal. (Average of fifty flashes.) (A) Electromyogram of triangularis of the lips; (B and C) electromyogram recorded at the level of the eyebrow arches. The frontorolandic response precedes the muscular one which is double: the first appears at 40 msec and the second at 69 msec.

of the frontal cortex. Its latency relative to the flash is then 40–42 msec, as if only early units have been facilitated since, for isolated evoked potentials, this latency usually exceeds 50 msec. Correlations with the occipital activity are more difficult to define since, at that moment, there often exists a response of a higher harmonic.

This muscular activity may not be directly related to the stimulation which precedes the response, but with the one prior to it. To study this possibility, we interrupted the ILS in order to average the end of the trains of flashes. After the last stimulation, there are as many frontal evoked potentials as myoclonic twitches—a potential with frequencies up to 15 cps and two later potentials; that is, for frequencies of 15 cps, one must deduct one evoked potential due to an "off" effect (see Figures 14 and 15). The actual latencies of a frontal potential and of the myoclonus corresponding to the last stimulation are 28–30 msec and 36–40 msec, respectively.

In all cases, the rhythmic facial myoclonic responses always precede the generalized myoclonic jerks which may appear, and these latter mainly

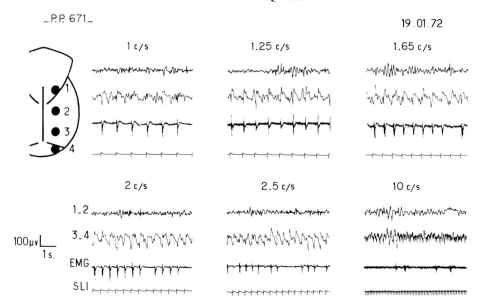

Figure 11. Myoclonic twitches of the triangularis of the lips appearing at different frequencies of flash stimulation (with same interval beginning at 1.65 cps). ILS induces regular myoclonic responses up to 2.5 cps.

occur with the most paroxysmal frontal responses. One of the animals demonstrated generalized tonic-clonic seizure after the end of ILS. Immediately after the seizure, during the period of EEG depression, light flashes (0.5–1 cps) induced facial myoclonic twitches of small amplitude which increased as the cortical activity returned to normal.

Cherubini and co-workers (10) and Carlier and co-workers (9) have thus confirmed some classic data, that is, the possibility of producing by a facial nerve lesion the appearance of a postparalytic peripheral spasm comparable to that described in man (1, 15, 49, 50) and in animals (2, 19, 24).

So far there is no obvious explanation for the differences in latency found between animals for the muscles from which myoclonus is recorded, but these differences may reflect different patterns of reinnervation of the facial muscles (50). However, Carlier and co-workers (9) demonstrated that this peripheral myoclonus could be modulated by central mechanisms.

As regards peripheral myoclonus:

a. Its induction by ILS at high frequencies is possible only in animals that have been previously photosensitive regardless of the degree of photosensitivity of the animal.

b. It is of a smaller intensity and more difficult to induce after a generalized seizure, even with flashes delivered at low frequencies.

c. In photosensitive animals, for a given stimulation at 25 cps, the myoclonus follows the frontorolandic paroxysmal discharges in the EEG, increasing when these latter increase and ceasing when they disappear. These latter may result from a disinhibition mechanism comparable to the one described by Kuhnt and Creutzfeldt (31) which would favor the appearance in the frontorolandic region and other subcortical structures (19) of responses evoked by light flashes. A similar mechanism may exist for the myoclonus (as a direct consequence of the light flash or of the resulting cortical potentials); the earliest units (40 msec) being facilitated over the latest ones. This would explain the reason why the myoclonus follow at 25 flashes per second.

EFFECT ON PHOTOSENSITIVITY AND ON THE VEPS OF DISCONNECTION
OF THE PERIOCULAR MUSCULATURE IN PHOTOSENSITIVE BABOONS (9, 13)

This study was carried out partly on the photosensitive animals used by Carlier and colleagues (9) after they had undergone the first stage of bilateral resection of the facial nerve and also on 4 animals who were photosensitive but had no peripheral or central lesions.

In the former, a few weeks or months after the facial nerve resection, a further operation was carried out. This consisted of disconnection of the insertion of all the periocular and periorbital musculature. This was performed after premedication with atropine and either under general anesthesia with pentobarbital or after Fluothane anesthesia, intubation, artificial respiration, Flaxedil immobilization, and additional local anesthesia. The technique of stimulation and implantation has been reported by Dimov and co-workers (13).

Study of the Animal's Photosensitivity. When the animals were tested after operation on the facial nerve and before any interference with the periocular musculature they still showed the same degree of photosensitivity, although as we mentioned above the clinical signs were somewhat different from those seen in intact animals (38, 41).

The paroxysmal EEG discharges still occurred in the form of spikes and polyspikes predominating in the frontorolandic region; virtually no differences were seen between the operated animals and the controls. Disconnection of the insertion of the periocular muscles did not affect photosensitivity, with the exception of a postoperative period of about 5 to 10 days when it was decreased or even abolished.

During the months following these two surgical operations the degree of photosensitivity did not vary but the EEG signs and the amount of myoclonus were accentuated and became more stable.

Study of the VEPs. In the control animals, as in the other *Papio papio* before surgery on the eyeballs, the VEPs had characteristics similar to those described by Menini and our group (34) both in the occipital and in the frontorolandic regions where they were of small amplitude.

Resection of both facial nerves had no effect, at least in the weeks and months immediately following the operation. Ten days after the operation

on the muscle, sporadic frontorolandic VEPs of large amplitude began to
occur. Their amplitude increased as time went by and, about $1\frac{1}{2}$ months
after the operations, they often looked like a spike-and-wave of which the
amplitude might reach 250–300 μV. The paroxysmal responses were fairly
stable but had the same variations as those previously described by Walter
and his group (53).

The average response recorded from bipolar derivations may be divided
into an early and a late part. The former consists of a negative wave of
larger amplitude (150–200 μV) with a latency of 20 to 24 msec, culminating
at 35 to 40 msec and followed by a positive wave of which the peak occurs
at 90 ($\pm$10) msec; the late part occurs in the form of three or four negative–positive oscillations, of which the respective latencies are 180 ($\pm$10),
210 ($\pm$20), and 220 ($\pm$40) msec. From one more posterior derivation this
VEP is found to have the same characteristics but to be of opposite polarity
(which suggests a focus of maximal activity at this level). When animals
were immobilized with Flaxedil the response showed no specific modifications and did not lose its paroxysmal nature. The occipital VEPs showed
no particular difference from those recorded from animals before surgery
or from controls.

In the operated animals the test response (R2) recorded from the frontorolandic region to paired flashes showed certain characteristics: the absolute refractory period was very brief since for a 20-msec interval the R2
response was present with all its components, which was followed by a
series of oscillations lasting sometimes up to 700 to 800 msec; for all the
intervals up to 200 msec, there was facilitation which could reach 450–500%
for the late components. The early components never reached the amplitude of R1 for the intervals used but their constant presence gave to the
global response (particularly from 60 to 80 msec) the appearance of polyspike and wave.

The excitability cycles of the occipital VEPs were similar to the responses
recorded from the same region in nonoperated animals. These results show
that over the course of time and regardless of any focal cerebral lesion,[*]
the frontal VEPs may increase in amplitude under certain experimental
conditions in animals selected for their extreme photosensitivity.

As yet nonphotosensitive animals have not been studied so it is difficult
to know what is involved in this modification of the VEPs. Our animals
underwent several surgical operations of various types and were anesthetized several times which generally has no effect. However, the periocular
operation may involve postoperative shock; one of the animals showed a
slowed EEG for several days after the operation, and a possible secondary
repercussion after surgery cannot be ruled out. If this were to be the case

[*] Walter and co-workers (53) have described large-amplitude frontal VEPs under certain
experimental conditions which can be explained only in some cases by cortical lesions unrelated
to the photosensitivity of the animals.

one might ask why the VEPs are modified only in the frontorolandic region and not occipitally. Disconnection of the insertion of the periocular muscles and the immobilization of the eyes so caused, also cannot be discounted. Conversely, the facial paralysis and the appearance of postparalytic facial spasm cannot by themselves explain this phenomenon (9). It is, however, possible that the combination of the two processes, disconnection of the insertion of the periocular muscles and the associated facial spasms may be the cause of these modifications which would thus initially have a purely peripheral origin. These peripheral lesions might then increase secondarily the excitability of the frontorolandic region, possibly through the intermediary of certain deep structures, notably the motor and sensory nuclei of the nerves involved (the third, fourth, fifth, sixth, and seventh). The hyperexcitability could be entirely due to phenomena of deafferentation involving liberation of these structures or to the association of phenomena of deafferentation (immobilization of eyes and eyelids, facial paralysis) and of excess of afferents (facial spasm).

RELATIONSHIPS BETWEEN PAROXYSMAL EEG DISCHARGES OBTAINED AFTER DISCONNECTION OF THE INSERTION OF THE PERIOCULAR MUSCULATURE AND THE FACIAL MYOCLONUS TRIGGERED BY STIMULATION AT DIFFERENT FREQUENCIES IN PHOTOSENSITIVE ANIMALS AFTER FACIAL NERVE RESECTION

A few weeks or months after the combined surgery on the facial nerve and the periocular muscles, the relationships between the paroxysmal EEG (frontorolandic) signs and the myoclonic signs became more and more obvious because of the considerable amplitude of the former and the appearance of facial spasm, which is very easy to study because of its exaggerated nature (Figure 12).

Stimulation at 5 cps caused frontorolandic VEPs of which the amplitude varied during the course of a train of stimuli and which sometimes looked like spike-and-wave. In the occipital region there was following at the same frequency—peribuccal myoclonus occurred at the same frequency as stimulation, whereas the frontorolandic VEPs were paroxysmal.

At 10 cps the frontorolandic EEG activity took the form of rhythmic spikes of large amplitude, synchronous with the photic stimulation. Occipital following was at the same frequency—each frontal spike was accompanied by a facial clonus. Between 15 and 20 cps, the same phenomenon persisted in the frontorolandic region but now the spikes were sometimes intermixed with slow waves. The paroxysmal discharges increased in amplitude. In the occipital region, following often shifted to a higher harmonic. The peribuccal myoclonus continued to follow the same rhythm as the frontorolandic discharges; these changed along with the EEG activity, affecting the face and the limbs more violently when the paroxysmal elements became larger and diminishing in the face and ceasing in the limbs during slow waves.

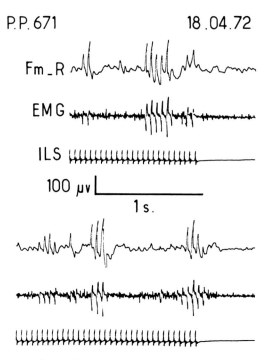

P.P. 671   18 . 04 . 72

Fm_R

EMG

ILS

100 μv

1 s.

Figure 12. Recording of the end of two trains of stimuli at 25 cps [intermittent light stimulus (ILS)] showing relationship between frontorolandic paroxysmal discharges (Fm-R) and the triangularis muscle of the lips [electromyogram (EMG)] in *Papio papio* 671.

At 25 cps the features recorded in the frontorolandic region became more paroxysmal but the spikes and polyspikes were very rapidly intermixed with slow waves; the more paroxysmal the spike elements were, the greater and slower were the slow waves (Figures 12 and 13). The occipital following remained unchanged at the higher harmonic; however, it was common for certain frontorolandic discharges and also for slow waves to spread to this region. The myoclonus was much more violent and more diffuse; it continued to keep step only with the paroxysmal elements, that is, it was interrupted by more obvious pauses than for the other frequencies. This is the frequency at which it is easiest to induce an afterdischarge, as previously demonstrated (27); when the latter occurs the relationships between the cortical discharge and the electromyographic (EMG) manifestations are completely different, at least during the tonic phase.

At 40 cps, photic stimulation may still trigger paroxysmal frontorolandic events in certain particularly photosensitive animals. Myoclonus, when it occurs, follows the same rhythm as the frontorolandic paroxysm; it is less violent than at 25 cps.

The averaged polygraphic recording of stimulus trains shows that an "off" resonse may occur when photic stimulation ceases. In general this appears only at frequencies above 20 cps. It becomes clearer as the fre-

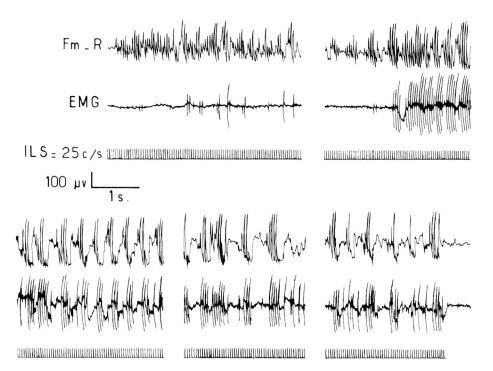

Figure 13. Relationship between the paroxysmal features recorded from the frontoro-landic region (Fm-R) and the electromyogram (EMG) of the triangularis during intermittent light stimulation (ILS = 25 cps) in a very photosensitive *Papio papio* that had undergone surgery for resection of both facial nerves and disconnection of the insertion of the periocular muscles. The paroxysmal frontorolandic features occur with the same fluctuations as the features recorded from the cortex; they decrease in amplitude or are blocked when cortical slow waves appear.

quency increases. This "off" response occurs in the form of a positive wave which is often paroxysmal. It occupies the frontorolandic region and pre-cedes a negative wave which involves the whole cortex and notably the occipital region where it is generally predominant. The beginning of the "off" response is followed, like the paroxysmal features recorded in the frontorolandic region during photic stimulation and with the same latency, by a facial clonus, whereas the subsequent slow wave is not accompanied by any muscular event. This phenomenon is very clear for frequencies close to 30 to 40 cps (Figures 14 and 15).

At the beginning of a new train of stimuli, the frontorolandic spikes, occipital following, and the myoclonic jerks reappear, but these depend on the length of the interval between two trains and on the degree of stability of photosensitivity of the animal in question. The first flash may sometimes trigger an "on" response of large amplitude followed by a myoclonus.

By using a preparation that produces exaggerated changes both in the EEG activity and in the facial myoclonic jerks caused by photic stimulation,

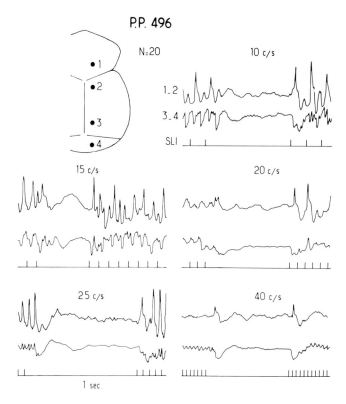

Figure 14. Relations between electroencephalogram spikes in the frontal cortex (1-2) and following in the occipital cortex (3-4) upon photic stimulation (ILS) at 10, 15, 20, 25, or 40 cps. Tracing corresponds to an average of 20 trains of flashes. See text.

it becomes easier to analyze the relationships existing between the frontal discharge and the peripheral myoclonus and also to examine the transformation of the polyspikes into polyspikes-and-waves.

We shall not elaborate on the numerous theories which have been put forward to explain how these slow waves are constituted and how the myoclonus is provoked, but it seems important to mention that these experiments show that the slow wave is most marked when the spikes preceding it are of greatest amplitude and that, under our experimental conditions, it appears only at certain frequencies of stimulation, generally high ones.

The occipital cortex is known to be necessary for the occurrence of the paroxysmal events provoked by photic stimulation in *Papio papio* (52) and is assumed to be instrumental in these, by a mechanism of disinhibition under the effect of certain stimulation frequencies (14, 31, 36); although the role of the occipital cortex should not be underestimated, our preparations put the accent back on the frontorolandic region and on its participation in photosensitive epilepsy in *Papio papio* (18, 35, 42, 43).

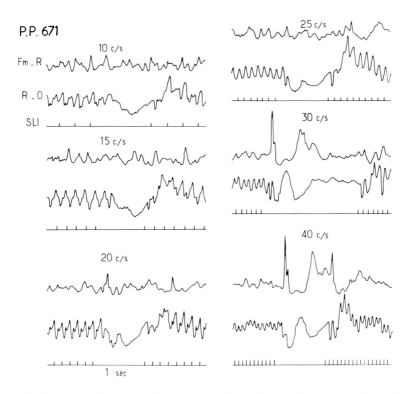

Figure 15. Relations between electroencephalographic spikes in the frontal cortex (Fm-R) and following in the occipital area (R-O) upon photic stimulation (ILS) at 10, 15, 20, 25, 30, and 40 cps in the *Papio papio* 671 after curarization. Tracing corresponds to an average of 20 trains of flashes. See text.

CORRELATIONS BETWEEN CLINICAL DATA AND EXPERIMENTAL RESULTS OBTAINED FROM *Papio papio*

There is nothing original about provoking a facial spasm during the month following an operation causing a lesion of the facial nerve in the baboon; however, the mechanism of triggering it with photic stimulation in photosensitive animals seems significant for several reasons.

This experimental model should allow a better appreciation of the importance of the facial nerve and the role played by the afferents from the face in the induction and maintenance of paroxysmal discharges induced by ILS in the photosensitive *Papio papio*.

From a clinical point of view the data supplied by this experimental model help us to understand the case published by Roger and his colleagues (46). It is now possible to consider, contrary to the opinion of these authors (22, 46) and Krebs (29), that this subject did, indeed, present a post-paralytic facial spasm (witness the facial hypotonia) of peripheral origin making it the classic facial spasm. Also, if we consider the EEG data reported by Roger and co-workers (46), their patient presented signs most suggestive of generalized epilepsy (for example, the occurrence at rest of spontaneous spike-and-wave discharges). His epilepsy was probably photosensitive in nature, first because photic stimulation triggered hemifacial myoclonus for a whole series of stimulation frequencies and, second, because the wearing of dark glasses alleviated the hemispasm.

Thus, this was not a special form of "diencephalic" epilepsy expressing itself as a facial spasm of peripheral origin, as these authors (46) thought (22). Rather we may now consider it to have been a postparalytic facial spasm of peripheral origin (39) occurring in a subject predisposed to generalized, photosensitive epilepsy of central origin, very probably familial. As in our photosensitive *Papio papio*, the facial spasm was very easily triggered and maintained by photic stimulation, hence the unilateral hemifacial nature of the myoclonus provoked by the latter.

The paroxysmal evoked responses in the twins with extreme photosensitivity are more difficult to explain. Such responses are exceptional in man. A similar case has recently been seen in a patient with amaurotic idiocy (3). Our findings in the *Papio papio* certainly suggest an orientation but at present it seems impossible to reach a conclusion. Aniridia certainly plays a role, and we have seen in *Papio papio* that pupil dilatation is one of the factors effective in triggering paroxysmal discharges under the effect of photic stimulation, the more so if the subjects are photosensitive.

If these conditions can be extrapolated to man (as to our twins), we can accept that aniridia is more effective when particularly extreme photosensitivity is associated with it.

However, the aniridia is not the whole explanation. This fact is supported by the data from the photosensitive baboons. The pupil dilatation obtained by periocular instillation of homatropine is not enough to provoke paroxysmal changes of the potentials evoked by isolated flashes and recorded in the frontorolandic region. It is possible that, apart from the aniridia, lesions of the retina may play a role; as mentioned above, in audiogenic epilepsy, cochlear lesions have been blamed. So far we have not been able to demonstrate any particular retinal characteristics in photosensitive animals. Our results are only fragmentary, from the histological point of view, but it seems that electroretinographically the responses from the photosensitive *Papio papio* do not have a specific morphology (17, 51). However, the possibility cannot be ruled out that the retina was injured during the various operations on the periocular region. Having no anatomical evidence as yet, it is difficult to conclude one way or the other about the possible role of retinal lesions in the occurrence of these paroxysmal evoked potentials in the *Papio papio* and in the twins.

It is possible that periocular lesions (notably of the muscles) may promote the occurrence of these paroxysmal frontorolandic responses. (At the present state of our experiments we must be cautious in interpreting data and so we must cite them only as a possibility in the *Papio papio*.) If the above is true, these lesions must produce hyperexcitability of certain deep structures, notably the motor and sensory nuclei of the nerves concerned in the lesions that were made.

It is within the realms of possibility that such hyperexcitability also exists in the twins, perhaps through a different mechanism, but due to a cerebellar syndrome.

Finally, it remains to be demonstrated what relationship might exist between such hyperexcitability of the brainstem nuclei and the paroxysmal frontorolandic response. Are they associated? Is one the consequence of the other? What are the respective roles of the visual cortex and frontorolandic cortex? Further experiments are necessary to answer these questions.

The account of the human clinical cases, the experimental observations collected from the photosensitive *Papio papio*, and their correlations bring out many facts which seem to us to be of importance.

The photosensitive *Papio papio* remains an excellent model (27) for the study of photosensitive epilepsy in general and particularly that of man. The points of comparison are many in regard to the common photosensitive epilepsy or the exceptional clinical cases which mimic it.

The data that we have at present about epilepsy in *Papio papio* are, however, still fragmentary. Numerous unknowns remain which necessitate (besides neurochemical and neuropharmacological investigations which we have not discussed here) the continuation of neurophysiological experimentation. In particular, the study of the effects of cerebral lesions (41) or peripheral lesions (if, indeed, it is they that are in question) should be pursued and in a more and more selective fashion to discover not only the resultant modifications of the degree of photosensitivity but also the electrographic (EEG, microelectrodes recordings, and so on) and clinical patterns evoked by ILS.

These results should be useful for research into the respective roles played by certain nuclei in the brainstem, on the one hand, and by the cerebral cortex (frontal? occipital?), on the other hand, in the pattern and the release of paroxysmal frontorolandic EEG discharges evoked by ILS.

These data, combined with neurochemical and neuropharmacological experimentation, should bring a better knowledge of the photosensitive epilepsy of *Papio papio* and that of man.

REFERENCES

1. Babinski, J., Hémispasme facial périphérique. *Rev. Neurol. (Paris)*, 1905, 13: 151–158.
2. Ballance, C., and Duel, A. B., *A Note on the Large Pyramidal Cell of Facial Area of the Left Rolandic Cortex Following Certain Experimental Op-*

erations Performed on the Right Facial Nerve. Thompson, Dundee, Scotland, 1934.

3. Ballis, T., and Beaumanoir, A., Self-provoked epilepsy in a case of the late infantile form of amaurotic idiocy. *Electroenceph. clin. Neurophysiol.,* 1972, **33**: 354.

4. Behrman, S., and Wyke, B., Vestibulogenic seizures. *Brain,* 1958, **81**: 529.

5. Bergamasco, B., Excitability cycle of the visual cortex in normal subjects during photosensory rest and cardiazol activation. *Brain Res.,* 1965, **2**: 51–60.

6. Bergamini, L., and Bergamasco, B. (Eds.), *Cortical Evoked Potentials in Man.* Thomas, Springfield, Illinois, 1967.

7. Bergamini, L., Bergamasco, B., and Mombelli, A., Visual evoked potentials in subjects with congenital aniridia, *Electroenceph. clin. Neurophysiol.,* 1965, **19**: 394–397.

8. Boynton, M., and Riggs, A., The effect of stimulus area and intensity upon the human retinal response. *J. Exp. Psychol.,* 1951, **42**: 217–226.

9. Carlier, E., Cherubini, E., Dimov, S., and Naquet, R., Résection des nerfs faciaux èt de la musculature périoculaire; leurs conséquences chez le *Papio papio* photosensible. *Electroenceph. clin. Neurophysiol.,* 1973, **35**: 13–23.

10. Cherubini, E., Carlier, E., and Naquet, R., L'azione della luce sullo spasmo del faciale post-paralitico nel *Papio papio* fotosensitile. *Riv. Neurol.,* 1972, **62**: 429–681.

11. Darrouzet, J., Niaussat, M., and Legouix, J. P., Etude histologique de l'organe de Corti de souris d'une lignée présentant des crises convulsives au son. *C.R. Acad. Sci. (Paris),* 1968, **266**: 1163–1165.

12. Dimov, S., Breffeilh, J. L., Menini, C., and Naquet, R., Etude des potentiels évoqués visuels chez des jumelles présentant une photosensibilité excessive. *Rev. EEG Neurophysiol.,* 1973, **2**: 308–311.

13. Dimov, S., Carlier, E., Cherubini, E., and Naquet, R., Effets de différentes lésions nerveuses et musculaires faciales chez le *Papio papio* photosensible *Rev. EEG Neurophysiol.,* 1973, in press.

14. Dimov, S., and Lanoir, J., Chronic epileptogenic foci in the photosensitive baboon *Papio papio. Electroenceph. clin. Neurophysiol.,* 1973, **34**: 353–367.

15. Feger, J., Boulu, R., and Rossignol, P., Le réflexe de clignement à la lumière étude de son trajet et de sa facilitation par la réserpine. *Electroenceph. clin. Neurophysiol.,* 1972, **32**: 247–258.

16. Fernandez-Guardiola, A., Harmony, T., and Roldan, E., Modulation of visual input by pupillary mechanisms. *Electroenceph. clin. Neurophysiol.,* 1964, **16**: 259–268.

17. Fernandez-Guardiola, A., Vuillon-Cacciuttolo, G., and Naquet, R., Résultats préliminaires sur l'étude de l'électrorétinogramme du singe *Papio papio. Acta Neurol. Lat. Am.,* 1968, **14**:.83–91.

18. Fischer-Williams, M., Poncet, M., Riche, D., and Naquet, R., Light-induced epilepsy in the baboon *Papio papio:* Cortical and depth recordings. *Electroenceph. clin. Neurophysiol.,* 1968, **25**: 557–569.

19. Fowler, E. P., Jr., Abnormal movements following injury to facial nerve. *JAMA*, 1939, **113**: 1003–1008.

20. Gastaut, H., Gastaut, Y., Roger, A., Corriol, J., and Naquet, R., Etude électrographique du cycle d'excitabilité cortical. *Electroenceph. clin. Neurophysiol.*, 1951, **3**: 401–428.

21. Gastaut, H., and Regis, H., Visually-evoked potentials recorded transcranially in man. In: *Symposium on the Analysis of Central Nervous System and Cardiovascular Data using Computer Methods.* (L. D. Proctor and W. R. Adey, Eds.). Natl. Acad. Sci., Washington, D.C., 1964: NASA, SP-72: 8–34.

22. Gastaut, H., and Roger, J., Une forme rare de l'épilepsie: Le spasme facial épileptique. *Rev. Neurol. (Paris)*, 1954, **90**: 158–159.

23. Hartline, H. K., The receptive field of the optic nerve fibers. *Am. J. Physiol.*, 1940, **130**: 690–699.

24. Howe, H. A., Tower, S. S., and Duel, A. B., Facial tic in relation to injury of facial nerve: Experimental study. *Arch. Neurol. Psychiat.*, 1937, **38**: 1190–1198.

25. Jesel, M., Hémispasme facial périphérique. Thèse Méd. Strasbourg, 1965.

26. Killam, K. F., Killam, E. K., and Naquet, R., Mise en évidence chez certains singes d'un syndrome photomyoclonique. *C.R. Acad. Sci. (Paris)*, 1966, **262**: 1010–1012.

27. Killam, K. F., Killam, E. K., and Naquet, R., An animal model of light sensitive epilepsy. *Electroenceph. clin. Neurophysiol.*, 1967, **22**: 497–513.

28. Killam, K. F., Naquet, R., and Bert, J., Paroxysmal responses to intermittent light stimulation in a population of baboon (*Papio papio*). *Epilepsia*, 1966, **7**: 215–219.

29. Krebs, M. E., Discussion of Gastaut and Roger (22).

30. Kuffler, S. W., Neurons in the retina: Organization, inhibition and excitation problems. *Cold Spr. Harb. Symp. Quant. Biol.*, 1952, **17**: 281–292.

31. Kuhnt, U., and Creutzfeldt, O. D., Decreased post-synaptic inhibition in the visual cortex during flicker stimulation. *Electroenceph. clin. Neurophysiol.* 1971, **30**: 79–82.

32. Lücking, C. H., Creutzfeldt, O. D., and Heinemann, U., Visual evoked potentials of patients with epilepsy and of a control group. *Electroenceph. clin. Neurophysiol.*, 1970, **29**: 557–566.

33. Marteret, H. G., Etude critique du tracé électromyographique du muscle orbicula ris oculi. Thèse Médecine, Paris, 1965.

34. Menini, C., Dimov, S., Vuillon-Cacciuttolo, G., and Naquet, R., Réponses corticales évoquées par la stimulation lumineuse chez le *Papio papio*. *Electroenceph. clin. Neurophysiol.*, 1970, **29**: 233–245.

35. Menini, C., and Naquet, R., Rôle des aires corticales prémotrices dans l'épilepsie photosensible du singe *Papio papio*. In: *Pathogenesis of Epilepsy* (Bulg. Acad. Sci., Ed.). Sofia, 1971: 303–317.

36. Menini, C., and Rostain, J. C., Activités unitaires évoquées par la stimulation lumineuse dans différents territoires corticaux chez le *Papio papio*. *J. Physiol. (Paris)*, 1970, **62**, Suppl. 3: 414–415.

37. Morocutti, C., Sommer-Smith, J. A., and Creutzfeldt, O., Das visuelle Reaktion Potential dei normalen Versuchspersonen und charakteristische Veränderungen bei Epileptikern. *Arch. Psychiat. Nervenkr.*, 1966, **208**: 234–254.

38. Naquet, R., Ames, F., Carlier, E., Charmasson, G., Catier, J., and Menini, C., Afférences périoculaires et photosensibilité du *Papio papio*. Etude clinique et électroencéphalographique. *Rev. EEG Neurophysiol.*, 1971, **1**: 430–431.

39. Naquet, R., Cherubini, E., Carlier, E., and Gastaut, H., Spasme facial et épilepsie photosensible chez le *Papio papio*. *Rev. Neurol. (Paris)*, 1973, **127**: 529–535.

40. Naquet, R., Killam, K. F., Killam, E. K., Bimar, J., and Poncet, M., Un nouveau "modèle animal" pour l'étude de l'épilepsie: Le *Papio papio*. *Actual. Neurophysiol. (Paris)* [8], 1968: 213–230.

41. Naquet, R., and Meldrum, B. S., Photogenic seizures in baboon. In: *Experimental Models of Epilepsy* (D. P. Purpura, K. F. Penry, D. Tower, D. M. Woodbury, and R. Walter Eds.). Raven Press, Hewlitt, New York, 1972: 373–406.

42. Naquet, R., and Menini, C., La photosensibilité excessive du *Papio papio*. Approaches neurophysiologiques et pharmacologiques de ses mécanismes. *Electroenceph. clin. Neurophysiol.*, 1972, **31**, Suppl.: 13–26.

43. Naquet, R., Menini, C., and Catier, J., Photically-induced epilepsy in *Papio papio*. The initiation of discharges and the role of the frontal cortex of the corpus callosum. In: *Synchronization of the EEG in the Epilepsies* (M. A. B. Brazier and H. Petsche, Eds.). Springer-Verlag, Vienna, 1972: 347–367.

44. Poncet, M., L'épilepsie photosensible du singe *Papio papio*. Etude clinique et électroencéphalographique. Structures corticales et profondes. Thèse Méd. Marseille, 1968.

45. Riche, D., Gambarelli-Dubois, D., Dam, M., and Naquet, R., Repeated seizures and cerebral lesions in photosensitive baboons (*Papio papio*). A preliminary report. In: *Brain Hypoxia* (J. B. Brierley and B. S. Meldrum, Eds.). Spastics Int. Med. Publ., London, 1971: 297–301.

46. Roger, H., Gastaut, H., and Roger, J., Hémispasme facial d'allure essentielle. Electroencéphalogramme à type d'épilepsie myoclonique. Action de la triméthadione sur le spasme et les tracés EEG. *Rev. Neurol. (Paris)* 1952, **87**: 422–424.

47. Rushworth, G., Observations on blink reflexes. *J. Neurol., Neurosurg. Psychiatry*, 1962, **25**: 93.

48. Serbanescu, T., Naquet, R., and Menini, C., Various physical parameters which influence photosensitive epilepsy in the *Papio papio*. *Brain Res.*, to be published.

49. Thiebaut, F., Isch, F., Isch-Treussard, C., and Maso-Subirana, E., Etude électromyographique de quelques cas d'hémispasmes faciaux. *Rev. Neurol. (Paris)*, 1954, **90**: 291–296.

50. Trojaborg, W., and Siemssen, S. O., Reinnervation after resection of the facial nerve. *Arch. Neurol.*, 1972, **26**: 17–24.

51. Vuillon-Cacciuttolo, G., Etude de la photosensibilité et des réponses évoquées le long de la voie visuelle chez le singe *Papio papio*. Thèse Neurophysiol., Marseille, 1970.
52. Wada, J. A., Terao, A., and Booker, H. E., Longitudinal correlative analysis of epileptic baboon *Papio papio*. *Neurology*, 1972, **22**: 1272–1285.
53. Walter, S., Menini, C., Foure, M., and Arfel, G., Aspect pseudo-paroxystique de certaines réponses évoquées visuelles recueillies au niveau frontal chez le babouin. *Rev. EEG Neurophysiol.*, in press.
54. Wartenberg, A., *Hemifacial Spasm: A Clinical and Pathophysiological Study*. Oxford Univ. Press, London and New York, 1952.

DEPTH RECORDINGS IN MAN IN TEMPORAL LOBE EPILEPSY

P. BUSER, J. BANCAUD, and J. TALAIRACH

Service de Neurochirurgie fonctionnelle et Unité 97 de l'INSERM (1)

Paris, France

A large number of studies on the temporal lobe epilepsies have been performed during the last 30 years, using corticographic or deeply inserted, gross recording electrodes or even microelectrodes, in order to determine the characteristics and the extent of the epileptic process and in order, if possible, to localize the epileptogenic focus (2, 3, 8–16, 20, 22, 23–25, 32, 34, 41, 44, 48, 50–52, 63–67, 71, 81).

Our observations reported here, although they are in the same general line, concern more specifically the functional relationships between various levels of the temporal lobe and the limbic system, as they can be assessed by oscilloscopic recordings performed during stereotaxic electrographic explorations (SEEG) [see Bancaud and co-workers (9)] in patients suffering from drug-resistant epilepsy. These explorations have been carried out with multiple, multilead electrodes, combining multichannel recordings with the clinical investigation of the patient. Two problems will be considered below: first, the time relationships between the abnormal spontaneous interictal activities in the epileptic temporal lobe and, second, connections between structures belonging to the limbic system, as they can be investigated by using the multilead system.

Approximately 60 patients were considered, with about 50% suffering from temporal lobe epilepsy, as determined through combined clinical, conventional electroencephalogram (EEG), and SEEG studies, and often confirmed by the subsequent neurosurgical approach. Moreover, and whenever this was possible, the temporal epilepsy was characterized as "unilateral" or "bilateral." For simplicity, we shall consider all these patients as belonging to a so-called T group. The other half of the patients were diagnosed as being not primarily of the T type, either because the epileptic focus was localized elsewhere or because its localization could not be determined. In these patients (termed here non-T), electrodes were nonetheless introduced in the temporal lobes in order to ascertain that these structures were not primarily involved in the epileptic process.

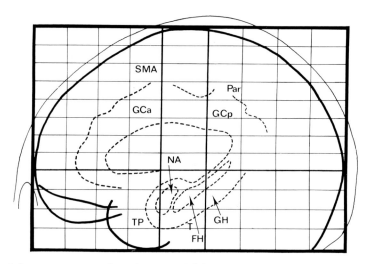

Figure 1. Schematic topography of temporal lobe and cingulate gyrus (GC) according to Talairach's standardized proportional system. Projection on sagittal plane, viewed from the left side. SMA—supplementary motor area; GCa, GCp—anterior and posterior division of GC; NA—amygdaloid nucleus; TP—tip of temporal lobe; GH—hippocampal gyrus; FH—hippocampal formation; Par—parietal cortex.

GENERAL METHODOLOGY

The stereotaxic technology used has been fully described elsewhere and does not need detailed mention here (75, 76). The stereotaxic apparatus permits the use of several deep electrodes, each with multiple leads, thus allowing simultaneous recording from and/or electrical stimulation of many sites in the brain. These electrodes are introduced through transcutaneoosseous trepanation holes under general anesthesia. Later, the patient lies comfortably, fairly vigilant throughout the electrophysiological exploration period (5–7 hours).

The anatomical locations of these electrodes can be determined with good accuracy using CA(anterior commissure)–CP(posterior commissure) landmarks, adjusted for the patient through a preliminary appropriate X-ray investigation with radiographs taken in frontal and sagittal planes.

Our discussion will concern the limbic system in a broad sense, comprising: (a) the amygdaloid nucleus* (NA); (b) hippocampal formation (*formatio hippocampi*, FH) mainly comprising the cornu Ammonis and gyrus dentatus; (c) hippocampal (or parahippocampal) gyrus (*gyrus hippocampi*, GH) with entorhinal cortex; (d) cingulate gyrus (*gyrus cinguli*, GC) with its anterior supracallosal (GCa), and posterior supracallosal (GCp) divisions. Figure 1 shows, in Talairach's standard coordinate system (76), these various structures projected on a sagittal plane.

---

* The amygdaloid area usually stimulated or recorded from was the basolateral portion of the nucleus.

An average of five to ten electrode shafts were introduced (diameter 2.5 mm); each had five to fifteen leads which were silver rings of 1.5 mm length, 1.5 mm apart. In order that each electrode could be used for either recording or electrical stimulation, all leads were connected to an input switchboard which allowed any appropriate combination of circuits.

Central electrical stimulations were delivered from a conventional, rectangular pulse generator. Their duration was usually adjusted between 0.1 and 1 msec and their intensity between 5 and 10 V. Because the electrodes had a rather constant interlead resistance (about 10,000 ohms), no measurement of the stimulating current was considered necessary. The stimulus frequency was adjusted depending on the particular needs; most often (and unless specified otherwise), shocks were given in isolation or at a repetition rate not exceeding 0.5/second. In other cases (for example, in order to elicit after-discharges), repetitive shocks were delivered at various frequencies (3–50/second).

Electrical activities were led into standard amplifiers and displayed on a scope with possibilities of "static" storage. (Tektronix 564). All records were taken between two adjacent leads (bipolar records).

More specific techniques, corresponding to each of the two studies undertaken herein will be described below in some detail.

Time Relationships between Interictal Spontaneous Discharges

It is well known that epileptic structures develop interictal, "synchronized" mass discharges, and a considerable number of investigations (including scalp EEG studies) contain detailed descriptions of their morphology (spikes, waves, sharp waves, and so on) and of their spatiotemporal distribution, to help localize the epileptic focus. Short-lasting spikes are usually considered of local origin ("stationary"), whereas waves of longer duration and complex shapes may be "propagated"; from the spatiotemporal relationships between such events recorded at different sites in the brain or on the scalp, conclusions have been drawn regarding the localization of the epileptic focus (8, 27, 47, 54–56).

It is beyond the scope of this presentation to discuss this methodology in general and its application to temporal lobe epilepsy. Instead we felt that the presence of a large number of electrodes could provide favorable conditions for examining the interictal paroxysmal activities (IPA) which almost always occur at different levels of the epileptic limbic system and for evaluating some aspects of their temporal relationships.

TECHNIQUES

Two distinct methods, of varying complexity, were employed in this study of IPAs.

The *first method,* that of instrumental superposition of activities, is very simple. One of the channels under inspection was led into an amplitude discriminator coupled with a pulse generator—a standard rectangular pulse was thus provided each time the amplitude of the incoming signal was higher than a certain determined value. The pulse was then used to trigger the sweep of the scope (external trigger). Repetition of several such sweeps (five to ten) triggered from one given channel (called *trigger channel*) could provide fairly good indication on the time-locking between events recorded from different brain locations.

We usually limited this simultaneous recording to two channels. Similar, but more elaborate methods (including tape recording, with later off-line playback of the tape with the addition of a trigger pulse preceding each selected spike occurring on the trigger channel) have been developed by others (68, 74, 77). Such techniques were not used here, as an on-line observation was considered preferable.

Because in our display system, the sweep started at a given moment in the rising phase* of the epileptic trigger spike, we could record only events following that spike, whereas the just-mentioned off-line techniques can start the recording sweep before it and so display the full phenomenon. Therefore, in our work, it became necessary in order to obtain complete information on time relationships for records to be taken with each channel being successively used as trigger channel for comparison.

The schematic drawing in Figure 2 summarizes this technique (I) and schematizes various typical situations which can be met when comparing two channels A and B; thus II represents complete time-locking with synchrony (a) or constant time-lag (b); (III) shows independence and (IV) is a case where B is or is not following A (at fixed delay). The trigger channel is always marked with an arrow.

The *second method* consisted in evaluating the cross-correlation function which, as is well known, indicates the general dependence between two time series of signals, x(t) and y(t). Ample use of this method has been made previously in EEG computations (17). In our particular case, the correlogram (Cxy) was computed for nonstationary random series. In order to be able to follow the transient changes of the correlation curve, the sampling time T was set rather short (1 second), a value which even so was well above the duration of the individual IPAs ("spikes," 50 msec on the average). The unit lag time τ (incremental delay) was usually set at 5×10^3 μsec; given that the correlation was performed over 100 points, this value fitted reasonably well with the duration of the observed phenomena. Moreover, our analyzer was computing the correlation function over fifty positive (τ to 50τ) and over fifty negative (-50τ to $-\tau$) values of the incremental delay, thus avoiding a tape recording and off-line playback to obtain that part of the curve corresponding to negative τ's.

---

* The system could theoretically be simplified by using the internal trigger of the scope. We found, however, that an external circuit for amplitude discrimination with a comparator amplifier gives more flexibility and accuracy.

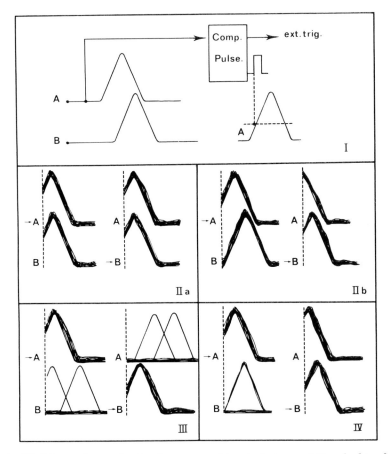

Figure 2. (I) Schema for study, by the superposition technique, of time-locking between paroxysmal events occurring at two brain sites. Trigger channel (A, arrow) is fed into voltage comparator with adjustable threshold, delivering trigger pulse to external trigger of scope (ext. trig.). (II, III, and IV) Cases most often encountered when comparing two channels, A and B (see explanations in text). Dashed vertical lines: start of sweep. Each diagram is supposed to consist of ten successive, superimposed sweeps.

A preliminary empirical study was carried out with "simulation" of epileptic spikes (consisting of rectangular pulses fed through appropriate RC circuits); this indicated which type of correlogram could be expected from such analysis of nonstationary phenomena with constant time-locking but variable delay. Figure 3 illustrates results obtained in this way with artificial spikes of either similar (left) or different (right) durations, each curve corresponding to a given interval between them. As can be seen, some indication may even be obtained concerning the interval between spikes occurring on the two channels under inspection, provided that the phenomena on each channel remain rather constant in shape and duration, which is very often the case for interictal epileptic phenomena, within certain limits.

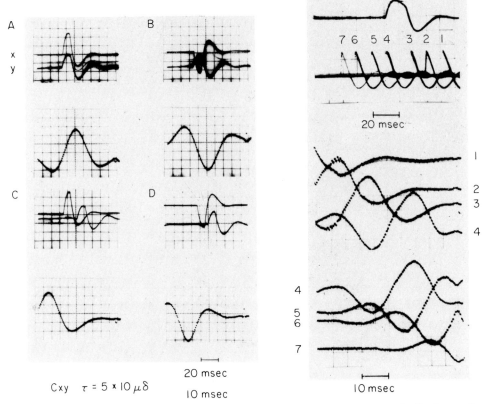

Figure 3. Cross-correlation studies using simulation with artificial "spikes" obtained with pulses and RC circuits. Spikes were of similar duration and different polarities and/or intervals in left group of pictures. In each case, A, B, C, and D, signals are shown at the top and correlogram at the bottom. In the right-hand picture, a given spike was correlated with a shorter one, with varying intervals between the two signals. A given correlogram labeled 1 to 7 corresponds to each position (1 through 7) of the short spike (top traces). In both experiments correlation was performed as x to y, and lag time τ was set at 50 μsec. Time scale on left picture: 20 msec for spike oscillograms, and 10 msec for correlograms. The two time scales are shown separately on the right-hand figure.

Because of the low values of T, the cross-correlation function was undergoing rapid changes, and it seemed interesting to be able to record the correlogram at discrete moments, when (and only when) a spike was occurring on one of the channels under study. For such purpose (Figure 4), one of the channels, in addition to being fed into the correlator, was passed through the amplitude discriminator and pulse generator circuit and the digital rectangular output pulse (of adequate duration) thus obtained was used to gate the correlator readout. Successive pictures of the correlation curve could thus be taken on the same polaroid frame, either superimposed or with slightly shifting the y position after each sweep. Clearly, then, the existence of a constant time-locking between paroxysmal events could immediately be deduced from inspection (Figure 5) of the

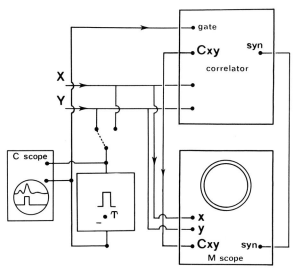

Figure 4. Diagram of the circuitry for cross-correlation operations. Channels x and y are fed into the correlator and eventually into the main oscilloscope (M. scope). The cross-correlogram (Cxy) is displayed on that same scope, whose sweep is synchronized (syn) by the correlator. One channel, selected as trigger channel (here y) is fed into the comparator and pulse generator. The pulse is then used to gate the correlator. Adjustment of the comparator to a selected amplitude of the paroxysmal spike is monitored on a control oscilloscope (C. scope).

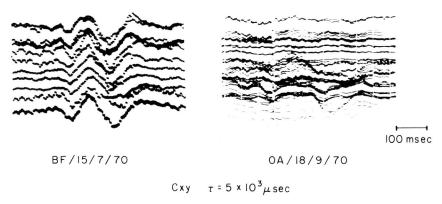

BF / 15 / 7 / 70   OA / 18 / 9 / 70

100 msec

Cxy $\tau = 5 \times 10^3 \mu$sec

Figure 5. Contrasting examples in two different patients of time-locking (left) and independence or variability in time relationships (right) between two cortical leads.

successive sweeps (left) and independence or variability in time relationships (right) as well.

RESULTS

We shall now give individual examples of this part of our study, namely, that of establishing correspondences between interictal paroxysmal activities appearing at various sites of the epileptic limbic structures, using one or the other methodology described above.

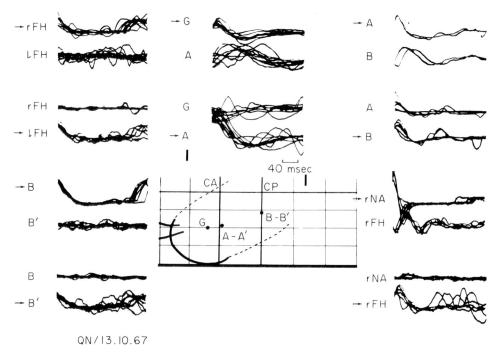

QN/13.10.67

Figure 6. Time relationships between interictal paroxysmal activities at various points in left and right temporal lobes. For electrode positions in sagittal plane, refer to Figure 1. Trigger channel is indicated by arrow. Voltage calibration: 100 μV (vertical bar). rFH—right hippocampal formation; lFH—left hippocampal formation; rNA—right amygdaloid nucleus; G—tip of right temporal lobe; A (right) and A′ (left)—anterior temporal cortex; B (right) and B′ (left)—posterior temporal cortex.

To begin with let us state that no systematic attention has been paid here to the shape of these activities. However, our general feeling [as pointed out earlier by Bancaud and co-workers (8)] is that, in direct bipolar recording from the vicinity of the active structures themselves, no systematic classes of IPAs can be distinguished (at variance with the classic EEG data). Most of the recorded phenomena were either monophasic or polyphasic, with diverse durations (10–100 msec.).

a. Case QN (Figure 6). This patient was suffering from bilateral temporal lobe epilepsy (as shown by clinical and SEEG examinations). Spikes were recorded from right FH (rFH) and left FH (lFH); from the superficial anterior temporal cortex, right (A) and left (A′); from the posterior temporal cortex, right (B) and left (B′); from the tip of right temporal lobe (G); and from the right NA (rNA).

The following conclusions may be drawn from the instrumental superposition technique: (1) lack of time-locking between rFH and lFH; (2) lack of time-locking between B and B′; (3) time-locking between G and A, between A and B, and between rNA and rFH (trigger channels are indicated by arrows). In addition, activity on the right side seems to be traveling frontocaudally with G leading A, A preceding B, and rNA, perhaps, preceding rFH (although latter statement is posing problems, as rFH activity is not necessarily preceded by rNA, whereas rNA activity is always followed by rFH).

b. Case CN (Figure 7). This is another good example of time-locking between left temporal points, as shown by superimposed cross-correlograms. Recordings were taken from the depth of the anterior temporal lobe (G'p), from a more posterior superficial temporal area (indicated here as A's), from NA (A'p), and from FH (B'p). Extremely good time-locking exists in such case between G' and A's, G' and NA, G' and FH, as emphasized by the constancy of the superimposed correlation curves.

c. Case RL (Figure 8). This is a third example of close relationships between phenomena in FH and GH; in this case both methodologies were used jointly.

In summary, to this point, we have presented one case of lack of time-locking between the two symmetrical temporal areas, in a case of bitemporal epilepsy (QN), and three examples of rather good correlation between firing of several areas within one temporal lobe. The first aspect was a very common observation in our group; actually, in no case have

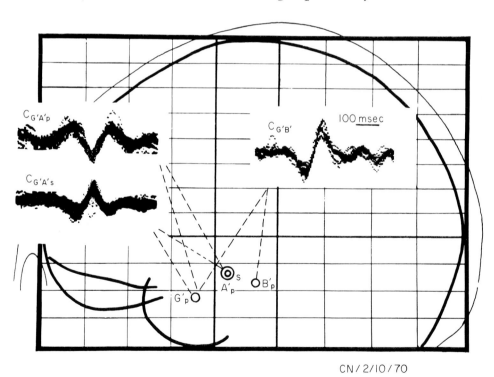

CN / 2 / 10 / 70

Figure 7. Successive correlograms (C) for interictal events in a patient, taken on the left side between temporal pole (G') and amygdala (A'p); temporal pole (G') and external temporal cortex (A's); temporal pole (G') and left hippocampal formation (B'p). τ, 5×10^3 μsec.

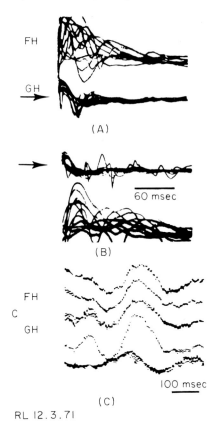

Figure 8. Simultaneous recording of paroxysmal waves from right hippocampal formation (FH) and right hippocampal gyrus (GH). (a, b) Superposition of records with GH being the trigger channel in figure a and FH in figure b (as indicated by arrows). (c) Successive cross-correlation (C) curves between FH and GH showing a fair constancy; slight shift of the y position of the CRO beam after each response; FH was trigger channel. τ, 5×10^3 μsec.

we noticed transhemispheric synchrony between FHs as yet. Concerning the time-locking within one temporal lobe, although it was observed very often, it cannot be considered as a constant feature. Let us now consider, in more detail, cases of greater complexity.

  d. Case SA (Figure 9). All electrodes were located on the left (left temporal lobe epilepsy); recordings were taken from FH and from three superficially lying points of the superior temporal lobe (G', K', H'). As can be seen, FH and G' are independent, as also G' and K', whereas G' and H' seem to be locked together.

  e. That a lack of correlation can exist within the same temporal lobe is also shown in Figure 10 (case RO). No time-locking exists between homonymous areas of the temporal lobes (lT_2e, rT_2e), but there is also no time-locking between left T_2e and lFH.

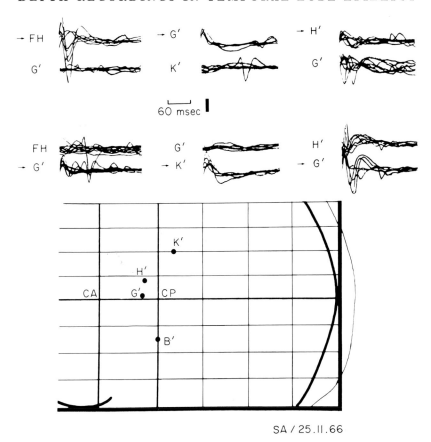

SA / 25.II.66

Figure 9. Time-locking study between various sites (G', H', K') in the left superficial temporal cortex (B') and left hippocampal formation (FH). Calibration: 200 μV (vertical line). CA—anterior commissure; CP—posterior commissure.

f. Cases PR (Figure 11) and FA (Figure 12). Patient PR was explored with electrodes in the right temporal lobe (two T_1 superficial leads, I and K, and one FH electrode, B_p), one electrode in the right supplementary motor area (M_p), and one in the posterior supracallosal gyrus (G_p).

It can be seen that a constancy in shape of the correlograms exists between the two neighboring superficial areas, I and K, between FH and GC (C_{BG}), but not between FH and the supplementary motor area, nor extremely well between K_s and B_p. In this case it is interesting to note that, again, a fairly good common relationship exists between points in one temporal lobe and the cingulate gyrus but not between the temporal lobe and a distant area such as the supplementary motor area.

Another aspect of this correlation between distant points of the "limbic system" is illustrated in Figure 12 (case FA). It can be noticed that a spike occurring in FH is followed almost every time by a late spike with a somewhat variable delay (about 150 to 200 msec) in GCp (upper frame);

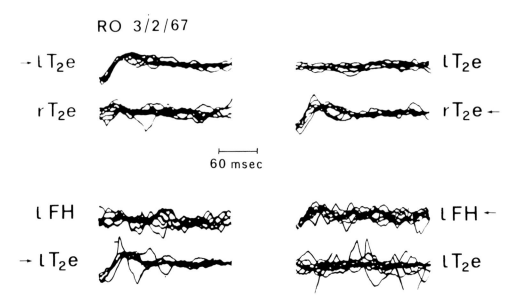

Figure 10. Time-locking study between left(l) and right(r) superficial temporal (T₂e) lobe sites and between lT₂e and hippocampal formation (lFH).

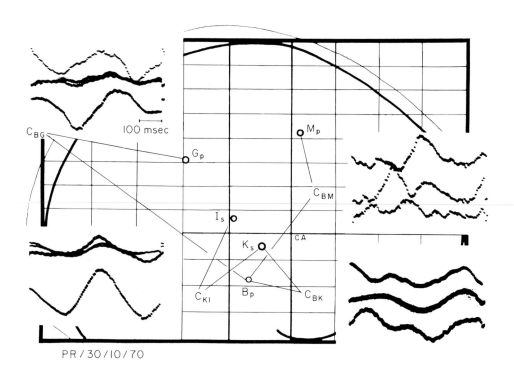

Figure 11. Cross-correlograms (C) between points in right temporal lobe (Iₛ and Kₛ), in right hippocampal formation (Bₚ), right supplementary motor area (Mₚ), and right posterior parietal cortex (Gₚ). τ, 5×10^3 μsec.

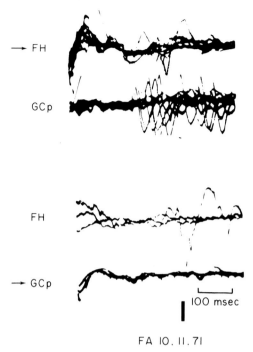

FA 10. 11. 71

Figure 12. Time-locking study between hippocampal formation (FH) and ipsilateral cingulate gyrus (GCp). Notice variable delay of spike in GCp when FH is the trigger channel. Calibration: 100 μV (vertical line).

as no identical correspondence could be obtained when GCp was the trigger channel (lower frame), it may be concluded that the spike "travels" from FH to GCp. Further indications of such connections between ventral and dorsal limbic structures will be given in the next section.

g. A time-locking between distant points can develop under certain conditions, as shown in Figure 13. In this case the superposition technique was used to compare right anterior GC (rGC) and left internal parietal cortex (lPar). The upper frame of this figure is relative to a period when no time-locking was observed between lPAs occurring at the two brain sites. Immediately afterward, the patient was given a small dose of Megimide (a dosage subthreshold for eliciting a seizure) and a clear "synchrony" could be observed for a period of time (second frame). The third frame illustrates the progressive fading out of this time-locking, as the action of Megimide dissipated.

Functional Connections within the Limbic System

The second aspect of our study was devoted to exploring connections between different structures belonging to the limbic system. Again, taking advantage of the presence of several multiple lead electrodes, we could

rGC lPar

→ rGC

lPar

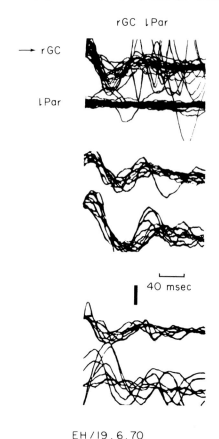

40 msec

EH / 19 . 6 . 70

Figure 13. Time dependence between right cingulate gyrus (rGC) and left parietal cortex (lPar); rGC was the trigger channel. Top: rGC firing, with no correspondence at lPar. Middle: After Megimide (subthreshold for seizure), excellent synchrony between the two brain sites. Bottom: Later on, tendency to return to control record. Calibration: 200 μV (vertical bar).

on many occasions stimulate between two leads of one electrode (say A) and record bipolarly from two leads of another one, B, at a certain distance from A. If a response was thus evoked, it would indicate the existence of some kind of connection (direct or indirect) from A to B.

It is well known that after-discharges or critical episodes can spread from one brain structure to others, through "preferential" interconnections which sometimes appear very complex (6, 7, 9, 13, 14, 20, 23, 26, 30, 33, 34, 38, 50, 53, 63, 82). Although interesting indications have come out of such studies, it seemed to us that more information on these interconnections could perhaps be gathered through a somewhat different approach, based on graded excitations of nerve tissue, using single shocks or short trains of pulses (although we were aware of the fact that electrical stimulation is, in any case, a very artificial way of activating central nervous structures).

TECHNIQUES

Our methodology here was quite simple: single pulses or short trains were delivered through two (in most cases adjacent) leads of one electrode shaft and recording was also performed bipolarly (again, almost always, from adjacent leads). As indicated above, shock intensities, durations, and frequencies were carefully controlled.

Activities were displayed on the oscilloscope and direct pictures taken of five to ten superimposed sweeps. As these recorded activities were usually very large, no averaging procedure was necessary.

RESULTS

Clearly, given a certain number of electrode shafts, say ten, with five to ten leads each, the total number of possible combinations was very high and a complete screening of all of them would have led to an overwhelming amount of information. Therefore, we generally restricted our exploration to stimulations and recordings at the following leads: (a) those that could be located (through X-ray control, or from inspection of the spontaneous electrical activity and from the effects of their repetitive stimulation) with a high probability in one of the basal rhinencephalic structures, NA, FH, anterior or posterior GH; (b) the deepest couple of leads of electrodes introduced perpendicularly to the sagittal plane, very close to or within GC (at various anteroposterior levels) (see Figure 1); and (c) the external leads of electrodes penetrating into the temporal lobe and, thus, located near the cortex of T_1 or T_2 gyri.

In many cases, as will be seen, two electrodes were introduced into symmetrical homonymous brain areas. Although the absolute physiological symmetry could never be completely ascertained, our data were sufficiently similar for many cases, so that we consider it justifiable to draw some functional conclusions, as will be seen below. Since the time has not yet arrived for giving a complete report of all our data, we shall limit this presentation to some characteristic observations.

Connections between Ipsilateral Structures of the Basal Rhinencephalon. Our studies of synchrony have indicated that NA, FH, and GH in the same hemisphere can, to some extent, behave "as an entity." As will be seen below, the single shock technique has revealed more selective connections.

a. Responses between Ipsilateral NA and FH. As a rule, in all patients considered here (T or non-T), a single shock applied to NA elicited a response in the ipsilateral FH. Its latency varied between 15 and 40 msec, depending on the subject, but it showed only little variation in one given subject; threshold voltages ranged from 4 to 10 V. No major change was observed when using short trains (50 msec, 50/second, 1 msec) except

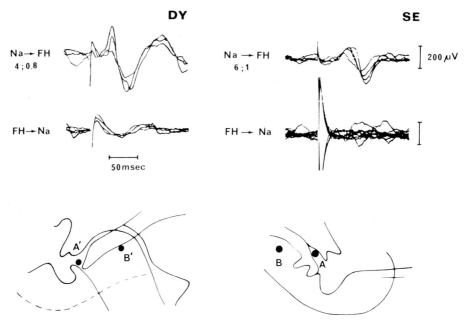

Figure 14. Relationships between ipsilateral amygdaloid nucleus (NA) and hippocampal formation (FH) in 2 patients without temporal lobe epilepsy (electrodes on left side in patient DY and on right side in patient SE). Stimulus parameters: 4 V, 0.8 msec (left) and 6 V, 1 msec (right). A (right) and A′ (left)—anterior temporal electrodes; B (right) and B′ (left)—posterior temporal electrodes.

for the threshold intensity. Figures 14, 15, and 16 give examples of these NA to FH responses.

A much greater variability was observed when looking for reverse connections, from FH to NA. Here we were led to divide our patients into two groups: (*a*) those with no clearly evoked NA activity to FH stimulation and (*b*) those showing a well-developed response with a variable latency, sometimes less than 20 msec. Our attention was essentially drawn to the fact that the latter cases all belonged to the T group, whereas most of the former cases were non-T patients. It thus appears that the backward-to-forward connection, that from FH to NA, is considerably facilitated in epileptic temporal lobes. Figures 15 and 16 illustrate such NA–FH two-way relationships, whereas Figure 17 shows that the FH → NA pathway is considerably facilitated shortly after administration of Megimide at a dose subthreshold for a seizure. This case (VG) was a T patient, but the FH shock was given at threshold value. Thus, some variability was observed before Megimide, then large responses developed just after administration of the drug, and they were again clearly reduced when tested 30 minutes later. Shocks were, of course, of constant parameters during these observations. Figure 18 also shows, in a more complex case, and with more tests, responses from NA to FH and vice versa from FH to NA.

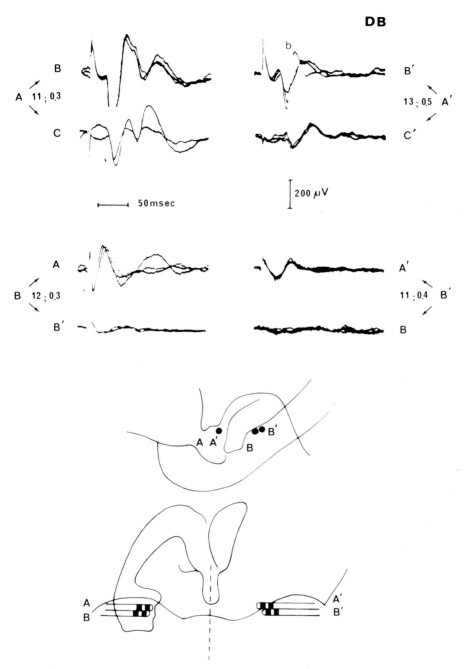

Figure 15. Patient with temporal epilepsy, presumably bilateral. A, (right) and A′ (left) amygdaloid nucleus (NA); B (right) and B′ (left) hippocampal formation (FH); C (right) and C′ (left) hippocampal gyrus. Electrodes A, A′, B, and B′ are shown on lateral aspect of hemisphere and also on a verticofrontal section in order to locate the two active leads in each case. Notice, in particular, NA → FH responses and FH → NA responses on right and left. There were no significant transhemispheric responses between the two FHs. The hippocampal gyrus was activated from ipsilateral NA on both sides.

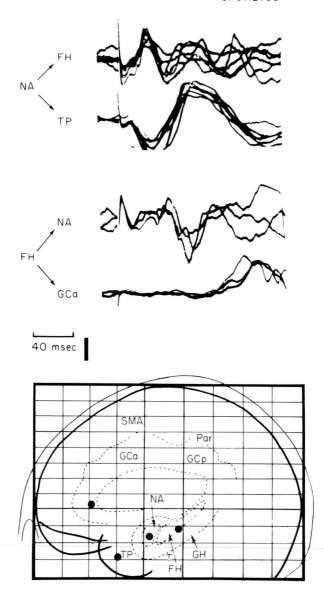

Figure 16. Temporal lobe epilepsy. Exploration on left side (see location at bottom). Stimulation of amygdaloid nucleus (NA) was activating hippocampal formation (FH) and the tip of temporal lobe (TP) as well, at longer latency. The FH stimulation elicited a response with rather long latency in NA and very long latency in anterior cingulate gyrus (GCa). Stimulus parameters: top, 10 V, 0.3 msec; bottom, 12 V, 0.3 msec. Calibration: 200 μV (vertical line). SMA—supplementary motor area; Par—parietal cortex; GCp—posterior GC; GH—hippocampal gyrus.

   b. Connections Tested between FH and GH or within GH. Anatomical data indicate that connections exist in both directions between FH and GH. This was in general confirmed in our stimulation studies: responses

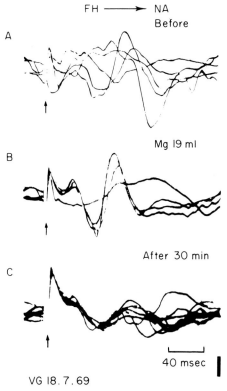

FH ⟶ NA

Before

A

Mg 19 ml

B

After 30 min

C

40 msec

VG 18.7.69

Figure 17. Case of left temporal lobe epilepsy with stimulation of hippocampal formation (FH). Recording from ipsilateral amygdaloid nucleus (NA). Effect of injecting Megimide. See explanations in text. Calibration: 200 μV (vertical line).

were in most cases obtained from FH and GH and also quite often in the reverse direction. At variance with the preceding case of NA and FH, we could not find a preferential pathway that would be facilitated in T patients.

Transrhinencephalic Connections. The anatomical literature emphasizes the existence of interhemispheric connections between the two NA (via anterior commissure) and between the two FHs (via both anterior commissure and *commissura fornicis*). Rather surprisingly, in our observations we could rarely elicit, by means of a single shock or short trains, transhemispheric homonymous responses between the two NAs or the two FHs.

The only exceptions were encountered in some patients belonging to a special group with bilateral temporal epilepsy. Actually reciprocal activations between NAs could be obtained in only 1 patient (out of 10 such bilateral cases); those between FHs were found in few cases and those between GHs were somewhat more frequent. Figure 18 illustrates a bilateral temporal case which was particularly favorable: there were no inter-NA responses; left FH was activated from the right, with no reciprocity; anterior (CC') and posterior (DD') GHs were eliciting reciprocal re-

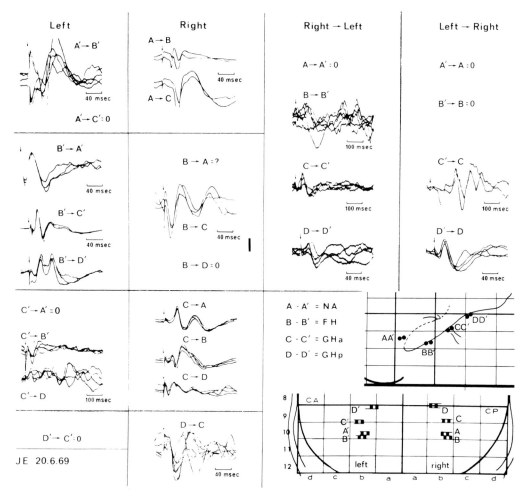

Figure 18. Complex example illustrating the systematic exploration of an epileptic with bitemporal signs. Electrodes were located in right (A) and left (A') amygdaloid nuclei (NA); right (B) and left (B') hippocampal formations (FH); right and left hippocampal gyri (GH), anterior (GHa, C and C') and posterior (GHp, D and D'). Electrode positions shown projected on sagittal plane and corresponding active leads also shown in verticofrontal projection. All stimuli used were of same parameters (8 V, 1 msec). Calibration: 200 μV (vertical line).

sponses in both directions. It should be noted, however, that the latencies were not quite identical for the left-to-right responses and those in the reverse direction.

An interesting fact is illustrated on Figure 19, where (as an exception in these investigations) repetitive stimuli at 3/second were delivered, instead of single shocks, and successive records were taken starting from the upper part of the frame. It can be seen that no response could be obtained from right to left NA or from left to right FH (left to right NA was not tested), whereas a response progressively developed from right

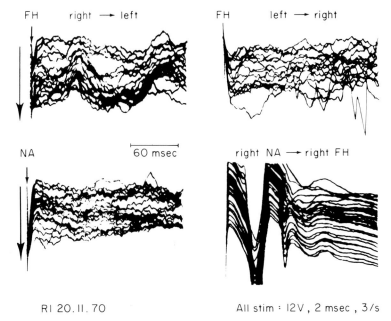

Figure 19. Facilitation of right hippocampal formation (FH) → left FH connection through 3/second repetitive stimulation of right FH. No facilitation was observed from left → right FH nor from right → left amygdaloid nucleus (NA). Right NA → right FH response was practically unchanged during such stimulation.

to left FH. Finally, it should be noted in the same figure that the right NA → FH responses remained practically unchanged with repetition of the shocks.

Connections between Rhinencephalon and Cingulate Gyrus. Anatomical data indicate that the GC projects to the hippocampus. On the other hand, it is a well known fact that temporal afterdischarges or seizures can spread to the cingulate in the reverse direction (see Discussion). So, our problem was to try to evaluate these connections with possibly a distinction between T and non-T patients.

The following data were obtained, with 17 T and 14 non-T patients.

a. Short latency responses could be elicited in the majority of patients, from one cingulate area to another (latency 10 msec) in both directions (GCa → GC or GCp → GCa), thus confirming the existence of (partially direct) connections within this structure (18).

b. Responses of variable latency were often obtained between GCp and the basal rhinencephalon. However, no general conclusions can be drawn as yet from inspection of these 31 cases, especially considering the distinction between T and non-T.

b1. In the great majority of our patients responses were obtained from FH to GC and no responses from GC to NA, FH, or even GH. The latencies of these responses usually ranged within the same values, that is 40–60 msec or even much more (Figure 16), thus indicating a complex but very "permeable" pathway. In a few cases (belonging to non-T's except for 1 patient), a rather spectacular type of response, with "spikes-and-waves" could be observed (Figure 20). This type of activity may have a pathological meaning, which has not as yet been determined.

b2. Let us now consider the connections from GC to the rhinencephalon. In most cases there was no response, as indicated above; but in some of our patients a response was observed with even very short latency. Our feeling for the time being is that these activities may behave somewhat like the connections from FH to NA, that is, be subject to considerable changes in threshold. As such cases could be observed in T and non-T patients as well, no conclusions can be reached, as yet, regarding their pathological significance.

DISCUSSION

Only some of the problems[*] which are posed by the above observations and by their interpretation will be considered herein.

Do Our Connection Data Fit the Literature?

The greater majority of our knowledge on interconnections at the rhinencephalic level in primates results from anatomical studies (4, 5, 18, 19, 21, 28, 31, 35, 45, 46, 61, 62, 69, 78–80, 84) and electrophysiological investigations in animals (29, 31, 32, 35–37, 42, 57, 58, 73).

1. When considering these data, it is hard to determine which pathway is involved in the connection from NA to FH, although it is probably polysynaptic. In the cat, NA responses to FH stimulation were observed by Gloor (31) and Steriade (73). Gloor suggested that they could pass either through entorhinal cortex (NA is known to project to the entorhinal area and the latter to FH), either through septum (via *stria terminalis*) and then to FH via septoammonic fibers which have been identified in the fornix (37, 79, 80). In the monkey, a direct path from NA to FH was postulated by Kaada (42) although Pribram and co-workers (57) found no evidence of such a pathway in their neuronographic studies.

The FH to NA pathways also remain speculative: anatomists claim that FH (and GH) project to entorhinal cortex and the latter to NA. Amygdaloid nucleus responses to FH stimulation have been observed in the cat by Steriade (73) and in the monkey by Green and Adey (37). However, Pribram and co-workers (57) again could not fire NA through strychninization of the hippocampus.

[*] Quite a number of important problems posed by the temporal lobe epilepsies will not be discussed here, as they are far beyond the scope of this presentation; in particular, the neurological aspects of the temporal accesses, and the clinical categories of temporal seizures (8, 9, 27, 39). Nor shall we discuss the problem of "epileptic focus" versus "lesioned area" and "irritative zone" as discussed in particular by Bancaud (8), Jasper (40), and Ajmone Marsan (1).

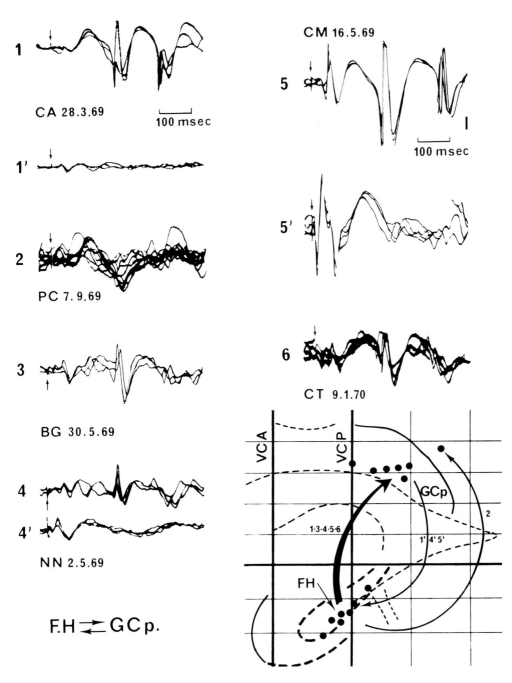

Figure 20. Interconnections between hippocampal formation (FH) and posterior cingulate gyrus (GCp) and neighboring parietal cortex in 6 different patients. Notice striking spike-and-wave pattern obtained for FH → GCp responses. Patient NN (4, 4′) was the only one in this group who had temporal lobe epilepsy. Calibration: 100 μV (vertical line). VCA—line passing through projection of anterior commisure; VCP—line passing through projection of posterior commisure.

2. The connections between the basal rhinencephalon and GC also deserve some comment.

The GC is composed of several zones (Brodmann areas 24, 25, 23, 29). Only relatively few studies have been devoted to its connections (37, 43, 61, 62, 70). Briefly, it is known to receive afferents from the anterior thalamic nuclei and from adjacent neocortical areas, and to send efferents to various thalamic areas, to the ipsilateral entorhinal cortex and to FH.

In our stimulation studies, the responses most commonly obtained were those from rhinencephalic areas to cingulate, in addition to the short-latency GC → GC responses. The latter can be explained by the well-demonstrated short corticocortical connections within this lobe (18); as for the FH → GC or GH → GC responses (including those, peculiar to the spike-and-wave type, as shown in Figure 20), the complex "Papez" route from FH to GC via hypothalamus and/or anterior nuclei of the thalamus could be a candidate, given the rather long latencies usually observed for these responses and also perhaps the "recurrent" aspect of some of them. But this is only speculative, the more so as, on some occasions, the FH → GC responses were of short latency. Rather surprisingly, reverse pathways, those predicted by the anatomy from GC to FH, were observed in only a few cases. It is certainly too early to draw definite conclusions as to the meaning of these results.

3. Even more surprising are the mainly negative results with activations of transrhinencephalic homonymous connections. At variance with the above observations, the classic anatomical data (28, 31, 35) this time provide positive indications, which, in a certain respect, were not confirmed by our electrophysiological findings: the difficulty in eliciting a contralateral homonymous response in most cases (even in bi-T patients except for some individual examples) is worth underlining.

In summary, there seems to be some disagreement between the anatomical documents and the functional data as they can be deduced from our stimulation and recording data. We shall come back to some aspect of this problem.

What Can Be the Significance of Time Relationships between Interictal Paroxysmal Activities?

It is known that a large number of studies in human, and to some extent also in animals, have dealt with the definition of the epileptic focus (in electrophysiological terms) and with the validity of this concept (1, 40, 59, 60, 83). These attempts were initially based on EEG scalp recordings, and later studies with focal, epicortical, or deep electrodes have indicated that a considerable proportion of the interictal paroxysmal activities cannot be recorded from the scalp (83). Therefore, conclusions drawn from scalp recordings, even if they are not theoretically wrong, may be biased because of insufficient information.

Now, supposing that we have enough deep electrodes available (even if this is not true in practice), what deductions can be made from such multiple interictal recordings? It is a rather widely accepted idea that interictal spikes have very complex spatiotemporal features and that, surrounding a lesioned area, several independent foci can develop with no time correlations (2, 8), and the conclusion may thus be that a study of these spatiotemporal correspondences would be of little value for localizing the focus.

Our present data confirm the impression that an epileptic temporal lobe can display several foci, with different interictal activities. However, they also indicate that the tendency toward time-locking within one temporal lobe is rather high, probably higher than in other cortical areas (frontal, parietal, occipital). This is at least what we feel when comparing our present findings with those, not mentioned here, performed on other types of epilepsies. Nevertheless, the asynchrony between the two temporal lobes is a well recognized fact (2).

How Can We Explain the Preferential Pathways Identified by Single Shocks?

We shall now consider the significance of single-shock responses and the modifications which some of them undergo in the epileptic temporal lobe, as compared with the normal one, and some of the discrepancies with anatomical data.

On a macroscopic scale, that of the interconnecting pathways between different structures, it is our feeling that the observed variability of responses is not due to incidental positioning of the electrodes but to significant changes in excitability. In other words, although we are not able, for the time being, to explain all our observations, we tend to lend significance to the fact that normal and epileptic limbic systems behave differently when explored with the single-shock technique. This assumption is again reinforced by other observations of our group regarding the existence or absence of transhemispheric responses between neocortical areas of the midline (frontal or parietal). A striking correlation could also be found between the existence of such (probably transcallosal) responses and the indications that the corresponding structures were involved in an epileptogenic process. It is also interesting here to recall the observation in Figure 17, where a temporary facilitation of the FH → NA pathway was elicited by Megimide.

At the synaptic level, the reasons for such changes in excitability (or responsiveness) of the FH → NA connections or of those between homonymous bilateral structures are beyond our competence. More studies should certainly be devoted to these long-term facilitation processes, which might be self-reinforcing (more bombardment facilitating more extension and so forth). Such studies would expand those "on mirror foci" (1, 49,

72). Although the mechanism of these facilitations remains unexplained, one could perhaps, suggest that there are different physiological categories of pathways (as described by anatomy)*: some are little sensitive to facilitation by the (unknown) epileptic process (including synaptic bombardment), such as NA → FH, whereas others, for instance FH → NA or transhemispheric connections, are very sensitive to repetition and so would be considerably facilitated and, thus, rendered "permeable," through either long-term interictal bombardment or the repetitive artificial excitation resulting from iterative electrical stimulation or pharmacological activation.

Can We Correlate Single-Shock Responses with Preferential Spread of IPAs and After-discharges?

It is a well accepted fact that after-discharges elicited in one of the rhinencephalic structures quickly spread to others, although some preferential propagation "lines" could be detected (6, 7, 9, 13, 14, 20, 23, 26, 30, 33, 34, 38, 50, 53, 63, 82). We may thus ask whether the facilitation of pathways—as indicated by the single-shock test—can explain the time-locking between spontaneous IPAs, or the spread of after-discharges, or self-sustained epileptic activities.

We may, here, refer to some of our observations, indicating that Megimide (or repetitive stimulation) can facilitate both the time-locking of IPAs (Figure 13) and the transfer of single-shock responses (Figures 17 and 19). Some common functional modifications may have appeared in the synaptic junctions of the system.

Returning to our previous hypothesis concerning the existence of two categories of pathways, we might even go a little further by considering that, among the "sensitive" ones, some may be in a state of facilitation sufficient for transmission of single IPAs; they would also respond to single-shock stimulation; other such sensitive systems would only transmit after repetitive excitation through either artificial electrical stimulation or an after-discharge. Thus, FH to NA would be of the first type, whereas transrhinencephalic pathways would in most cases remain of the second type, requiring a repetitive firing to become "functional." So that, depending on the particular conditions, an interictal exploration would detect some spikes, those which are of local origin or transmitted through the most sensitive synaptic systems,† but other connections would remain inoperative and detectable only after activation through pharmacological treatment or strong repetitive stimulation. Of course, this hypothesis is purely formal and does not take into consideration the synaptic peculiarities of these connections. Whether their differences in behavior are due only to the number of synaptic junctions involved or to their specific reactions to the pathogenic

---

* By "pathway," of course, we do not necessarily mean monosynaptic connections.

† We did not discuss here the possibility of morphological differences (if any) between local or transmitted spikes.

process remains for future investigations. For the time being, it can be expected that, depending on the individual case and the brain area which is involved, localization of the epileptogenic focus may or may not be possible by inspection of the spatiotemporal characteristics of the recorded IPAs.

REFERENCES

1. Ajmone Marsan, C., Acute effects of topical epileptogenic agents. In: *Basic Mechanisms in the Epilepsies* (H. H. Jasper, A. A. Ward, and A. Pope, Eds.). Churchill, London, and Little, Brown, Boston, 1969: 299–319.
2. Ajmone Marsan, C., and Baldwin, M., Surgical series in temporal lobe epilepsies. Electrocorticography. In: *Temporal Lobe Epilepsy* (M. Baldwin and P. Bailey, Eds.). Thomas, Springfield, Illinois, 1958: 368–395.
3. Ajmone Marsan, C., and van Buren, J., Epileptiform activity in cortical and subcortical structures in the temporal lobe of man. In: *Temporal Lobe Epilepsy* (M. Baldwin and P. Bailey, Eds.). Thomas, Springfield, Illinois, 1958: 78–108.
4. Adey, W. R., and Meyer, M., An experimental study of hippocampal afferent pathways from prefrontal and cingulate areas in the monkey. *J. Anat.*, 1952, 86: 58–74.
5. Adey, W. R., and Meyer, M., Hippocampal and hypothalamic connections of the temporal lobe in the monkey. *Brain*, 1952, 75: 358–384.
6. Andy, O. J., and Akert, K., Electroencephalographic and behavioral changes during seizures induced by stimulation of Ammon's formation in the cat and monkey. *Electroenceph. clin. Neurophysiol.*, 1953, Suppl. 3, 48.
7. Arana-Iniguez, R., Reis, D., Naquet, R., and Magoun, H. W., Propagation of amygdaloid seizures. *Acta Neurol. Lat. Am.* 1955, 1: 109.
8. Bancaud, J., Talairach, J., Bonis, A., Schaub, C., Szikla, G., Morel, P., and Bordas-Ferrer, M., *La stéréo-électroencéphalographie dans l'épilepsie.* Masson, Paris, 1965.
9. Bancaud, J., Talairach, J., Morel, P., and Bresson, M., La corne d'Ammon et le noyau amygdalien: Effets cliniques et électriques de leur stimulation chez l'Homme. *Rev. Neurol. (Paris)*, 1966, 115: 329–352.
10. Bickford, R. G., The application of depth electrography in some varieties of epilepsy. *Electroenceph. clin. Neurophysiol.*, 1956, 8: 526–527.
11. Bickford, R. G., MacDonald, H. N. A., Dodge, H. W., and MacCarty, C. S., Distant evoked responses to depth stimulation in patients with neurologic disease. *Electroenceph. clin. Neurophysiol.*, 1957, 9: 176.
12. Bickford, R. G., Petersen, M. C., Dodge, H. W., and Sem-Jacobsen, C. W., Observations on depth stimulation of the human brain through implanted electrographic leads. *Proc. Staff Meet. Mayo Clin.*, 1953, 28: 181–187.
13. Bogen, J., Sperry, R., and Vogel, P., Commissural section and propagation of seizures. In: *Basic Mechanisms in the Epilepsies* (H. H. Jasper, A. A. Ward, and A. Pope, Eds.). Churchill, London, and Little, Brown, Boston, 1969: 439.

14. Brazier, M. A. B., Depth recordings from the amygdaloid region in patients with temporal lobe epilepsy. *Electroenceph. clin. Neurophysiol.*, 1956, **8**: 532–533.

15. Brazier, M. A. B., An application of computer aid to a problem in clinical electroencephalography. *Electroenceph. clin. Neurophysiol.*, 1965, **18**: 522.

16. Brazier, M. A. B., An application of computer analysis to a problem in epilepsy. *Excerpta Med. Int. Congr. Ser.*, 1966, **124**: 112–128.

17. Brazier, M. A. B., and Casby, J. U., Cross correlation and autocorrelation studies of EEG potentials. *Electroenceph. clin. Neurophysiol.*, 1952, **4**: 201–211.

18. Cajal, S. Ramón, *Histologie du système nerveux de l'Homme et des Vertébrés*. Maloine, Paris, 1911.

19. Cowan, W. M., Raisman, G., and Powell, T. P. S., The connections of the amygdala. *J. Neurol., Neurosurg. Psychiatry*, 1965, **28**: 137–151.

20. Delgado, J. M. R., and Hamlin, H., Direct recordings of spontaneous and evoked seizures in epileptics. *Electroenceph. clin. Neurophysiol.*, 1958, **10**: 463–486.

21. De Vito, J. L., and White, L. E., Projections from fornix to the hippocampal formation in the squirrel monkey, *J. Comp. Neurol.*, 1966, **127**: 389–398.

22. Dodge, H. W., Bailey, A. A., Bickford, R. G., Petersen, M. C., Sem-Jacobsen, C. W., and Miller, R. H., Neurosurgical and neurologic applications of depth electrography. *Proc. Staff Meet. Mayo Clin.*, 1953, **28**: 188–191.

23. Feath, W. H., Walker, E. A., and Andy, O. J., Propagation of cortical and subcortical epileptic discharge. *Epilepsia*, 1954, **3**: 37–48.

24. Feindel, W., and Penfield, W., Localization of discharges in temporal lobe automatism. *Arch. Neurol. Psychiat.*, 1954, **72**: 605–630.

25. Feindel, W., Penfield, W., and Jasper, H. H., Localization of epileptic discharge in temporal lobe automatism. *Trans. Am. Neurol. Assoc.*, 1952, **77**: 14–17.

26. Frost, L. L., Baldwin, M., and Wood, C. D., Investigation of primate amygdala; movements of face and jaws: After discharge and anterior commissure. *Neurology*, 1958, **8**: 543–547.

27. Gastaut, H., Clinical and electroencephalographical classification of epileptic seizures. *Epilepsia*, 1970, **11**: 102–113.

28. Gastaut, H., and Lammers, H. J., Anatomie du rhinencéphale, In: *Les Grandes Activités du Rhinencéphale*. Masson, Paris, 1960: 1–166.

29. Gloor, P., Electrophysiological studies on the connections of the amygdaloid nucleus in the cat. I. Neuronal organization of the amygdaloid projection system. *Electroenceph. clin. Neurophysiol.*, 1955, **7**: 223–242.

30. Gloor, P., The pattern of conduction of amygdaloid seizure discharge. *Arch. Neurol. Psychiat.*, 1957, **77**: 247–248.

31. Gloor, P., Amygdala. In *Handbook of Physiology* (Am. Physiol. Soc., J. Field, Ed.). Williams & Wilkins, Baltimore, 1960: Sect. 1, Vol. II: 1395–1420.

32. Gloor, P., Temporal lobe epilepsy: Its possible contribution to the understanding of the functional significance of the amygdala and of its interaction with neocortical-temporal mechanisms. In *The Neurobiology of the Amygdala* (B. Eleftheriou, Ed.). Plenum, New York, 1972: 423–457.

33. Gloor, P., Vera, C. L., Sperti, L., and Ray, S. N., Investigations on the mechanism of epileptic discharge in the hippocampus. *Epilepsia,* 1961, **2**: 42–62.

34. Green, J. D., Significance of the hippocampus in temporal lobe epilepsy. In: *Temporal Lobe Epilepsy* (M. Baldwin and P. Bailey, Eds.). Thomas, Springfield, Illinois, 1958: 58–68.

35. Green, J. D., The hippocampus. In: *Handbook of Physiology* (Am. Physiol. Soc., J. Field, Ed.), Williams & Wilkins, Baltimore, 1960: Sect. 1, Vol. II: 1373–1389.

36. Green, J. D., The hippocampus. *Physiol. Rev.* 1964, **44**: 561–608.

37. Green, J. D., and Adey, R., Electrophysiological studies of hippocampal connections and excitability. *Electroenceph. clin. Neurophysiol.,* 1956, **8**: 245–262.

38. Green, J. D., and Shimamoto, T., Hippocampal seizures and their propagation, *Arch. Neurol. Psychiat.,* 1953, **70**: 687–702.

39. Jasper, H. H., Functional subdivisions of the temporal region in relation to seizure patterns and subcortical connections, In: *Temporal Lobe Epilepsy* (M. Baldwin and P. Bailey, Eds.). Thomas, Springfield, Illinois, 1958: 40–57.

40. Jasper, H. H., Mechanisms of propagation: Extracellular studies. In: *Basic Mechanisms in the Epilepsies* (H. H. Jasper, A. A. Ward, and A. Pope, Eds.). Churchill, London, and Little, Brown, Boston, 1969: 421–438.

41. Jasper, H. H., and Rasmussen, T., Studies of clinical and electrical responses to deep temporal stimulation in man with some considerations of functional anatomy. *Res. Publ., Assoc. Res. Nerv. Ment. Dis.,* 1958, **36**: 316–334.

42. Kaada, B. R., Somatomotor, autonomic and electrographic responses to electrical stimulation of rhinencephalic and other structures in Primates, Cat and Dog. *Acta Physiol. Scand.,* 1951, **23**, Suppl. 83: 1–285.

43. Kaada, B. R., Cingulate, posterior orbital, anterior insular and temporal pole cortex. In: *Handbook of Physiology* (Am. Physiol. Soc., J. Field, Ed.), Williams & Wilkins, Baltimore, 1960: Sect. 1, Vol. II: 1345–1372.

44. Kellaway, P., Depth recording in focal epilepsy. *Electroenceph. clin. Neurophysiol.,* 1956, **8**: 527–528.

45. Klingler, J., and Gloor, P., The connections of the amygdala and of the anterior temporal cortex of the human brain. *J. Comp. Neurol.,* 1960, **115**: 333–370.

46. Lorente de Nó, R., Studies on the structure of the cerebral cortex. I. The area entorhinalis. *J. Psychol. Neurol.,* 1933, **45**: 381–438.

47. Magnus, O., and Naquet, R. Physiologie et pathologie du rhinencéphale. In: *Les grandes activités du rhinencéphale.* Masson, Paris, 1961: 191–221.

48. Mark, V. H., Ervin, F. R., Sweet, W. H., and Delgado, J. M. R., Remote telemeter stimulation and recording from implanted temporal lobe electrodes. *Confin. Neurol.,* 1969, **31**: 86–93.

49. Morrell, F., Physiology and histochemistry of the mirror focus. In: *Basic Mechanisms in the Epilepsies* (H. H. Jasper, A. A. Ward, and A. Pope, Eds.). Churchill, London, and Little, Brown, Boston, 1969: 357–370.

50. Pagni, C. A., and Morossero, M. D., Some observations on the human rhinen-
    cephalon. A stereoencephalographic study. *Electroenceph. clin. Neuro-
    physiol.*, 1965, **18**: 260–271.

51. Paillas, J. E., Vigouroux, R., Corriol, J., and Bonnal, J., Intérêt de l'en-
    registrement électrographique du noyau amygdalien au cours des opéra-
    tions pour épilepsie temporale. *Rev. Neurol. (Paris)*, 1952, 86: 19–54.

52. Pampiglione, G., and Falconer, M. A., Phénomènes subjectifs et objectifs
    provoqués par la stimulation de l'hippocampe chez l'homme. *Physiologie
    de l'hippocampe*. CNRS, Paris, 1962: 399–408.

53. Passouant, P., Gros, C., Cadilhac J., and Vlahovitch, B., Les postdécharges
    par stimulation électrique de la corne d'Ammon chez l'homme. *Rev.
    Neurol. (Paris)*, 1954, **90**: 265–274.

54. Penfield, W., and Erickson, T., *Epilepsy and Cerebral Localization*. Thomas,
    Springfield, Illinois, 1941.

55. Penfield, W., and Jasper, H. H., *Epilepsy and the Functional Anatomy of the
    Human Brain*. Little, Brown, Boston, 1954.

56. Penfield, W., and Rasmussen, T., *The Cerebral Cortex of Man. A Clinical
    Study of Localization of Function*. Macmillan, New York, 1957.

57. Pribram, K., Lennox, M., and Dunsmore, R., Some connections of the orbito-
    fronto-temporal, limbic and hippocampal areas of Macaca mulatta. *J.
    Neurophysiol.*, 1950, **13**: 127–133.

58. Pribram, K. H., and Maclean, P. D., Neuronographic analysis of medical and
    basal cortex. II. Monkey. *J. Neurophysiol.*, 1953, **16**: 324–340.

59. Prince, D., Microelectrode studies of penicillin foci. In: *Basic Mechanisms
    in the Epilepsies* (H. H. Jasper, A. A. Ward, and A. Pope, Eds.). Chur-
    hill, London, and Little, Brown, Boston, 1969: 320–328.

60. Purpura, D. P., Mechanisms of propagation: Intracellular studies. In: *Basic
    Mechanisms in the Epilepsies* (H. H. Jasper, A. A. Ward, and A. Pope,
    Eds.). Churchill, London, and Little, Brown, Boston, 1969: 481–505.

61. Raisman, G., Cowan, W. M., and Powell, T. P. S. The extrinsic afferent,
    commissural and association fibres of the hippocampus. *Brain*, 1965,
    88: 963–996.

62. Raisman, G., Cowan, W. M., and Powell, T. P. S., An experimental analysis
    of the efferent projection of the hippocampus. *Brain*, 1966, 89: 83–108.

63. Rand, R. W., Crandall, P. H., and Walter, R., Chronic stereotactic implanta-
    tion of depth electrodes for psychomotor epilepsy. *Acta Neurochir.
    (Wien)*, 1964, **11**: 609–630.

64. Rayport, M., Buser, P., Bancaud, J., and Talairach, J., Single neurone activity
    in hippocampus and amygdala of man. *Bull. N.Y. Acad. Med.*, 1967,
    43: 420–428.

65. Rayport, M., and Waller, J. M., Microelectrode analysis of the human epi-
    leptiform spike. *Excerpta Med. Int. Congr. Ser.*, 1961, **37**: 17.

66. Ribstein, M., Exploration du cerveau humain par électrodes profondes.
    Electroenceph. clin. Neurophysiol., 1960, 16, Supp.: 1–130.

67. Riechert, T., and Umbach, W., Cortical and subcortical EEG patterns during
    stereotaxic operations in subcortical structures of the human brain. *Elec-
    troenceph. clin. Neurophysiol.*, 1955, 7: 663–664.

68. Rossi, G. F., Problems of analysis and interpretation of electrocerebral signals in human epilepsy. A neurosurgeon's view. In: *Epilepsy: Its Phenomena in Man* (M. A. B. Brazier, Ed.), Academic Press, New York, 1973: 259–285.

69. Schneider, R. C., Crosby, E. C., and Kahn, E. A., Certain afferent cortical connections of the rhinencephalon. *Progr. Brain Res.*, 1963, **3**: 191–217.

70. Showers, M. J., The cingulate gyrus: Additional motor area and cortical autonomic regulator. *J. Comp. Neurol.*, 1959, **112**: 231–302.

71. Sloan, N., Pool, J. L., and Ransohoff, J., EEG responses to electrical stimulations of the periamygdaloid, anterior temporal, posterior orbital and anterior cingulate cortices in non epileptic man. *Electroenceph. clin. Neurophysiol.*, 1952, **4**: 243.

72. Spencer, W. A., and Kandel, E. R., Synaptic inhibition in seizures. In: *Basic Mechanisms in the Epilepsies* (H. H. Jasper, A. A. Ward, and A. Pope, Eds.). Churchill, London, and Little, Brown, Boston, 1969: 575–603.

73. Steriade, M., Development of evoked responses into self-sustained activity within amygdalo hippocampal circuits. *Electroenceph. clin. Neurophysiol.*, 1964: 221–236.

74. Storm van Leeuwen, W., Kamp, A., and Reneman, R. S., Activités électriques périodiques lors de l'abaissement de température à 16–20°C chez le Chien. *Rev. EEG Neurophysiol.*, 1971, **1**: 106–108.

75. Talairach, J., David, M., Tournoux, P., Corredor, H., and Kvasina, T., *Atlas d'anatomie stéréotaxique*. Masson, Paris, 1957.

76. Talairach, J., and Szikla, G., *Atlas d'anatomie stéréotaxique du télencéphale. Etudes anatomo-radiologiques*. Masson, Paris, 1967.

77. Torres, F., An averaging method for determination of temporal relationship between epileptogenic foci. *Electroenceph. clin. Neurophysiol.*, 1967, **22**: 270–272.

78. Valverde, F., Amygdaloid projection field. Rhinencephalon. *Progr. Brain. Res.*, 1963, **3**: 20–30.

79. Votaw, C. L., Certain functional and anatomical relations of the Cornu Ammonis of the Macaque. I. Functional relations. *J. Comp. Neurol.*, 1959, **112**: 353–382.

80. Votaw, C. L., Certain functional and anatomical relation of the Cornu Ammonis of the Macaque monkey. 2. Anatomical relations. *J. Comp. Neurol.*, 1960, **114**: 283–293.

81. Walker, E. A., and Ribstein, M., Enregistrements et stimulations des formations rhinencéphaliques avec electrodes profondes à demeure chez l'homme. *Rev. Neurol. (Paris)*, 1957, **96**: 453–459.

82. Walker, E. A., and Udvarhelyi, G. B., Dissemination of acute focal seizures in the monkey. *Arch. Neurol.*, 1965, **12**: 357–380.

83. Ward, A. A., The epileptic neuron: Chronic foci in animal and man. In: *Basic Mechanisms in the Epilepsies* (H. H. Jasper, A. A. Ward, and A. Pope, Eds.). Churchill, London, and Little, Brown, Boston, 1969: 263–288.

84. Whitlock, D., and Nauta, W., Subcortical projections from the temporal neocortex in Macaca. *J. Comp. Neurol.*, 1956, **106**: 183–212.

TACTICAL CONSIDERATIONS LEADING TO SURGICAL
TREATMENT OF LIMBIC EPILEPSY

RICHARD D. WALTER

Brain Research Institute, University of California, Los Angeles, California

The clinician or clinical neurophysiologist involved in the evaluation of patients with limbic epilepsy for appropriate surgical treatment is confronted with a variety of decisions that relate to a successful outcome. These decisions might be looked upon as a tactical problem leading to the solution of the individual patient's seizure disorder. In this context, this chapter will be based on the pragmatic experience of evaluating 48 patients with limbic or temporal lobe epilepsy under the auspices of the Clinical Neurophysiology Project at UCLA Medical Center.* The presentation will be more in the nature of a clinical discourse, emphasizing practical decisions, rather than a basic science treatise on temporal lobe epilepsy.

There are a number of detailed reports relating to the surgical treatment of temporal lobe epilepsy based on scalp electroencephalograms (EEG) and electrocorticographic recordings (2, 10, 13, 18). Other reports (3, 8, 20) have described the use of depth electrodes in connection with surgical treatment. A growing international interest appears to be developing in the surgical treatment of convulsive disorders based on the use of chronic depth electrode implantation. Groups of neurologists, neurosurgeons, and clinical neurophysiologists are being formed in various medical centers throughout the world to undertake this type of study and treatment. The following information is presented to offer the experience of one such group, hoping that it will be helpful to others. The decisions involved in the evaluation of patients for possible surgical treatment will be described under headings in the sequence encountered in the clinic or hospital setting.

DECISIONS IN SELECTING PATIENTS FOR SURGICAL CONSIDERATION

Assuming that the patient's clinical seizure history is compatible with partial epilepsy originating in the temporal lobe, the primary concern at this point is in regard to the nature of the lesion responsible for the seizure

* Supported by Grant NS 02808 of the National Institute of Neurological Diseases and Stroke. The research was carried out in the UCLA Neuropsychiatric Institute and the Brain Research Institute.

disorder. The clinical presentation of limbic epilepsy is now recognized to be quite diverse, and the subtle details of the aura, autonomic phenomena, automatisms, and amnesia will not be elaborated further in this chapter. In our clinic, the evaluation of such a patient would develop along the following broad outline.

Duration of Seizure History

In the past, we had a tendency to accept with relative complacency the fact that a seizure history extending over many years was incompatible with a dangerous, life-threatening, space-occupying lesion. During the past 12 years of evaluating such patients, however, we have been surprised and dismayed to uncover intracranial lesions in patients with long seizure history with such frequency that our complacency is no longer justified. These lesions generally fall into the category of tumors in the glial series, occasionally meningiomata, and A-V malformations other than the microscopic findings in resected specimens, as reported by W. Jann Brown (this volume) in our own series of patients and the findings of others (5, 11, 15, 16). Our policy, then, is to evaluate fairly extensively each patient presenting with limbic epilepsy, regardless of the duration of the seizure history.

Clinical Assessment of the Patient

Although generally unrewarding, the detailed neurological examination and historical review will occasionally demonstrate significant clues indicating such ominous lesions. In keeping with general experience, olfactory or gustatory phenomena in the seizure history are particularly associated with structural lesions other than hippocampal sclerosis. Change in seizure patterns, the development of neurological signs, and the appearance of the traditional sign of increased intracranial pressure naturally force the decision in the direction of surgical consideration.

Radiographic Procedures

We have taken advantage of the tremendous development in neuroradiology, both in regard to the reduction of morbidity and mortality that such procedures entail, and in view of the growth of increased precision. Without exception, our patients with limbic epilepsy undergo an evaluation of routine radiological examination of the skull, specifically looking for calcification in the temporal area, difference in the size of the middle fossa, as well as any of the other traditional radiological abnormalities. In the last 10 years we have also routinely secured brain scans. Though the yield is low, the procedure is innocuous and is occasionally rewarded by a finding that completely changes the decision-making about such a patient.

The use of contrast procedures has a tendency to be more individualized. At a time when these procedures appeared more formidable, we were less inclined to use them—unless a significant clue was present in the patient's clinical examination. Now, both as a function of our having missed lesions and with the reduction in morbidity, we routinely secure both a pneumo-encephalographic study and bilateral carotid arteriographic studies. Of the two procedures, pneumoencephalography has the highest yield in terms of lateralization by the demonstration of distortion, displacements, or dilatation of the temporal horn. However, we feel that the examination is not complete unless we also perform arteriography. The yield for abnormality is not as high, but the rewards are in the demonstration of an occasional tumor or arteriovenous malformation.

Electroencephalographic Studies

Clinical electroencephalography has advanced to a point, and the standard of practice is such that it is recognized now that a single recording during the waking state is an inadequate examination for limbic epilepsy. The diagnosis of limbic seizures is not made on an electroencephalographic basis, in that all patients who have limbic epilepsy do not have surface electrical abnormalities and all that spikes in the temporal region is not epilepsy.

On a present empirical basis, we prefer to have three separate wake–sleep recordings in any patient who is being considered for surgical treatment. As in other electroencephalographic–clinical correlations, a consistent slow wave focus is more indicative of an ominous structural lesion and can be used in itself as an argument for the decision to proceed with contrast studies.

Notoriously, what appears to be a focal, unilateral spiking focus on one single examination is found to be more complicated in terms of bilaterality when serial recordings are made. If there is no, or inconclusive evidence for a focal abnormality in the routine EEG, then we utilize the option of recording with special electrodes designed to assay the electrical activity being generated in proximity to the temporal lobe. In the first 25 patients being considered for surgical treatment in our series, we routinely used sphenoidal electrodes and recorded both during the waking state and during sleep. A review of the findings from these sphenoidal electrode studies, correlating with surface electrical abnormalities, and the results obtained from depth electrode studies, demonstrated a low yield of significant localizing information. We have, therefore, discontinued the use of sphenoidal electrodes.

In recent years, nasopharyngeal electrodes have supplanted the use of sphenoidal leads. The ease of application, the lack of discomfort, and the detection of electrical abnormalities is about the same for nasopharyngeal as for sphenoidal electrodes. Our current strategy in the use of these electrodes, however, is based on the fact that they assist us in demonstrating electrical abnormalities that can be added to the body of clinical data. The results of nasopharyngeal recordings, however, are not adequate for considering surgery on this information alone. The crucial question is, does this focal EEG abnormality—regardless of the method of its detection, whether by surface recording or sphenoidal or nasopharyngeal leads—represent the origin of this patient's clinical seizures? We feel that with currently available techniques this question cannot be answered by any means other than recording during a spontaneous clinical seizure from depth electrodes.

There are two situations that present clinically with a frequency that deserves special comment. The first is the patient with the clinical diagnosis of what appears to be limbic epilepsy, based on the details of the seizure pattern, but who, electroencephalographically demonstrates generalized, bilaterally synchronous spike-and-wave complexes from the surface. In practice, these may range from persistent bilateral symmetry to subtle episodes of an apparent focal discharge. The diagnosis of limbic epilepsy may well be questioned on the basis of this finding, as it is now recognized that many of the clinical features of limbic seizures may also appear in generalized epilepsy.

The second situation is the electrographic appearance of independent, bilateral, temporal spiking either on the surface or in the nasopharyngeal leads. A range is encountered from absolute parity between the two sides, persisting over time, to rare transient abnormalities demonstrated on one side, in contrast to frequent and persistent discharges on the other side.

Decisions regarding the eligibility for possible surgical treatment are obviously difficult in these two general situations. What clinical neurophysiological techniques, outside of depth electrode implantation, are available for the resolution of the problem? There are, at the present time, two general techniques that have been used to provide answers regarding "true" electrographic localization.

One technique involves the use of a convulsant agent, such as pentylenetetrazol, to dissect out a focal electrical event that is responsible for the patient's clinical seizures. Obviously the mere activation of an electrical focus in this context is inadequate, and the drug must be administered by a method and at a dosage such that a clinical seizure, hopefully duplicating the "spontaneous" event, occurs. In the early part of this study we used pentylenetetrazol for this specific purpose. First, our results were clouded by the technical difficulties of matching the spontaneous seizure by the right amount of drug, in that generalized seizures were very apt to occur, and by the tremendous amount of artifact obscuring the recording using conventional EEG techniques. Second, the theoretical possibilities remained that the focus, activated by this technique, did not truly represent the events occurring in a spontaneous seizure. We have since abandoned this procedure.

Another strategy is that of using drugs in the barbiturate series in a manner as reported by Lombroso (14) using thiopental, Musella (17) and

Wilder (23) using methohexital, or the intracarotid technique reported by Gloor (12). With these techniques, we have studied patients who have bilateral or independent right and left spiking foci but at the present time have not had sufficient experience to correlate the results of either the localization resulting from depth electrode implantation or the eventual outcome following surgery. Again, the theoretical possibility remains that the localizations derived from these techniques may not correspond to the site responsible for the patient's seizures. Conversely, we are currently reluctant to consider for possible surgical treatment any patient who consistently shows generalized abnormalities in response to any of the barbiturate-type techniques. (We are aware that there is growing evidence that what appears to be generalized in surface recordings may actually be focal and cortical in origin, but this is beyond the specific discussion of limbic epilepsy).

THE CRITERIA ADOPTED FOR DEPTH ELECTRODE IMPLANTATION

Recognizing that generalizations may be both inadequate and unnecessarily leading to constraint, we have adopted the following criteria leading to chronic depth electrode implantation.

1. The patient does have limbic epilepsy. This judgment is based on the best clinical and clinical–neurophysiological determination possible. Other types of partial seizures may be considered for depth electrode studies, and our experience of these cases is described by Dr. P. H. Crandall in this volume.

2. The patient does not have a demonstrated lesion that would in itself require surgical treatment. Although in our experience surprises still occur after the most careful clinical and radiographical evaluation, the procedures must be carried out.

3. Anticonvulsant therapy has been ineffective in controlling the seizures. The admission of medical failure may be a more difficult decision than the presence or absence of a space-occupying lesion. Time is required to test the effectiveness of the major categories of anticonvulsants both in regard to an appropriate dose and to combination. It is beyond the scope of this presentation to outline the medical therapies used in the convulsive disorders. It may well be that the increasing availability of gas–liquid chromatography for the determination of blood levels of multiple anticonvulsants may improve seizure control so that surgery is not warranted. Another possibility is that a shorter period of time may be required to indicate a medical failure.

4. The seizure frequency is incapacitating. Perhaps, at best, this is a qualitative type of determination with a great deal of variation between patients. One seizure per month may be a disaster to one patient but may represent fairly good seizure control for another and have little effect on his socioeconomic status.

5. The patient's mental status is such that the procedure can be tolerated. A major practical consideration is the patient's ability to undergo chronic depth electrode studies without doing harm to himself. The head dressing may be violated and the electrode removed by the patient, either as a result of psychosis or mental retardation. Judgments may be difficult in this area, and we have relied on psychiatric and psychological consultation. A certain degree of mental retardation is not, in itself, a contraindication to the procedures, but we are reluctant to study grossly psychotic patients with depth recordings.

6. The age of the patient should be considered. We are not, at this time, able to offer absolute generalizations regarding the ideal age range for considering this procedure. Some of the older patients in our series have experienced more difficulties in the area of rehabilitation after successful surgical treatment. Patients in the age range of 10 to 15 years are less likely to be considered as candidates. Aside from a natural reluctance to implant electrodes in such young patients, there is an empirical argument that with further central nervous system maturation and endocrine stabilization the seizure disorder may become less of a problem and be brought under medical control. We are aware of two arguments advanced in favor of early surgery. The first is that the possibly harmful effects of long-term anticonvulsant medication may be avoided, and, second, the overall period of disability in the young patient's life will be diminished by early surgery. At the present time we have no statistical data to support or deny these proposals.

DECISIONS ENCOUNTERED IN CONNECTION WITH DEPTH ELECTRODE IMPLANTATION

If the patient meets the previously described criteria and implantation is the procedure of choice prior to surgical excision, there are a number of problems that develop as a result of this course of action.

Selection of Electrode Sites

Based on the extensive experience of others who have been active in the surgical treatment of limbic epilepsy and based on the well-documented neuropathological changes in this disorder, one can select targets that would reasonably be anticipated to be deep epileptogenic foci. The surgical implantation techniques used in this study have already been reported (6, 8, 20). Although unilateral targets can be selected, based on this past experience, some difficulty arises in the decision of unilateral versus bilateral temporal lobe implantation. When the patient demonstrates bilateral, independent electrical abnormalities from either the surface or nasopharyngeal leads, then it is an easy decision to implant both temporal lobes. However, if the patient has consistently demonstrated a unilateral problem on his surface and nasopharyngeal recordings and, to argue the extreme case, has some radiographical localization, such as an enlarged temporal horn on the same side as the electrical abnormality, then one may ask, Why implant electrodes in that patient and why not proceed directly to surgical treatment?

In the early part of our program, we circumvented implantation and proceeded directly to surgery, as was the standard strategy at that time. In some circumstances, but very rarely, we implanted electrodes only on the side of greatest suspicion. During the last 5 years, however, we have elected to implant both deep temporal areas in all patients suspected of having limbic epilepsy. The justification, for what may appear to be an arbitrary decision, is that in spite of "surface" evidence, be it from the scalp, nasopharyngeal electrode, or barbiturate studies, there still may be a possibility that this evidence is erroneous and not related to the patient's clinical seizures. A review of our tentative localizations based on surface evidence, compared with the more definitive depth electrode localization indicates an error of at least 10%. In other words, the unsuspected side may be responsible for the patient's seizures at least 10% of the time.

An additional argument in favor of bilateral implantation is the adequacy of the normal side to sustain the function of recent memory, if the abnormal side is removed. A method of evaluating this possibility will be mentioned later.

Finally, in regard to target selection, there is always a real possibility that the problem is not strictly "limbic" in origin. Epileptogenic foci outside of the classic limbic system have been reported to present as limbic epilepsy. The inevitable sampling problems inherent in depth electrode studies in man preclude the development of a universal strategy that will correctly identify all cases.

Interictal Recordings

It has been our policy to begin recordings from the depth sites and the electrodes implanted in the calvarium as soon as the patient is reasonably comfortable following the implantation procedure. This is generally the first postoperative day. Our initial concern was that the recordings obtained in this early postoperative period might be marred by artifacts resulting from the implantation procedure itself. What might be termed "injury potentials"—brief bursts of extremely high-frequency spiking, occurring at only one depth electrode site—have been observed in only 3 patients, and this pattern subsided after a 3-day period. The more generalized slowing, a result of the prolonged anesthesia and/or the contrast procedures necessary for implantation, also subsides over a 24–48 hour period. Although these early tracings may be regarded with some degree of suspicion, they may be useful and often indicate the ultimate localization confirmed by several weeks of recordings.

The basic question involved in the evaluation of the simultaneous depth and surface recordings is, Which particular signal or pattern is most indicative of the site of origin of the patient's seizure? We have observed the following categories of interictal recordings during this period of study.

a. Spike and/or spike–wave sequences:

1. Bilaterally synchronous, nonfocal discharges from all depth sites. The details of this finding have been reported by Rossi and co-workers (21).

2. Independent discharges appearing with nearly equal prevalence from both the right and left deep temporal structures.

3. Primarily focal or regional discharge from one temporal lobe. This might be considered to be the "ideal case" from the viewpoint of interictal recordings. We have not found, however, a single example of spike and/or waves confined exclusively, over several weeks of recordings, to one side. Parenthetically, it has also been our experience to observe some degree of spiking in all patients with convulsive disorders who have been studied to date. This not unexpected finding is undoubtedly a result of our inclusion for depth electrode evaluation those patients who have independent spiking of a bilateral type in their surface EEG recordings.

b. Areas of slowing or regions of nonreactivity:

1. Focal areas or regions of slowing have been observed when compared to the homologous sites. It is difficult to evaluate, in terms of abnormality, slow background frequencies appearing at a single depth electrode site. It is impossible to be absolutely sure about the symmetry of the bilateral placements, particularly with the high probability of pathological changes. If, however, the area is more regional, for example, appearing in all three or four depth electrodes implanted in one hippocampus, then it is more reasonable to assume that this represents a valid and possibly significant observation.

This regional slowing may range from its gross appearance during the waking state to more subtle manifestations, such as a suppression of sleep spindles during sleep or an absence of the characteristic fast activity induced by barbiturates.

2. Generalized slow frequencies in both right and left temporal lobes. This is an uncommon finding and obviously of no assistance in localization. The decisions regarding critical localization, then, in dealing with interictal recordings, is that they are unreliable because they are interictal. All the authors who have used depth electrode techniques in patients with convulsive disorders have observed the wealth of apparent electrical abnormality from the depth that is without apparent clinical significance.

Ictal Recordings

Certainly the logical answer to definitive localization of the site of origin of the patient's seizure is to record during a seizure. There are a number of factors that influence the securing of such recordings, and we now consider our depth electrode study to be inadequate unless we have obtained this information.

TECHNICAL ASPECTS

Chronically implanted depth electrodes are less apt to be subject to movement artifact, and electromyographic contamination does not occur. Artifacts induced by head movement can be further reduced by using telemetering techniques [the system we are currently using has been described previously (1, 9)]. Telemetering also has the distinct advantage of increasing the total recording time without the constraints, either physical or psychological, induced by hard wire-on-line methods. We are confident that we have significantly increased the probability of recording during a "spontaneous" clinical seizure.

SEIZURE DENSITY IN POSTIMPLANTATION PERIOD

In keeping with the age-old clinical observation that a change in environmental set may reduce the frequency of seizure, such is the general case following implantation. For the same reasons outlined in the section on activation procedures prior to implantation, we are reluctant to use currently available convulsants. Our current policy is to begin gradually withdrawing the anticonvulsant agents which the patient continues following the operative procedure. Our concern about producing status epilepticus has not been justified to date. This reduction in medication is now begun 2 or 3 days after implantation.

HOW MANY CLINICAL SEIZURES ARE REQUIRED FOR
DEFINITE LOCALIZATIONS?

If one accepts the observation that hippocampal sclerosis is the most common pathological substrate for limbic epilepsy and that this may be a bilateral process, then it is reasonable to propose that there may be patients with independent foci on each side, each capable of resulting in clinical seizure activity. Ideally, then, we prefer to record a number of clinical seizure events to check against this bilateral possibility. How large a number of seizures are to be recorded for absolute reliability has not been determined by us, but we feel more comfortable with more than three, but practical considerations regarding the duration of implantation may make a larger number difficult to obtain. To date, we have encountered two patients with limbic epilepsy who clearly had bilaterally independent foci responsible for clinical seizures and who, therefore, were excluded for subsequent surgical resection.

TYPES OF ELECTROGRAPHIC FINDINGS DURING THE ICTUS

We have not experienced great difficulty in making decisions regarding focal or regional onset during an aura or other manifestations of the patient's clinical seizure (7). In the context of this paper we are not concerned with the sequence of propagation of the seizure as revealed by the depth recordings, but only in the judgment based on the apparent site of origin. In the domain of practical consideration, three possibilities have been encountered.

a. Precise Focal Origin. In this situation (see Figure 1) the seizure discharge can be seen to originate in one or possibly two single bipolar recordings, propagate to nearby sites, and perhaps eventually appear in areas in the opposite hemisphere. In our experience, this finding is uncommon, that is, the apparent origin from what appears to be a small volume of brain.

b. Regional Focal Origin. An example of this finding is presented in Figure 2A–C. The more commonly encountered finding is that the electrical abnormality leading to a clinical seizure—but preceding the clinical event—appears in more than one bipolar recording electrode, suggesting the possibility of a much larger volume being involved at the time of initiation.

c. Generalized Discharges at the Onset. We have observed this situation to be less common in those patients carefully selected for "limbic epilepsy"

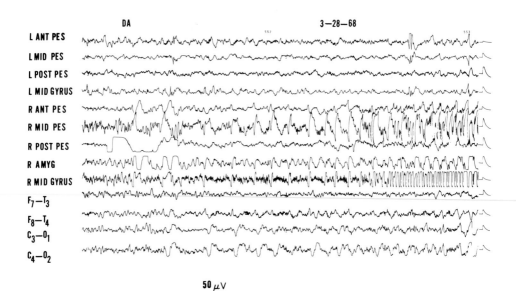

50 μV

Figure 1. Focal spontaneous seizure from right (R) mid-hippocampal gyrus. This 20-second depth and surface recording demonstrates the focal onset of a clinical limbic seizure beginning in the right mid-hippocampal gyrus. The onset is marked by fast 26–30 cps activity in the bipolar leads, with concurrent spiking and sharp wave activity in the right mid-pes hippocampi. An artifact appears in the right posterior pes hippocampus recording. There is no gross reflection of this deep discharge in the surface recordings in the lower four channels. L—left; ANT—anterior; POST—posterior, AMYG—amygdala.

and more common in those patients suspected of having a focal origin out-side of the limbic system.

There is a basic problem in determining the true focal origin of seizure activity using depth electrode recordings in man. This is the sampling prob-lem which may never be completely or adequately solved. We obviously do not know what is taking place in the regions in which we have no elec-trodes. Therefore, what may appear to be regional, at the time of seizure onset, may be in reality the projection or propagation of a small epilepto-genic focus at a nonrecorded site to the regions that are being recorded. In the chapter in this volume by W. Jann Brown this situation is illustrated by the schematic plot of both the extent of the pathological changes in a resected specimen and the electrode sites.

Electrical Stimulation Studies

Our policy has been to stimulate electrically each available depth elec-trode site in an effort to provide additional localizing information that would be of help in the treatment of the specific patient under study. In the early phase of this program we anticipated that the practical yield derived from stimulation would be very high.

Some of the outcomes that seemed theoretically possible were (a) a quantifiable difference in the threshold for after-discharge, the lowest value being at the site responsible for the patient's seizures; (b) a consistent duplication of the patient's spontaneous seizure by electrical stimulation in every patient; (c) some feature of the after-discharge, duration, wave form, or facility of propagation, that would be unique for the true seizure focus.

In our experience, these hopeful possibilities have not been realized. It may well be that an electrode surrounded by gliosis found in hippocampal sclerosis will have a higher threshold for after-discharge—indeed, if an after-discharge can be obtained at all. We have not been able to duplicate either a fragment or the complete spontaneous seizure sequence in all of our pa-tients. A review of the afterdischarges induced in areas initiating the spon-taneous clinical seizures are not morphologically or quantitatively different from other after-discharges.

Nevertheless, we continue to perform electrical stimulation studies, in that there may be a practical yield in two dimensions of the patient's evalu-ation. There is at least a 50% probability of obtaining an electrically in-duced after-discharge that is correlated with a report by the patient or ob-served behavioral change that relates to the patient's seizure disorder. Duplicated reports of an aura matching the spontaneous variety can be used to bolster the evidence for definitive localization. There are reports from patients about subjective experiences that do not appear to relate to their seizure pattern, and these have been partially reported by Chapman and co-workers (4).

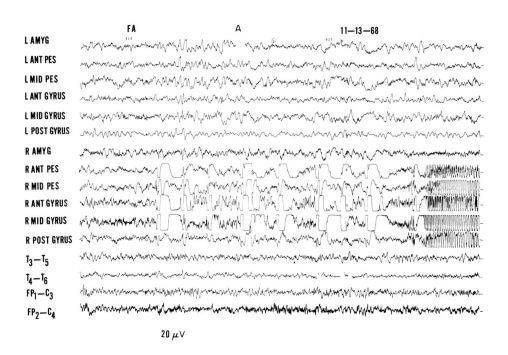

L AMYG
L ANT PES
L MID PES
L ANT GYRUS
L MID GYRUS
L POST GYRUS
R AMYG
R ANT PES
R MID PES
R ANT GYRUS
R MID GYRUS
R POST GYRUS
$T_3 - T_5$
$T_4 - T_6$
$FP_1 - C_3$
$FP_2 - C_4$

FA   A   11—13—68

20 μV

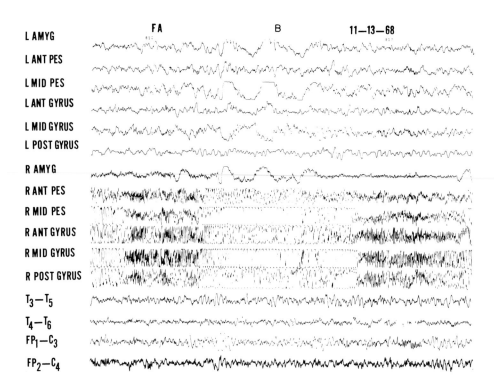

L AMYG
L ANT PES
L MID PES
L ANT GYRUS
L MID GYRUS
L POST GYRUS
R AMYG
R ANT PES
R MID PES
R ANT GYRUS
R MID GYRUS
R POST GYRUS
$T_3 - T_5$
$T_4 - T_6$
$FP_1 - C_3$
$FP_2 - C_4$

FA   B   11—13—68

20 μV

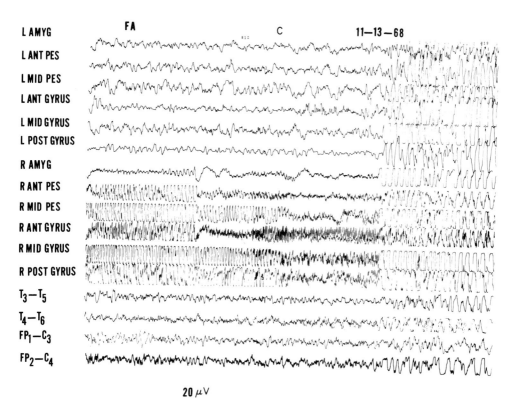

Figure 2. Regional onset of spontaneous seizure in right (R) depth sites. (A) In this 20-second recording, high-amplitude discharges appear in all of the right depth areas at a repetition rate of about 1.5 seconds. There is a slight reflection of this activity at its onset in the right surface recording, $T_4 - T_6$. Near the end of the 20 seconds, the depth activity demonstrates high-frequency, high-amplitude spiking activity. (B) During the next 20-second period, the spiking continues as a region in the right depth, with the exception of the right amygdala (AMYG). There are no signs of a clinical seizure or any subjective reports from the patient at this time. (C) The high-frequency spiking continues to be regional, and then abruptly the discharge appears in all depth sites. At this point, the patient demonstrated the beginning of his usual clinical seizure pattern. L—left; ANT—anterior; POST—posterior.

There are situations that we have encountered that are more complex than the initiation of a clinical seizure by electrically stimulating a site at or close to the focus responsible for the patient's clinical seizure. Figure 3A–D illustrates one such example of false localization, and another complex situation is illustrated in Figure 4A–E. We are reasonably sure that the patient's focus was correctly identified and resected, based on an 8-year seizure-free follow-up. Electrical stimulation of the temporal lobe sites that were involved in the initiation of the spontaneous clinical seizures were ineffective in producing an after-discharge. This may have been a function of electrode implantation in largely glial areas. Stimulation of the opposite side, however, resulted in after-discharges that were clinically silent when

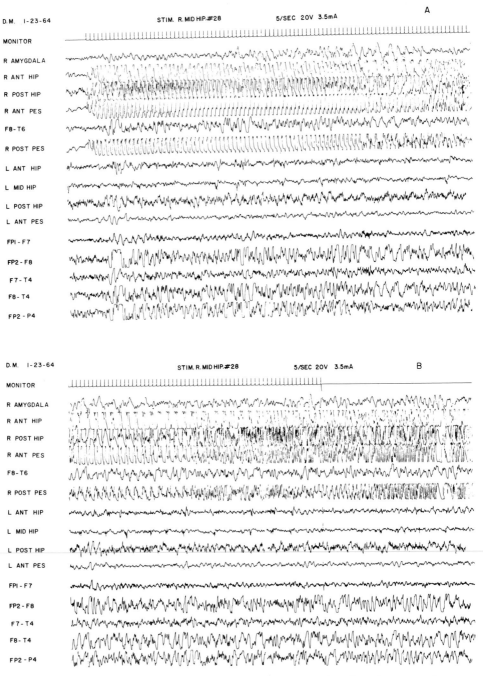

Figure 3. An example of an after-discharge resulting in the clinical report of a past aura. (A) Electrical stimulation at a rate of 5/second at 3.5 mA delivered to the right (R) middle hippocampal gyrus resulted in the appearance of evoked potentials, time locked with the stimulus in all of the right depth leads except the right amygdala. (B) In the next 20 seconds of recording after trace A, the evoked depth activity no longer is related to the stimulus. An after-discharge was produced that remained confined to the same area demonstrating the evoked activity. (C) The

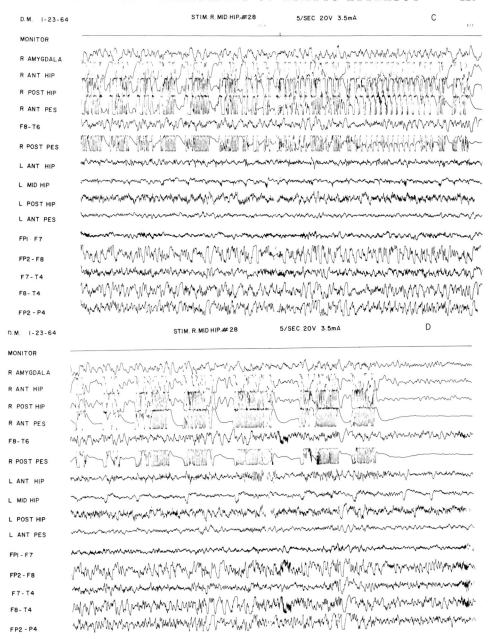

D.M. 1-23-64   STIM. R. MID HIP.#28   5/SEC 20V 3.5mA   C

MONITOR

R AMYGDALA

R ANT HIP

R POST HIP

R ANT PES

F8-T6

R POST PES

L ANT HIP

L MID HIP

L POST HIP

L ANT PES

FPI - F7

FP2 - F8

F7 - T4

F8 - T4

FP2 - P4

D.M. 1-23-64   STIM. R. MID HIP.# 28   5/SEC 20V 3.5mA   D

MONITOR

R AMYGDALA

R ANT HIP

R POST HIP

R ANT PES

F8-T6

R POST PES

L ANT HIP

L MID HIP

L POST HIP

L ANT PES

FPI - F7

FP2 - F8

F7 - T4

F8 - T4

FP2 - P4

after-discharge continued confined to the deep temporal structures as illustrated in this continuous tracing. Although only the right surface leads are included, slowing has been apparent since the onset of the electrical stimulation. (D) Prominent electrical flattening appeared in both the right anterior (ANT) and posterior (POST) pes hippocampus (HIP) at the termination of the afterdischarge. Note the deflection in the left (L) mid-hippocampal gyrus synchronous with the onset of each burst on the opposite side. At the termination of the after-discharge, the patient reported having experienced a vaguely recalled aura—not her typical type—which may have been present at the onset of her seizure disorder. She was also transiently confused. Because the spontaneous clinical seizure began on the left side, a left temporal lobe resection was performed 8 years ago, and the patient remains seizure-free.

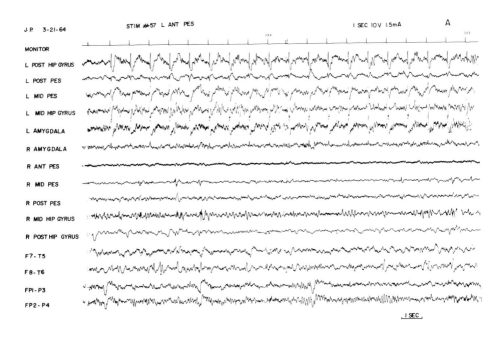

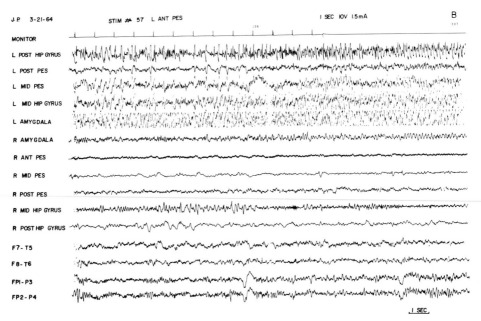

Figure 4. An after-discharge, initiated in the "good" left (L) depth sites propagated to the opposite side resulting in a clinical seizure. (A) Electrical stimulation of the left anterior (ANT) pes hippocampus (HIP) at 1/second, 1.5 mA resulted in an evoked potential appearing in all left-sided depth sites. [Right (R) anterior pes hippocampal lead in this and subsequent figures is artifactual (B)]. The evoked activity in the left depth structures in the next 20 seconds of recording after trace A no longer is time locked to the stimulus and an after-discharge is produced.

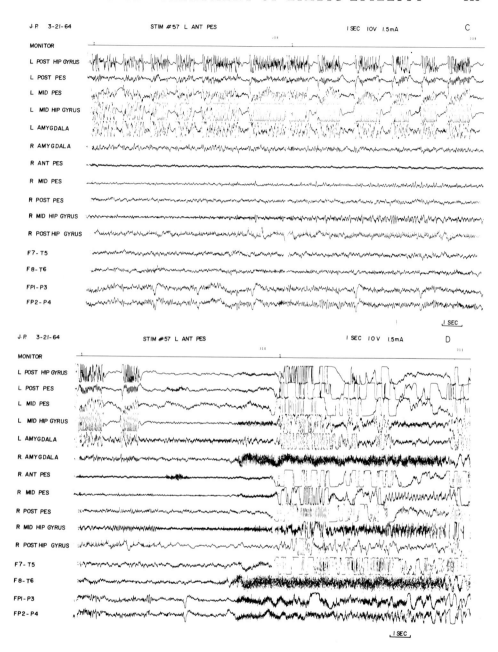

(C) In the following 20 seconds of recording after trace B, the after-discharge continues in the left depth sites. Low-amplitude rhythmical spiking appears more prominently in the right posterior hippocampal gyrus electrode. No clinical seizure activity was observed nor reported by the patient up to this time. (D) The subsequent 20 seconds of recording illustrate the apparent termination of the left-sided after-discharge, with a generalized suppression of electrical activity in all leads. Although the right posterior hippocampal gyrus lead continues to show low-amplitude spiking, this spiking stops at the time of general suppression; however, the right middle hippocampal gyrus demonstrates very low-amplitude fast frequencies. The electromyographic artifact appearing in the surface leads marks the beginning of the patient's usual clinical limbic

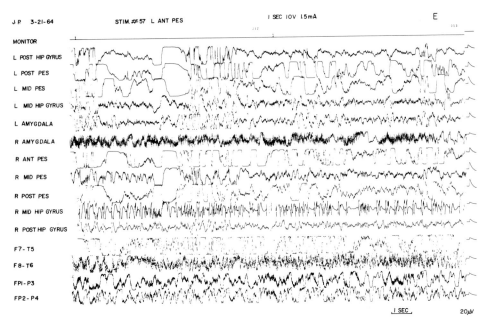

J.P.   3-21-64   STIM.# 57 L ANT PES   I SEC IOV I.5mA   E

MONITOR

L POST HIP GYRUS

L POST PES

L MID PES

L MID HIP GYRUS

L AMYGDALA

R AMYGDALA

R ANT PES

R MID PES

R POST PES

R MID HIP GYRUS

R POST HIP GYRUS

F7-T5

F8-T6

FPI-P3

FP2-P4

                                                                    I SEC   20μV

seizure. (E) During the clinical seizure, the apparent site most active in terms of spiking activity is the right middle hippocampal gyrus. This same finding was duplicated on three occasions during the study of this patient. A right-sided temporal lobe resection was performed 8 years ago, and the patient has remained seizure-free.

confined to this temporal lobe, but when propagated to the opposite side, a clinical seizure was produced, matching the spontaneous variety.

It has been possible in 8 of our patients to provide some information by electrical stimulation on the integrity of what might be termed the "good" temporal lobe. These patients have demonstrated transient confusion and an amnestic state for several minutes for 2 hours after unilateral, electrically induced after-discharges. Clinically, the syndrome is suggestive of transient global amnesia. Our explanation for this phenomenon is that one hippocampus is sclerotic and is the area responsible for the seizure disorder; the other hippocampus is ordinarily functionally intact but, when subjected to the after-discharge, becomes temporarily nonfunctional. For a time, then, the hippocampus in each hemisphere is inoperative and this amnestic syndrome is produced. This proposal, in part, is based on the reports of others (19, 22) describing the effects of bilateral hippocampal pathology.

In the area of practical decision-making, we have used this observation to indicate that (1) the hippocampus on the "good" side is adequate for memory functions should the opposite hippocampus be removed; (2) it would be quite inadvisable to resect the temporal region from which this syndrome can be demonstrated; and (3) by inference the pathology of the hippocampus on the "bad" side must be fairly extensive.

Our material at this point, however, is not complete enough to confirm statistically the validity of these suppositions. Finally, the determination that the appropriate decision has been made regarding the individual patient's seizure focus can be made only after years of continued observation.

ADDITIONAL METHODS OF LOCALIZATION

Although at the present time we see no way to circumvent the localization obtained by recording during a spontaneous clinical seizure, other methods have been and are currently being utilized. The depth electrode implantation procedure has the obvious disadvantage of a certain element of risk to the patient, requires at least a month of hospitalization, is exceedingly expensive, and can only be performed in large medical centers. Two directions of research are currently being undertaken to solve this practical problem, but they will be outlined only briefly in this presentation.

Techniques Eliminating Depth Electrode Implantation

It may be feasible in the future to rely more heavily on the localization obtained from surface recordings alone. This accomplishment is dependent on the demonstration of a consistently detectable signal in the surface recordings that reflects the abnormal events occurring within the depth. With computer techniques, it is hoped that a study of surface–depth relationships, as obtained in these patients, will eventually replace implantation in the future. The surface signals to be studied could still be obtained by telemetry and be based on interictal as well as ictal events occurring spontaneously and by activation.

Other Techniques Utilizing Depth Electrodes

Other physiological parameters are being measured from within the depth structure, such as impedance, blood flow, oxygen consumption, CO_2, and pH. Again it is premature to speculate on the possible replacement of the reliability of the ictal EEG by these determinations. The study of latencies and propagation within the depth structure by computer techniques, as performed by Dr. Brazier (and reported in this volume), also has great promise.

SUMMARY

The tactical considerations involved in the use of chronically implanted depth electrodes for localization leading to the surgical treatment of limbic epilepsy are initially those of patient selection. A patient who has medically intractable limbic epilepsy, who has been screened for gross pathological lesions, who is incapacitated by his seizure disorder, and who is not severely psychotic or retarded may be considered favorably for depth electrode evaluation regardless of his surface EEG abnormality.

Second, a different class of decisions appears during the course of the implantation study, all of which are directed toward a definitive localization of the seizure process. Information is obtained based on the interictal recordings, during clinical seizures, and in response to electrical stimulation of the depth sites. In our experience, the most reliable and useful information is derived from the ictal recordings that can be technically facilitated using telemetry techniques. The electrical stimulation studies may, but not always, provide confirmatory evidence for localization as well as clues relating to the intactness of the noninvolved temporal lobe.

REFERENCES

1. Adey, W. R., Hanley, J., Kado, R. T., and Zweizig, J. R., A multichannel telemetry system for EEG recording. *Proc. Symp. Biomed. Eng. Marquette Univ.,* 1966, 1: 36–39.
2. Bailey, P., and Gibbs, F. A., The surgical treatment of psychomotor epilepsy. *JAMA,* 1951, 145: 365–370.
3. Bancaud, J., Talairach, J., Bonis, A., Schaub, C., Szikla, G., Morel, P., and Bordas-Ferrer, M., *La stéréo-électroéncephalographie dans l'épilepsie.* Masson, Paris, 1965.
4. Chapman, L. F., Walter, R. D., Markham, C. H., Rand, R. W., and Crandall, P. H., Memory changes induced by stimulation of hippocampus or amygdala in epilepsy patients with implanted electrodes. *Trans. Am. Neurol. Assoc.,* 1967, 92: 50–56.
5. Corsellis, J. A. N., The incidence of Ammon's horn sclerosis. *Brain,* 1957, 80: 193–208.
6. Crandall, P. H., Brown, W. J., and Brinza, K., Stereotaxic accuracy in vivo of Talairach method in temporal lobes. *Confin. Neurol.,* 1966, 27: 14–153.
7. Crandall, P. H., and Walter, R. D., The ictal electroencephalographic signal identifying limbic system seizure foci. *Proc. Amer. Assoc. Neurol. Surg.,* 1971.
8. Crandall, P. H., Walter, R. D., and Rand, R. W., Clinical application of studies of stereotactically implanted electrodes in temporal-lobe epilepsy. *J. Neurosurg.,* 1963, 21: 827–840.
9. Dymond, A. M., Zweizig, J. R., Crandall, P. H., and Hanley, J., Clinical application of an EEG radiotelemetery system. *8th Annu. Rocky Mt. Bioeng. Symp.,* 1971: 16–20.
10. Falconer, M. A., and Serafetinides, E. A., A follow-up study of surgery in temporal lobe epilepsy. *J. Neurol., Neurosurg. Psychiatry,* 1963, 26: 154–165.
11. Falconer, M. A., Serafetinides, E. A., and Corsellis, J. A. N., Etiology and pathogenesis of temporal lobe epilepsy. *Arch. Neurol.,* 1964, 10: 233–248.
12. Gloor, P., Rasmussen, T., and Garretson, H., Fractionalized intracarotid metrazol injection. A new diagnostic method in electroencephalography. *Electroenceph. clin. Neurophysiol.,* 1964, 17: 322–327.
13. Green, J. R., and Scheetz, D. G., Surgery of epileptogenic lesions of the temporal lobe. *Arch. Neurol.,* 1964, 10: 135–148.

14. Lombroso, C., and Erba, G., Primary and secondary bilateral synchrony in epilepsy. *Arch. Neurol.*, 1970, **22:** 321–334.
15. Margerison, J. H., and Corsellis, J. A. N., Epilepsy and the temporal lobe. *Brain*, 1966, **89:** 499–530.
16. Meyer, A., Falconer, M. A., and Beck, E., Pathological findings in temporal lobe epilepsy. *J. Neurol., Neurosurg. Psychiatry*, 1954, **17:** 276–285.
17. Musella, L., Wilder, B. J., and Schmidt, R. P., EEG activation with intravenous methohexital in psychomotor epilepsy. *Neurology (Minneap.)*, 1971, **21:** 594–602.
18. Penfield, W. P., and Flanigan, H., Surgical therapy of temporal lobe seizures. *Arch. Neurol. Psychiat.*, 1950, **64:** 491–500.
19. Penfield, W. P., and Milner, B., Memory deficits produced by bilateral lesions in the hippocampal zone. *Arch. Neurol. Psychiat.*, 1958, **79:** 475–497.
20. Rand, R. W., Crandall, P. H., and Walter, R. D., Chronic stereotactic implantation of depth electrodes for psychomotor epilepsy. *Acta Neurochir. (Wien)*, 1964, **11:** 609–630.
21. Rossi, G. F., Walter, R. D., and Crandall, P. H., Generalized spike and wave discharges and nonspecific thalamic nuclei. *Arch. Neurol.*, 1968, **19:** 174–183.
22. Scoville, W. B., and Milner, B., Loss of recent memory after bilateral hippocampal lesions. *J. Neurol., Neurosurg. Psychiatry*, 1957, **20:** 11–21.
23. Wilder, B. J., Electroencephalographic activation in medically intractable epileptic patients. *Arch. Neurol.*, 1971, **25:** 415–426.

THE PROBLEM OF SYNCHRONIZATION IN THE SPREAD OF EPILEPTIC DISCHARGES LEADING TO SEIZURES IN MAN[*]

H. PETSCHE and **P. RAPPELSBERGER**

Institut für Hirnforschung, Österreichische Akademie der
Wissenschaften, and Neurologisches Institut, Universität
Vienna, Austria

The following arguments are mainly concerned with estimating and underlining the role of the cerebral cortex in the eruption and maintaining of the epileptic seizure. For years it has been obvious to neurologists that the cortex with its highly complex structure must be the main theater of epileptic activity. However, the great discoveries in the pioneer epoch of the electroencephalogram (EEG) (32) and more advanced techniques of investigating deep brain regions stressed the importance of the large subcortical regions as the center of primary activity. This point of view was supported unequivocally by Penfield and Jasper (36): "The cortex seems to be responding passively to impulses arriving over projection pathways from discharges arising in the higher brain stem." This statement and the ideas previously expressed by Penfield (35) about the convergence of neural activities, the stratum of consciousness, and his coinage of the concept "centrencephalon" propagated the concept—still adhered to by many electroencephalographers—of the cortex as only a kind of passive projection screen for events originally taking place in the upper brainstem. Even when the classic centrencephalic pattern, spike-and-wave, was shown to have a directional spread over the whole cortex instead of occurring simultaneously on all electrodes (39), a type of "hose-pipe" effect from the part of the thalamus was proposed to explain this phenomenon.

More recently, however, the increasing number of studies on the activity of the cortex with multiple electrodes together with greater experience in depth recordings in humans (4, 58) have provided additional evidence for a rather autonomous role of the cortex even in generalized seizures. Together with this new interest in the cortex, the demand for a better understanding of cortical structure has become increasingly urgent.

The studies presented here reflect this shift in interest from the neurophysiological mechanisms in the deep structures to cortical mechanisms

[*] This work was carried out with support from the Fonds zur Förderung der wissenschaftlichen Forschung (No. 770, 1118, 1402). We also wish to thank Mr. A. Kaiser for his technical assistance.

and, finally, to the fine structure of the cortex; i.e., from a discussion of the clinical EEG, to neurophysiological phenomena observed by multiple semimicroelectrodes within the cortex, and, finally, to electron-microscopical findings pertinent to the question of synchronization and the spread of seizures.

DEFINITION OF THE CONCEPT OF SYNCHRONIZATION

One of the greatest difficulties in defining this concept is that those working in different fields have quite different ideas about synchronization. There is general agreement that the EEG phenomena, if they are to be considered as *synchronized,* have to be caused by a summation of some basic processes which, however, are still unknown in almost all their aspects. At the Vienna Symposium (1971), dedicated particularly to this subject, general agreement was attained only insofar as the present term does not reflect well enough the fact that, in synchronized activities, EEG patterns of more-or-less homogeneous shape are observed on extended areas of the cortex. Therefore, the term *synmorphism* was proposed instead. This word could better achieve its purpose since it does not anticipate any statement about time (which is implicit in the word "synchronous"). But even this new word does not account for one inherent attribute that we think is among the most significant, namely, its gradual character. It is obvious that there are different degrees of synchronization between, say, the alpha rhythm and a generalized delta wave pattern.

The term *synchronization* in its strict sense implies that two EEG patterns occur exactly simultaneously over different areas. Nevertheless, the greater part of our work shows that during synchronization just the contrary is happening, since one of its most significant features is that synchronized EEG events show a directional spreading. Actually, it takes some time for another area of the cortex to build up an EEG pattern that is similar to the one recorded in the adjacent region. Therefore, in the following, we use the word "synchronization" merely for those unknown mechanisms that make two EEG patterns look almost alike to two different recording electrodes. This aspect of synchronization was also chosen because it makes the phenomenon measurable and thus quantifiable. Coherence, which represents the normalized cross-power spectrum of two time-series, turned out to be a useful measure of the degree of similarity between such series. Coherence readings range from 0 (no relationship whatsoever) to 1 (identity of the two EEG traces) (7, 8, 59).

In the following, it will also be shown that this way of describing the electrical interconnectivity of different brain areas seems an appropriate method of determining structural differences in the cortex.

OBSERVATIONS ON HUMANS

The reasons why we started studying this phenomenon go back to 1952, when we were puzzled by the fact that unipolar and bipolar recordings, when made simultaneously, did not yield the results expected, as the voltage in the bipolar record only rarely corresponded to the voltage difference of the two unipolar traces. There were also often considerable differences in wave shape between unipolar and bipolar records. These discrepancies were shown to be caused by phase differences which were first demonstrated by a vector technique (38) and later by a toposcopic method (29). It soon became obvious that even the most regular and apparently synchronous electrical event, such as the regular spike-and-wave pattern of children during absences, are composed of potential fields spreading over the scalp at different speeds, the spikes faster than the waves (4–15 vs 2–7 m/second (39).

Among the observations made on this subject only a few are presented here.

Several preferred points of origin were found both for spikes and for waves, particularly at the boundary between frontal and parietal cortex and near both the frontal and the occipital poles. Although spikes and waves are closely time-related, there is no mutual dependence so far as their starting points are concerned: they may start at quite different points. Thus the two phenomena proved to be quite different events. The most frequent points of origin of both spikes and waves as well as their spreading behavior are shown in Figure 1. It was found that the speed of both spikes and waves was different in the frontal and the parietal cortex and that there was no correlation between the direction of spread and the site of maximum voltage observed (which was usually in the frontal region near the vertex). Usually the direction of spread was longitudinal. Since then, some of these findings have been confirmed by Cohn and Leader (10) and by Lehmann (27).

All these observations coincided with the hypothesis, proposed with some hesitation at that time, that the cortex plays a significant role in the phenomenon of synchronization.

In order to strengthen this view, a closer study of the cortical regions concerned was needed. Therefore an attempt was made to compare the EEG findings with data drawn from Economo and Koskinas' (12) work on the structure of the human cortex. A comparison between EEG and anatomical data showed that the region where the most distinct changes of traveling speed occurred and where spikes and waves also started preferentially (35% of the waves and 33% of the spikes) was identical with the place where the two cortical areas that are structurally most dissimilar meet, namely, the sulcus centralis. Moreover, a comparison between the speeds of both the spikes and the waves over the precentral and postcentral cortex, on the one hand, and the cortical structure, on the other, showed no relationship between speeds and the thickness of the single cortical layers, but a distinct inverse relationship emerged between the traveling speed and the cellular density in layer V only. The cellular densities of layer V of the parietal and frontal cortex have a ratio of 1:2.55, whereas

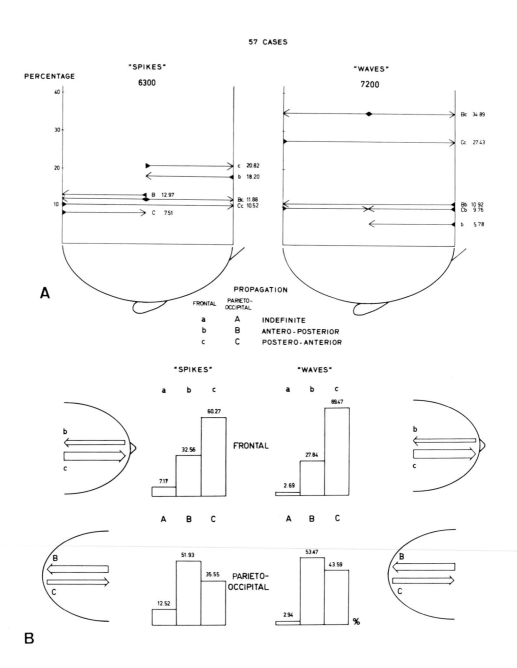

Figure 1. (A) Percentage of points of origin and direction of propagation for spikes and waves of 57 cases of petit mal epilepsy. In each case, one petit mal seizure ("absence") was analyzed. Most of the waves start at the vertex, i.e., the boundary between the frontal and the parietal cortex. (B) Although spikes and waves propagate independently from each other, the preferred direction of propagation is roughly the same on the frontal half (upper part of the diagram) and the parieto-occipital half of the skull (lower part of the diagram). 6300 spikes and 7200 waves were analyzed.

the speeds have a ratio of 2.4:1 on the average. Thus, the more densely the pyramidal cells of layer V are packed, the slower is the propagation of spikes and waves. It seems, therefore, as if the arrangement and the number of cells within the pyramidal layer are closely connected with the phenomenon of spreading, i.e., synchronization, and, furthermore, that synchronization is caused in some way by an activation of one cell by an adjacent one.

Generally, these findings of cortical mechanisms underlying synchronization were supported by observations on other normal and pathological cases, such as in 1 case of a brain tumor (14) and in 2 cases of subacute encephalitis Van Bogaert (43).

In humans, however, it is difficult, often even impossible, to prove the traveling character of brain activity for other than regular and generalized phenomena. One of the main reasons for this is the rich folding of the layer that produces the EEG, namely, the cortex. Furthermore, the overlying tissues and fluids, particularly the cerebrospinal fluid (CSF), help to conceal these phenomena to a large extent in the EEG. Therefore, the following experiments have all been made on the lissencephalic rabbit in which the above findings have been fully confirmed, even for less regular and more localized patterns.

The significance of the point from which a certain wave pattern spreads was not yet defined at the time when the above-mentioned studies were undertaken. Thus, the following experiments concentrated upon determining the origin of the hippocampus theta wave which proved to be the proper model activity for the study of spreading characteristics. Two main findings are to be mentioned from these results. (1) The theta rhythm is triggered by the cellular activity of a zone in the middle of the septum (nucleus of the diagonal band; Figure 2) (17, 46). The rhythmical firing of these cells stimulates the anterior parts of the dorsal hippocampus to produce the theta wave. It was shown that the shape of theta wave is identical with the discharging pattern of the diagonal band cells. Thus, the theta waves seem to be built up by excitatory postsynaptic potentials (EPSPs) elicited by the firing of cells in the diagonal band. The theta waves themselves were shown to spread along the dorsal hippocampus in a rostrocaudal direction with an average speed of 34 cm/second. This spreading seems to be caused by an excitation of functional slices [see Andersen and coworkers (2)] which are arranged perpendicularly to the direction of spread. (2) Moreover, it was shown that a linear relationship exists between theta speed and frequency (45).

Experimental Results on Cortical Synchronization

It was decided to establish first the possible role deep brain structures may play in maintaining synchronized activities. To clarify this problem, a series of isolated hemispheres was studied (44). Several days before the

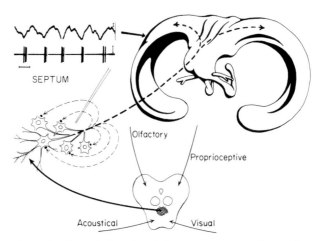

Figure 2. The theta rhythm of the dorsal hippocampus in the rabbit is triggered by cells discharging rhythmically in bursts in the nucleus of the diagonal band in the septum. The burst frequency is proportional to the degree of sensory excitation of the animal. Theta waves start from the most anterior parts of the dorsal hippocampus from whence they propagate symmetrically in a rostrocaudal direction. Time, 100 msec; calibration: 100 μV for the upper trace (hippocampal theta activity), 1 mV for the lower trace (septal burst cells).

experiments proper, the corpus callosum and the capsula interna were separated in rabbits under pentobarbital narcosis. Then, a few days later, toposcopical recordings with multiple surface electrodes were made from these animals. Seizures were elicited with Metrazol and by electrical stimulation. It was found that both the spreading characteristics and the wave patterns did not differ from those recorded before the isolation. The only difference was that very regular patterns, such as spike-and-wave, did occur more often and last longer after isolation than they did before the operation (Figure 3).

These experiments demonstrated that, for synchronization in seizure patterns, obviously the thalamus is not indispensable.

The next step was to find out how the cortex would be able to propagate the complex wave patterns observed in seizures. The toposcopical recording used hitherto proved inadequate to solve this question, and a method of a two-dimensional representation of potential fields was developed (42).

These studies confirmed the results previously obtained with the toposcope and gave more precise results regarding the shape of the potential fields and their transformation when moving. Elementary seizure waves were found to be due to circular potential fields moving in the 10^{-1}-m/second range over the cortex. More complex graphoelements proved to be caused by the superposition of potential fields of different characteristics. The polarity of the field that moves corresponds to the polarity of the more "peaked" phase (the steeper phase of the graphoelement of the EEG). These were in most cases the positive fields (Figure 4). More-

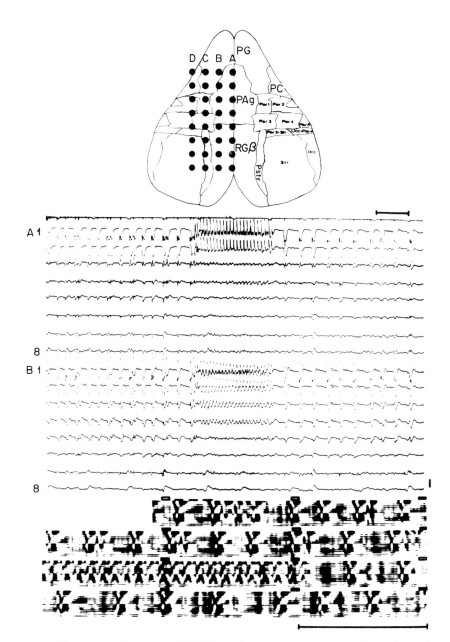

Figure 3. Electroencephalogram (EEG) and topogram of a regular spike-and-wave and polyspike-and-wave activity in neuronally isolated hemispheres. The seizure was elicited by electrical stimulation at B1–B8. Unipolar recordings; the EEG was recorded at 6 cm/second, the respective topogram at 10 cm/second. Time marks in the EEG record and in the topogram are synchronous, to make correlation possible. Spikes and waves are composed of a great variety of potential fields with different localizations and propagation characteristics. PG, Area praecentralis granularis; PC, area postcentalis; PAg, area praecentralis agranularis; Par 1-5, area parietalis 1-5; Str, area striata; **Pstr,** area parastriata; Occ, area occipitalis; RG β, area retrosplenialis granularis β. Calibration 500 μV.

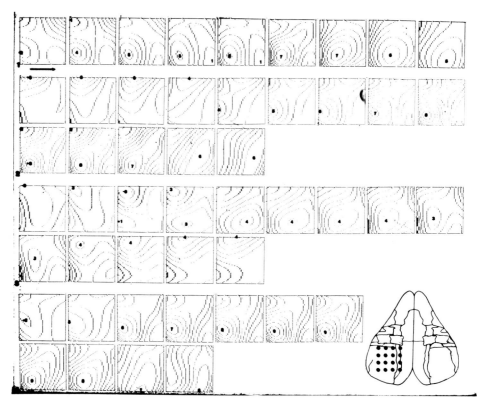

Figure 4. Propagation of seizure waves over the striatal area of rabbits. Four samples were chosen. The equipotential fields were printed every 6 msec. The numbers indicate both the location and the voltage of the field maximum (between two subsequent numbers there is a voltage step of 267 μV). These four seizure waves arise in the lateral parts of the area striata and propagate in a lateromedial or a caudorostral direction. See Fig. 3 legend for key to areas of the topogram.

over, at cytoarchitectonic borderlines, the potential fields became distorted or faded out or elicited other potential fields in contiguous areas.

These experiments confirmed the findings on the closed human skull and supplied more detailed information on traveling wave patterns. The strong influence of cytoarchitectonic boundaries on the traveling characteristics of the potential fields stands out particularly clearly. This fact once more indicates an intricate connection between cortex and wave propagation.

In order to clarify further the relation of cortical structure to the phenomenon of spread, a study by making transverse incisions into the cortex down to the white matter was undertaken (40). By this procedure the blood supply of the cortex was left intact and no edema developed. Sufficiently long incisions that extended as far as the white matter changed homogeneous seizure patterns to heterogeneous ones with regard to both wave shape and frequency and resulted in completely independent patterns on either side of the incision. When such preparations were stimulated electrically or when Metrazol was applied, seizure patterns developed on either or on both parts of the hemisphere divided by the incision. In the latter case, however, the patterns were clearly different in shape and duration. But, even when the frequency patterns seemed identical, the coherences measured simultaneously between adjacent electrodes clearly indicated the presence of two independent patterns.

These results are illustrated in Figure 5A. Unipolar records were taken from electrodes C1–C7 (nose bone as reference). At a higher recording speed of 6 cm/second (Figure 5B), it may be seen with the naked eye that the seizure pattern which was produced by contralateral electrical stimulation is least coherent between electrodes 3 and 4, whereas the other patterns seem more or less alike. The place of least coherence coincides roughly with the boundary between area praecentralis granularis and area

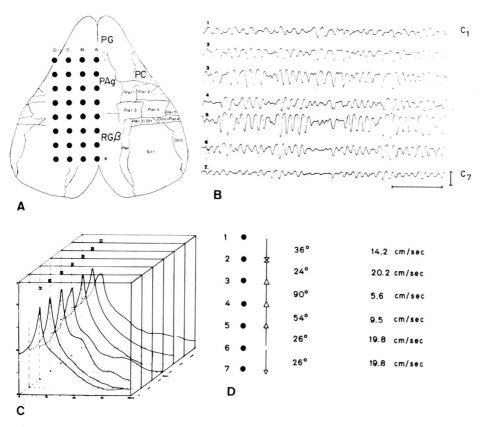

Figure 5. Seizure activity of the intact cortex of the rabbit. (A) Position of electrodes (2 mm distances) on the rabbit's cortex. PG, Area praecentralis granularis; PC, area postcentralis; PAg, area praecentralis agranularis; Par 1-5, area parietalis 1 - 5; Str, area striata; Pstr, area parastriata; Occ, area occipitalis; RG β, area retrosplenialis granularis β. (B) Seizure pattern, produced by contralateral electrical stimulation, recorded unipolarly from electrodes C1–C7. Calibration, 500 μV, 1 second. (C) Power spectra of channels 1–7. (D) Direction of propagation, phase, and average speed of the waves. The differences of wave shape, frequency, and spreading characteristics are thought to depend on structural differences of the cortex.

parietalis according to Rose (49). Figure 5C shows the seven power spectra of the normalized EEG data (recording time, 6 seconds). These spectra were estimated by means of an autoregressive model (between seven and ten regression parameters were sufficient to attain an approximation of more than 99% to the power of the EEG sample). The spectra of these records have almost equal shapes, except that the peaks of several spectra appear somewhat broader, indicating a greater variability of the basic frequency in this channel. This holds particularly true of spectra 1–4. In these records, the lower frequencies are also more pronounced than in the records taken from the posterior regions. This difference is seen in the EEG sample too. We assume that the different speeds of propagation, calculated from the phase differences, are also caused by the structural differences in the cortical areas from which recordings were made.

Figure 5D shows the average phases and spreading directions. Electrode 6 seems a preferred point of origin, whereas at electrode 2 waves seem to arrive from the opposite direction. Coherences of this sample are shown in Figure 7A.) Between electrodes 3 and 4, there is a distinct sink in the main frequency. This region coincides with the transition from A. praecentralis granularis to A. parietalis and is also characterized by a delay of the waves (the average propagation speed slows down to 5.6 cm/second).

Figure 6 shows the results after a vertical incision into the cortex. The length of the incision is indicated in Figure 6A. The flattening of record 5 (Figure 6B) is obviously caused by the incision. But in front of and behind the incision the activities seem to be alike—even their power spectra do not reveal any considerable differences. The spreading pattern, however (Figure 6D), has changed: all activity now seems to propagate toward the lesion and none originates at the lesion. These events are not unexpected because, as a result of the lesion, some cortical activities that are needed as a functional pacemaker seem to be discontinued.

The effect of the lesion is best seen when coherences are compared (Figure 7A and B) before and after the incision. The differences in coherence, which we believe are caused by differences in cortical structure (Figure 7A), are indicated by a more-or-less deep sink at the main frequency. In contrast, after the incision there is only a small peak visible where the main frequency crosses the incision (probably by volume conduction). This coherence of 53% between electrodes 4 and 5 and 63% between electrodes 5 and 6 decreases to 16% when the coherence between records 4 and 6 is calculated.

This was a consistent finding in preparations in which the incisions were long enough to prevent interaction between the events in front of and behind the incision around the ends of the incision. In cases with shorter incisions (about 10 mm and not reaching down to the deep extension of the retrosplenial cortex near the midline), coherent activities in the two separated areas alternated with activities showing no coherence in an un-

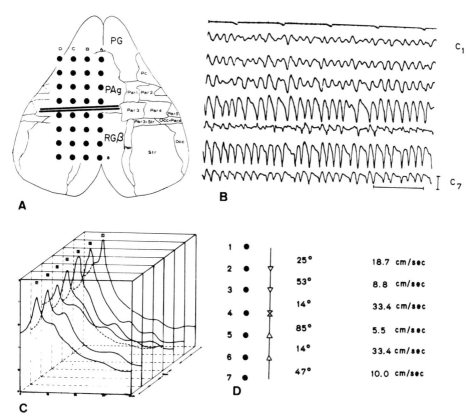

Figure 6. Seizure activity in rabbit cortex after vertical incision between electrode rows 4 and 5. (A) Position of electrodes (2 mm distances); the two parallel lines show the vertical incision. PG, Area praecentralis granularis; PC, area postcentralis; PAg, area praecentralis agranularis; Par 1-5, area parietalis 1 - 5; Str, area striata; Pstr, area parastriata; Occ, area occipitalis; RG β, area retrosplenialis granularis β. (B) Seizure pattern, produced by contralateral stimulation, recorded unipolarly from electrodes C1–C7. Calibration: 500 μV, 1 second. (C) Power spectra of channels 1–7. (D) Direction of propagation, phase, and average speed of the waves.

predictable way that needs further investigation. This observation shows that during the same seizure the degree of interconnectivity and, therefore, of synchronization between two areas may permanently change and, seems to be composed of a great many different events.

Other observations, such as the apparently non-Gaussian character of the seizure patterns recorded from the surface of the brain, and the fact that the deepest cortical layers seem to be indispensable for propagation of seizure activities, and, finally, the differences depending on cortical structure, called for an expansion of these studies in the third dimension of the cortex, its depth. This was performed by using four multiple microelectrodes which were inserted through 0.5-mm steel metal tubes resting on the cortical surface at a distance of 2 mm. Under microscopical control, both the

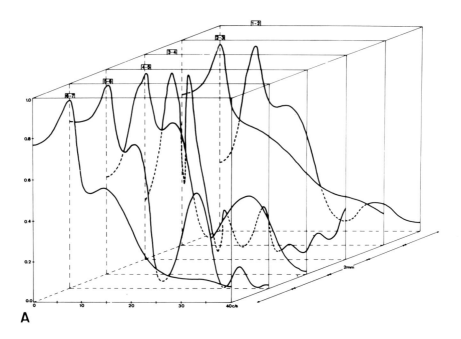

A

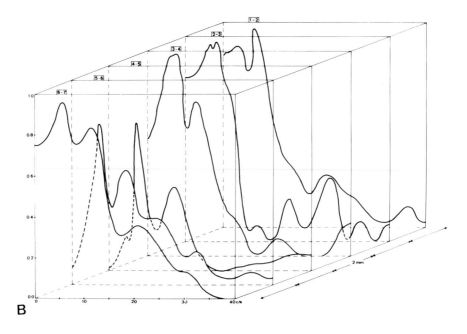

B

Figure 7. (A) Coherences between two adjacent records of the electroencephalogram sample of Figure 5 before the incision. (B) Same measurements as in A after a vertical incision, as shown in Figure 6. The incision results in a decrease of the coherence between channels 4 and 5 and 5 and 6.

steel tubes and the tips of the respective microelectrodes were arranged separately by independent microdrives so as to touch the cortex. Next, the microelectrodes were simultaneously lowered by a microdrive. By this device it was possible to study the events recorded from an equidistant row of microelectrodes in different cortical layers and to compare them with the corresponding epicortical electrodes.

Amplitude Histograms with Depth

The first studies using probability density function (pdf) were mainly concerned with the question whether or not the EEG is Gaussian. If only epicortical activities are studied, and particularly the human EEG, the pdf shows a nearly Gaussian distribution. This, however, is not true of seizure activities, particularly when recorded from intracortical levels, as shown in Figure 8.

Amplitude histograms of tape-recorded normal EEGs and seizure patterns of 30 second duration have been made by the analogue-to-digital converter of the CAT 1000 (Computer of Average Transients, Technical Measurement Corporation, New Haven, Connecticut) at steps of 200 μm. First the activity of the unanesthetized, artificially respirated animal was recorded throughout all levels of the cortex. This activity is the same as in rabbits without artificial respiration and consists mainly of periods of spindle activity alternating with irregular slow waves of less than 500 μV amplitude. Next, Metrazol was injected intravenously (20 mg/kg). A depth profile of the intracortical–epicortical voltage ratios is shown for both spontaneous and seizure activity, in two cortical regions, 4 mm apart, the parietal region (Figure 8A) and the striata (Figure 8B). At both sites the activity in the deep cortical areas is characterized by its voltage attaining several times the reading of the EEG voltage when measured epicortically. Usually, there is a rather steep rise in voltage ratios starting in layer IV.

In contrast to these findings, spontaneous activity does not show this phenomenon. There is only a slight rise in amplitude with increasing depth, but nowhere was there any hint that, for normal activity, the deep pyramidal layer has a role similar to the one it seems to play in seizures.

The two dashed lines of Figure 8 indicate the difference of the skewness of the epicortical and intracortical histograms. These curves demonstrate that, on both areas, skewness has an opposite polarity in superficial and deep layers, with a crossing over at 500 μm in the striata and at 600 μm parietally. To some extent, this change from positive (when recorded from more superficial levels) to negative skewness (when recorded from deeper layers) reflects the phase reversal found in wave patterns at about layers II–III. In contrast to this finding, spontaneous activity shows neither a phase reversal with depth nor a crossing over in its difference of skewness.

The histograms of both normal and seizure patterns are also presented for several intracortical levels in Figure 8. The large deviation from a Gaus-

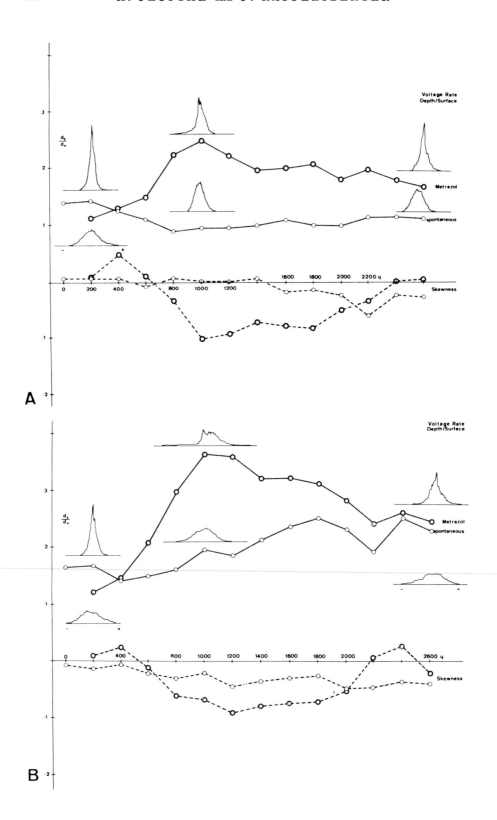

sian distribution in seizures is a consistent finding, as is the almost Gaussian distribution for normal activities.

These differences may also be explained in terms of the concept of synchronization. During seizures, the cortex seems to be involved throughout its whole vertical extent in producing only a few kinds of patterns among which the most prominent and probably also functionally most significant seems to be slow rhythmic waves which may act as a functional link throughout all layers. These slow waves may be caused by an alternating polarization of the basal and the most apical dendritic arborizations of the pyramidal cells of layer V. This pattern is superimposed, at different levels, by smaller, faster events (local spikes), the existence of which is obviously due to tiny generators, namely, different nerve cells at different layers. In normal activity, only these tiny generators seem to be active, without a generalizing factor being present and conducting the activity throughout the cortex. This kind of activity has a much lower degree of synchronization; the amplitude histograms, therefore, correspond much more to the case of noise passed through a filter and the many tiny uncorrelated generators may be considered to be the source of this noise.

Figure 8 demonstrates another consistent finding: the maximum amplitude coincides with layer V of deep pyramidal cells; the zone of phase reversals, on the other hand, is usually found within layers II and III which, however, according to Rose (49) cannot be clearly distinguished in these regions. This observation demonstrates once more that layer V is intimately connected to the generation of seizure activity, a finding first proposed by Adrian (1).

It should be mentioned, however, that these results concerning voltage are true of the lower frequencies of the seizure only. The higher frequencies (spikes, e.g., those produced by penicillin) follow other laws and are to be dealt with later on.

Shape of Seizure Waves Recorded Intracortically

Apart from the above-mentioned differences in voltage, there are a few more distinct features by which intracortical activities are characterized. One general experience when recording from the deeper parts of the cortex is the low degree of volume conduction, so that in some cases voltage gradi-

---

Figure 8. Amplitude histograms from electroencephalogram samples of 30 second duration, recorded simultaneously epi- and intracortically at steps of 200 μm. dt/do, Ratio between interpercentile ranges $X_{.95}$ to $X_{.05}$ of amplitude histograms of intracortical and epicortical activities. (A) Parietal area; (B) striatal area. Spontaneous activity has a less steep voltage rise with depth than seizure activity (Metrazol). The histograms of spontaneous activity are more likely to represent a Gaussian distribution than the histograms of seizure activity. This is also visible in the difference of skewnesses (skewness of epicortical histogram minus skewness of intracortical histogram which is, in spontaneous activity, closer to zero than it is in seizure activity.

ents up to 10 mV/mm are found in the vertical direction. In the horizontal direction the reading is somewhat less, but there is a significant difference between more superficial and deeper layers: within the latter, steeper horizontal voltage gradients are found than on the surface (4 mV/mm vs 2 mV/mm) (41). This observation seems to indicate that at more superficial levels the excitation is more inclined to disperse than in deeper layers of the cortex where it seems to be more confined. Several further observations contribute to this assumption, such as the general finding that in intracortical recordings below a certain depth the amount of higher frequencies is usually larger than in epicortical recordings. This is clearly seen in a comparison between the power spectra and coherences of two simultaneous intracortical recordings (at 1600 μm) and the two corresponding surface recordings (Figure 9A and B). For the power spectra (Figure 9A, the four diagrams at the corners of the square) the readings are considerably higher in deep cortical layers than at the surface, and the higher-frequency components are more pronounced in the deep recordings. The difference in the mutual interconnectivity (which was previously assumed from observations on the voltage gradients), appears very clearly in the coherence measurements: coherence is high between the two surface electrodes (90%), less between the two deep electrodes (36%), and least between surface and depth recordings (24 and 11%).

Figure 9B presents, for the same sample, the phase diagrams. For both surface and depth electrodes, there is a linear relationship between phase and frequency, indicating that the envelope of the group of waves of this frequency band travels with constant speed. Usually, from the existence of group velocity, a propagation of energy can be concluded. Therefore, the cortex may be compared with a delay-line. The same conclusions were drawn by Peronnet and co-workers (37) in their studies on spontaneous cortical activity in humans.

However, the phase diagram between surface and depth electrodes presents an almost horizontal line at the main frequency range. The phase readings of 108° and 126°, respectively, demonstrate a vertical spreading of these higher-frequency components (spikes) originating in deep cortical regions. The spreading velocities calculated from these readings (5.8 cm/second for the propagation between electrodes 11–1 and 5.6 cm/second for propagation between electrodes 12–2) confirm our observations on the intracortical vertical spreading rates of penicillin spikes.

The general finding that the shape of the potential shows less variation when recorded from the surface than when recorded from deep regions, together with the above-mentioned observations of steep horizontal potential gradients in the deep cortical layers, lead one to assume that the more superficial cortical layers act as a kind of a low-pass filter for the activities of deeper layers.

Before trying to summarize these findings into a hypothesis, several more findings concerning the spikes, that is, the faster components of a seizure, are described.

These spikes were studied on spike-and-wave patterns elicited by contralateral electrical stimulation, Metrazol seizure activities, and penicillin foci (41). Two samples are used for illustration. One is a regular spike-and-wave activity which, for this rabbit, was its consistent form of afterdischarge upon electrical stimulation of the contralateral cortex (Figure 10). This pattern was studied throughout all cortical layers of the striata. The wave remained roughly in-phase with respect to surface down to a depth of about 1100 μm, and from then on it reversed its phase. But the spike behaved in a quite different way: starting from the surface and proceeding toward deeper layers, it seemed to climb further and further up to the crest of the wave and, thus, to be more and more phase-shifted with respect to the surface spike. At a depth of 1100 μm the spike voltage reached a maximum. The waves may be presented by a vertical dipole with an electric zero zone in between, whereas the spikes propagate in a vertical direction to the cortex surface, in this case at 5 cm/second.

The same is true of penicillin spikes which offer, by their fairly constant shape, the best and most constant conditions for investigating this spreading. They too were found to attain their maximum voltage in the deep pyramidal layer (up to 7 mV) where they originate and are propagated with a speed in the centimeter per second range up to the cortical surface (41). This propagation may be explained by an active conduction along dendrites, as was proposed by Green and Petsche (19) for hippocampal seizures ("pips") and confirmed by Purpura and co-workers (48). The above-mentioned findings—the filter effect of the more superficial layers and the relatively high degree of independence (in spite of synchronization) of different electrodes—are particularly evident in penicillin spikes, as shown in Figure 11. The figure presents nine subsequent spikes, recorded from the surface (first trace), and from three microelectrodes at a depth of 1000 μm. Trace 3 is from the microelectrode corresponding to the surface recording, trace 1 from the one 2 mm rostrad, and trace 4 from the one 2 mm caudad. The potentials are extended in length in order to show variations in shape more clearly; the exact time relationship is maintained between surface and depth.

Figure 11 clearly demonstrates that the shape of penicillin spikes remains almost the same at the surface, but it changes with depth. Also, with depth, multiple spikes may occur, whereas on the surface only single spikes are recorded. Moreover (not to be seen in this figure), the time relationship between the different spikes in the depth electrodes changes to a high degree, whereas the surface spike seems to present a more-or-less average activity. All these findings gave rise to the concept of a columnar structure of the cortex, beginning at a depth of about 400 to 500 μm. This columnar structure causes a partial isolation of the electrical events in the deeper

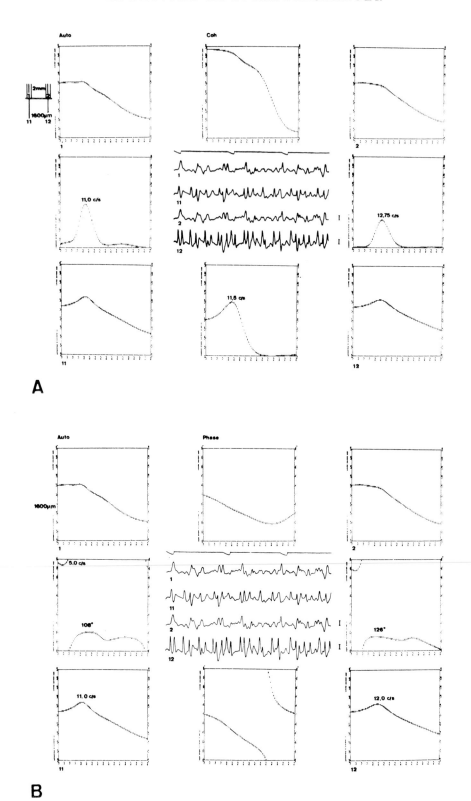

A

B

layers of the cortex. The vertical spreading of several fast electrophysiological events, such as penicillin spikes, suggest the possibility of a system of vertical channels in the cortex.

ANATOMICAL FINDINGS SUPPORTING COLUMNAR ORGANIZATION OF THE CORTEX

It has been known for a long time that in myelin stainings of the cortex, a radial structure may be seen reaching from the white matter far up into the gray matter. This structure was dealt with in a careful monograph by Kaes (24) in 1907. Kaes studied the architectonic differences of the myelin radiation but was unable to present any explanation of its functional significance. One of the first who claimed that the functional units of cortical circuitry must be vertical ranges of nerve cells was Lorente de Nó (28), who postulated such columns extending between layers II and VI. Because of the accumulation of evidence on the part of neurophysiologists (23, 33), recently the question of columns was investigated anew by several authors. Colonnier (11), however, did not arrive at unequivocal results as to the morphological substrate of columns. The same is true of Szentágothai (55) who contributed some evidence for a functional organization in columns by his findings of a limited range of collaterals and of axon endings of the Golgi Type II neurons connected to a pyramidal cell. Von Bonin and Mehler (6) again studied this question on Golgi material but recognized a columnar cellular structure only in the cortex of humans and higher vertebrates, denying such a structure in rabbits and, therefore, not conferring on it a possible physiological role.

One of the few uncontested demonstrations of a discontinuous organization of a cortical area was given by Woolsey and van der Loos (61) who found, on tangential sections through area S1 in layer IV of the parietal cortex of the mouse, structures which they called "barrels." These barrels have diameters of between 100 and 400 μm and seem to be composed of a ring of nerve cells encircling a central region more or less void of cells. A layer with few cells surrounds each of these rings. In region S1, about 200 of such barrels are found. According to the experiments of Welker (60) with cluster microelectrodes, each of these barrels seems to be coordinated to one vibrissa.

Based on our neurophysiological findings and the resultant hypothesis of a columnar structure, Fleischhauer and co-workers (13) studied the cor-

Figure 9. (A) Autospectra and coherences between respective surface and intracortical electrodes (1600 μm). Metrazol seizures. Coherence is largest between the surface electrodes, less between the intracortical recordings, and least between surface and intracortical recordings. (B) Phase diagrams of same sample as in A. The linear intracortical records indicate the presence of a pattern propagating with constant group velocity. The relatively large phase shift between surface and intracortical electrodes at the frequency of the spikes, as seen in the electroencephalogram, are caused by the vertical propagation of the spikes.

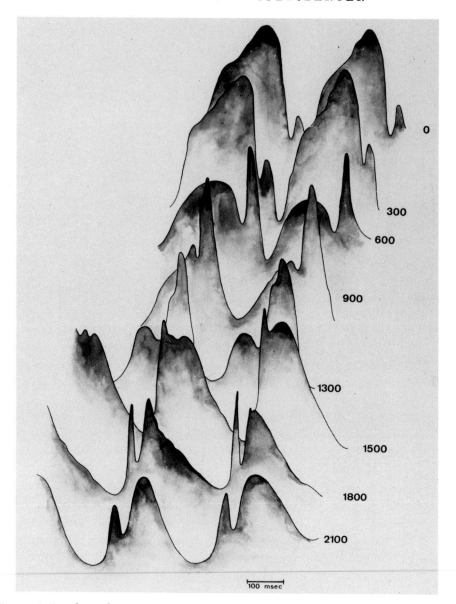

Figure 10. Regular spike-and-wave activity, elicited by contralateral electrical stimulation and recorded at steps of 300 μm (0 = surface). The spike-and-wave complexes are arranged so as to be in correct time relation with the pattern recorded at the surface. The spike seems to climb further and further up the crest of the wave the deeper the recorded layer. Between 900 and 1500 μm, the phase of the wave reverses. The spikes are propagated from deep pyramidal layers toward the cortical surface, whereas the pattern of the waves supports the concept of a vertical intracortical dipole.

tical areas from which these results were obtained. By using a special staining process (Luxol-fast-blue followed by Goldner's trichrome, or by periodic acid-Schiff test and counterstaining with hematoxylin) and carefully choosing the direction of cutting and the thickness of the slices, these au-

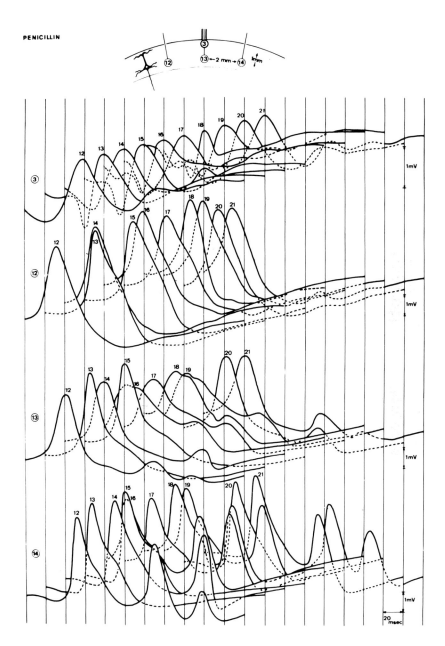

Figure 11. Penicillin spikes recorded from the surface (electrode 3) and from three intracortical electrodes (12, 13, and 14) at a depth of 1000 μm. Nine subsequent surface spikes and their respective intracortical discharges are arranged at equal intervals. The spikes when recorded intracortically are a high voltage and show a great variability in both voltage and shape. Moreover, the frequency of multiple spikes is high intracortically and the time relationships between the intracortical spikes change to a high degree. The surface spikes, therefore, seem to present more-or-less averaged activities.

thors found that all apical dendrites of the pyramids of layer V, instead of being randomly distributed as in nerve cells, form bundles consisting of up to more than ten main dendrites (Figure 12). This distances between these bundles are 40–50 μm. The picture changes at the border between layers IV and III where the dendrites begin bifurcating and splitting up in order to form the feltwork of the upper cortical layers. A comparison of frontal with tangential sections (Figure 12b) and of serial sections reveals that within a given vertical bundle the individual dendrites are constantly changing position with respect to each other.

In electron micrographs, the dendrites of a bundle are seen to be separated by numerous very small profiles and small myelinated fibers. The

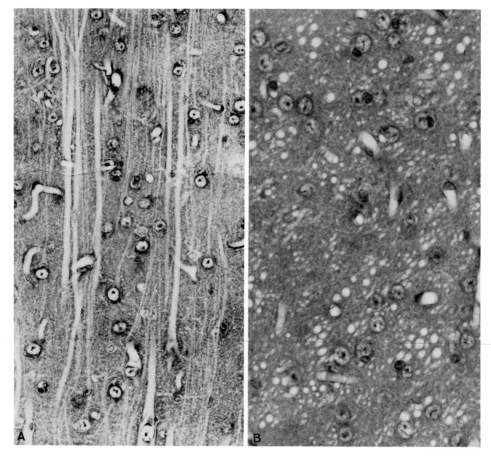

Figure 12. (A) Frontal section through layers II–IV of the parietal cortex of the rabbit. (Stains: Kluver; periodic acid-Schiff; hematoxylin. Magnification: ×335). The large apical dendrites of several pyramidal cells approach each other and continue side by side until they bifurcate in layer III or II and form bundles. (B) Horizontal section through layer IV of the same object (Magnification: ×245). The apical dendrites are arranged in groups with distances of about 40 to 50 μm in between. (By kind permission of Professor K. Fleischhauer, Anatomical Institute of the University, Bonn, West Germany.)

bundle shown in Figure 13 shows also dendrites in such close contact that for a great part of their circumference the two plasma membranes are separated only by the extracellular space. In subsequent sections of the same bundle, the cross sections of two dendrites are seen to approach in this way and to separate several times so as to form several close appositions. Between these dendrites in close apposition, special membrane structures such as dendrodendritic synapses or tight junctions (52) have not been observed, but further and more detailed electron-microscopic studies are being performed. Nevertheless, at some places, the membranes of adjacent dendrites were characterized by a multitude of mitochondria. A schematic drawing of the structure and interlacing of the dendrites of two bundles is shown in Figure 14.

In this context it seems worthwhile to consider the possible functional meaning of such close appositions of dendrites. Since 1937 it has been demonstrated several times that the large dendrites of motoneurons are arranged in bundles (26). The Scheibels (50) studied Golgi material from mature cats and monkeys and found that the majority of the motoneuron dendrites are on the rostrocaudal axis, organized in densely packed bundles. Each bundle was shown to be composed of dendrites from neurons of different motor cell columns, representing different functional groups, and also from propriospinal neurons.

An electron-microscopical study of these bundles of dendrites in the spinal cord of cats was published by Matthews and co-workers (31). These authors describe findings similar to the ones by Fleischhauer and others (13). The bundles consist of five to twenty closely packed dendrites and vary between 20 and 60 μm. The length of a bundle varies from a hundred to several hundred micrometers. The population of dendrites within a bundle changes as individual dendrites are added or subtracted. As in the cortex, the spinal cord dendrites are also partly separated by thin astrocyte processes, partly in direct apposition without any specialization of the adjacent plasma membranes. In a few cases, however, these authors found that the gap of 180 Å between two adjacent dendrites contained small amounts of flocculent, electron-dense material. Such material also occurs along the cytoplasm of the apposing membranes. In one of these junctional complexes, several mitochondria were found.

Stensaas and Stensaas (53) made the same observation on dendrites of frog motoneurons and found that some 15% of the dendritic surface area is involved in this apposition.

Matthews and co-workers (31) conclude from these findings that these narrow contacts between dendrites probably play some role in the synchronization of motoneurons by altering the threshold in adjacent dendrites during excitation. A similar assumption is suggested by the Scheibels (50), who believe that these bundles, utilizing both synaptic and extrasynaptic mechanisms, constitute subcenters for the integration of motor output.

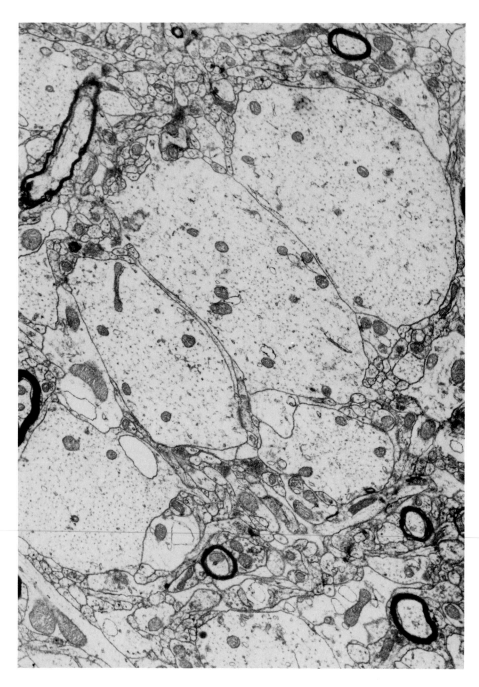

Figure 13. Electron micrograph of a dendrite bundle (horizontal section). The cross sections of two dendrites contact for a great part of their circumference at several times so that the two plasma membranes are separated only by the extracellular space. Magnification: ×14,025. (By kind permission of Professor K. Fleischhauer, Anatomical Institute of the University, Bonn, West Germany.)

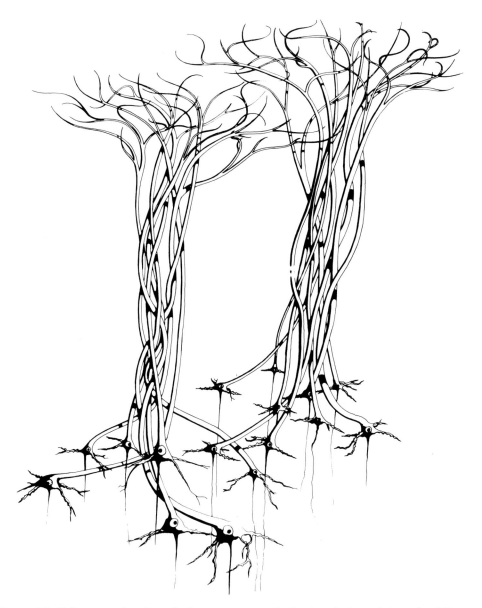

Figure 14. Schematic drawing of the structure and the interlacing of two dendrite bundles.

In this context it is wise to remember the experimental findings on direct electrical interactions between nerve cells in teleost spinal neurons (5), in the crayfish (15), in Mauthner cells of the goldfish (16), in the leech ganglion (21), in the lobster cardiac ganglion (22), in the ciliary ganglion of the chick (30), and in the frog spinal cord (20). But even without any particularly organized membrane structure, interaction between peripheral nerves has been demonstrated experimentally (3, 18, 25, 51, 54). Terzuolo and Bullock (56) demonstrated that extracellular voltage gradients of only 1 mV/mm were able to modify firing rates in the stretch receptor neurons of the crayfish. Nelson (34) demonstrated in threshold studied on the spinal cord that a synchronous antidromic activation of many adjacent motoneurons results in a short-latency facilitation of the single motoneuron that was being studied, the facilitation resulting in a lowering of threshold by as much as 30%. Because of this short latency, field effects, but not recurrent collaterals, can be implicated.

According to these studies and the analogous anatomical findings in the cortex, the possibility of an electrotonic transfer of excitation and inhibition in the cortex has to be also considered. The existence of this mechanism for spreading would have extensive implications, because an electrotonic synapse differs basically in two ways from a chemical reaction of the transmitters: (1) a transfer in both ways is possible and (2) steady oscillations of current may also be transferred, whereas, on the common synapses, only an all-or-none-transfer is possible.

Both the anatomical findings on the cortex and the observations of the relatively high gradients of the field potentials observed in seizures suggest the possibility of a nonsynaptic transfer of both excitation and inhibition in the cortex, at least so far as spreading of epileptic events is concerned.

PROPAGATION OF SEIZURE WAVES IN THE CORTEX: SYNCHRONIZATION

At the center of the functional columns postulated by the neurophysiological findings is a dendritic bundle that arborizes in the upperst two cortical lamina. Up to more than ten pyramidal cells may act together to form such a bundle. Its single shafts are thought to be in electrical interaction depending on the degree of excitation. Each pyramidal cell is connected, by recurrent collaterals, to several Golgi Type II neurons the function of which is most probably inhibitory (55). According to Szentágothai, the zone of collateral inhibition extends to about 0.5 mm. Nothing is known so far about the effects of these bundles in normal activity. In seizure activity, however, they seem to be excited to act as discharging units. This is suggested by our findings on penicillin spikes propagating in a vertical direction, is further supported by the findings of Green and Petsche (19) in hippocampal seizures and by Purpura and co-workers (48) who demonstrated that, under certain conditions of high excitation, the apical dendrites behave like axons in propagating spikes. It is expected that in the case of a synchronized discharge within a bundle of dendrites, the inhibitory effect of the surrounding Golgi Type II cells is also maximal. This potent inhibitory effect was shown by Prince and Wilder (47) who found a distinct "surround" inhibition extending as far as 8 mm from the center of the penicillin focus. This surround inhibition involved all cortical levels similarly: in this zone, inhibitory postsynaptic potentials (IPSPs) were found in 88% of the cells, whereas depolarization shifts (DS) were found in only

12%; but, within the focus, DS were found in 76% of the cells and IPSPs in only 24% of the cells. As soon as this surround inhibition breaks down and the seizure develops, the greater part of the cells change from producing IPSPs to DS.

According to the above-mentioned experiments with vertical incisions into the cortex, the deepest layers seem to play the most significant role in the propagation of seizure patterns. This is quite in accordance with the experiments of Burns (9) and also with Adrian's (1) concept about the propagation of the "deep response." He observed propagation without decrement and attributed this to "elements the active region of which is situated somewhat under the surface, their inactive one being situated near the surface." Spread, in the case of self-sustained after-discharges, was inferred by Adrian to occur at a level corresponding to the layer of basal pyramidal dendrites. Also Burns (9) speaks of "deep cells" that appear to form an "infinitive network beneath, and parallel to the cortical surface." A possible anatomical substratum for the spreading of excitation maintaining seizure activity is the dense horizontal fiber plexus of the pyramidal cells of layer VI, described by Tömböl (57) from Golgi studies of the sensorimotor cortex in the rabbit. There is another dense fiber plexus in layer I, and Tömböl discusses the probable significance of this and the strong vertical connections between these two plexuses with respect to synchronization. According to our findings with vertical incisions, however, the plexus of layer I does not seem to have any great significance for synchronization.

If conclusions drawn from neurophysiological findings in the spinal cord may be transferred to the cortex where the same dendritic structures are present, a transfer of excitation not only occurs at synapses via the layer VI, horizontal axonal plexus, but may also take place by electric excitation via the apical dendrites within the bundles—if one pyramidal cell, belonging to the same dendritic bundle discharges, then the probability increases that the other cells in the group will also be brought into firing (via dendrites). Moreover, if a bundle, consisting of dendrites of up to more than ten large pyramidal cells, discharges as a whole, there is a strong probability that several adjacent cells, even if they send their apical dendrites to other bundles, are also driven to discharge, either via recurrent collaterals or via the closely intermingled dendritic arborization in the uppermost layers. In this way, the range of excitation becomes larger and larger and the seizure spreads.

There are several observations, however, that deserve further consideration, e.g., that spikes also propagate in a vertical direction; that several types of seizure patterns may occur superposed without influencing one another; that seizure patterns may occur in certain cortical layers only; and, finally, that an inverse relationship seems to exist between wave duration and speed of propagation, thus indicating a basic role of potential gradients for spreading. It is to be hoped that on the basis of the above hypothetical concepts, these phenomena may also be explained in the future.

REFERENCES

1. Adrian, E. D., The spread of activity in the cerebral cortex. *J. Physiol.* (*Lon.*), 1936, **88**: 127–161.
2. Andersen, P., Bliss, T. V. P., and Skrede, K. K., Lamellar organization of hippocampal excitatory pathways. *Exp. Brain Res.*, 1971, **13**: 222–238.
3. Arvanitaki, A., Effects evoked on an axon by the activity of a contiguous one. *J. Neurophysiol.*, 1942, **5**: 89–108.
4. Bancaud, J., Physiopathogenesis of generalized epilepsies of organic nature (stereoencephalographic study). In: *The Physiopathogenesis of the Epilepsies* (H. Gastaut *et al.*, Eds.). Thomas, Springfield, Illinois, 1969: 158–185.
5. Bennett, M. V. L., Aljure, E., Nakajima, Y., and Pappas, G. D., Electronic junctions between teleost spinal neurons: Electrophysiology and ultrastructure. *Science*, 1963, **141**: 262–264.
6. Bonin, G. von, and Mehler, W. R., On columnar arrangement of nerve cells in cerebral cortex. *Brain Res.*, 1971, **27**: 1–9.
7. Brazier, M. A. B., Electrical activity recorded simultaneously from the scalp and deep structures of the human brain. A computer study of their relationships. *J. Nerv. Ment. Dis.*, 1968, **147**: 31–39.
8. Brazier, M. A. B., Interactions of deep structures during seizures in man. In: *Synchronization of EEG Activity in Epilepsies* (H. Petsche and M. A. B. Brazier, Eds.). Springer-Verlag, Berlin and New York, 1972: 409–427.
9. Burns, B. D., *The Mammalian Cortex*. Arnold, London, 1950.
10. Cohn, R., and Leader, H. S., Synchronization characteristics of paroxysmal EEG activity. *Electroenceph. clin. Neurophysiol.*, 1967, **22**: 421–428.
11. Colonnier, M. L., The structural design of the neocortex. In: *Brain and Conscious Experience* (J. C. Eccles, ed.). Springer-Verlag, Berlin and New York, 1966: 1–23.
12. Economo, C. V., and Koskinas, G. N., *Die Cytoarchitektonik der Hirnrinde des erwachsenen Menschen*. Springer-Verlag, Berlin and New York, 1925.
13. Fleischhauer, K., Petsche, H., and Wittkowski, W., Vertical bundles of dendrites in the neocortex. *Z. Anat. Entwicklungsgesch.*, 1972, **136**: 213–223.
14. Foitl, G., and Petsche, H., Das Verhalten der biolelektrischen Felder an einem Fall von Hirntumor. *Arch. Psychiatr. Nervenkr.*, 1959, **200**: 36–51.
15. Furshpan, E. J., and Potter, D. D., Transmission at the giant motor synapses of the crayfish. *J. Physiol.* (*Lon.*), 1959, **145**: 289–325.
16. Furukawa, T., and Furshpan, E. J., Two inhibitory mechanisms in the Mauthner neurons of goldfish. *J. Neurophysiol.*, 1963, **26**: 140–176.
17. Gogolák, G., Stumpf, C., Petsche, H., and Sterc, J., The firing pattern of septal neurons and the form of the hippocampal theta wave. *Brain Res.*, 1968, **7**: 201–207.

18. Granit, R., and Skoglund, C. R., Facilitation, inhibition and depression at the "artificial synapse" formed by the cut end of a mammalian nerve. *J. Physiol. (Lon.)*, 1945, **103**: 435–448.

19. Green, J. D., and Petsche, H., Hippocampal electrical activity. IV. Unitary events and genesis of hippocampal seizures. *Electroenceph. clin. Neurophysiol.*, 1961, **13**: 868–879.

20. Grinnel, A. D., A study of the interaction between motoneurons in the frog spinal cord. *J. Physiol. (Lon.)*, 1966, **182**: 612–648.

21. Hagiwara, S., and Morita, H., Electrotonic transmission between two nerve cells in the leech ganglion. *J. Neurophysiol.*, 1962, **25**: 721–731.

22. Hagiwara, S., Watanabe, A., and Sato, N., Potential changes in syncytial neurons of lobster cardiac ganglion. *J. Neurophysiol.*, 1959, **22**: 554–572.

23. Hubel, D. H., and Wiesel, T. N., Receptive fields, binocular interaction and functional architecture in the cat's visual cortex. *J. Physiol. (Lon.)*, 1962, **160**: 106–154.

24. Kaes, T., *Die Grosshirnrinde des Menschen in ihren Massen und in ihrem Fasergehalt*. Fischer, Jena, 1907.

25. Katz, B., and Schmitt, O. H., A note on interaction between nerve fibres. *J. Physiol. (Lon.)*, 1942, **100**: 369–371.

26. Laruelie, L., La structure de la moelle épinière en coupes longitudinales. *Rev. Neurol. (Paris)*, 1937, **67**: 695–725.

27. Lehmann, D., Human scalp EEG fields: Evoked, alpha, sleep, and spike-wave patterns. In: *Synchronization of EEG Activity in Epilepsies* (H. Petsche and M. A. B. Brazier, eds.). Springer-Verlag, Berlin and New York, 1972: 307–326.

28. Lorente de Nó, R., Architectonics and structure of the cerebral cortex. In: *Physiology of the Nervous System* (J. F. Fulton, ed.). Oxford Univ. Press, London and New York, 1938: 288–330.

29. Marko, A., and Petsche, H., The multivibrator-toposcope, an electronic multiple recorder. *Electroenceph. clin. Neurophysiol.*, 1960, **12**: 209–211.

30. Martin, A. R., and Pilar, G., Transmission through the ciliary ganglion of the chick. *J. Physiol. (Lon.)*, 1963, **168**: 464–475.

31. Matthews, M. A., Willis, W. D., and Williams, V., Dendrite bundles in lamina IX of cat spinal cord: A possible source for electrical interaction between motoneurons? *Anat. Rec.*, 1972, **171**: 313–328.

32. Moruzzi, G., and Magoun, H. W., Brain stem reticular formation and activation of the EEG. *Electroenceph. clin. Neurophysiol.*, 1949, **1**: 455–473.

33. Mountcastle, V. B., Modality and topographic properties of single neurons of cat's somatic sensory cortex. *J. Neurophysiol.*, 1957, **20**: 408–434.

34. Nelson, P. G., Interaction between spinal motoneurons of the cat. *J. Neurophysiol.*, 1966, **29**: 275–287.

35. Penfield, W., The cerebral cortex and consciousness. *Arch. Neurol. Psychiatry* 1938, **40**: 417–442.

36. Penfield, W., and Jasper, H. H., *Epilepsy and the Functional Anatomy of the Human Brain*. Little, Brown, Boston, 1954.

37. Peronnet, F., Sindou, M., Laviron, A., Quoex, F., and Gerin, P., Human cortical electrogenesis: Stratigraphy and spectral analysis. In: *Synchroni-*

zation of EEG Activities in Epilepsies (H. Petsche and M. A. B. Brazier, eds.). Springer-Verlag, Berlin and New York, 1972: 235–262.

38. Petsche, H., Das Vektor-EEG. Wien. Z. Nervenheilkd., 1952, **5**: 304–320.

39. Petsche, H., Pathophysiologie und Klinik des Petit Mal. Toposkopische Untersuchungen zur Phänomenologie des Spike-Wave-Musters. Wien. Z. Nervenheilkd., 1962, **19**: 345–442.

40. Petsche, H., and Rappelsberger, P., Influence of cortical incisions on synchronization pattern and travelling waves. Electroenceph. clin. Neurophysiol., 1970, **28**: 592–600.

41. Petsche, H., Rappelsberger, P., and Frey, Zs., Intracortical aspects of the synchronization of self-sustained bioelectrical activities. In: Synchronization of EEG Activities in Epilepsies (H. Petsche and M. A. B. Brazier, Eds.). Springer-Verlag, Berlin and New York, 1972: 263–284.

42. Petsche, H., Rappelsberger, P., and Trappl, R., Properties of cortical seizure potential fields. Electroenceph. clin. Neurophysiol., 1970, **29**: 567–578.

43. Petsche, H., Schinko, H., and Seitelberger, F., Neuropathological studies on Van Bogaert's subacute sclerosing leucoencephalitis. In: Encephalitides (L. Van Bogaert et al., Eds.). Elsevier, Amsterdam, 1961: 363–385.

44. Petsche, H., and Sterc, J., The significance of the cortex for the travelling phenomenon of brain waves. Electroenceph. clin. Neurophysiol., 1968, **25**: 11–22.

45. Petsche, H., and Stumpf, C., Topographic and toposcopic study of origin and spread of the regular synchronized arousal pattern in the rabbit. Electroenceph. clin. Neurophysiol., 1960, **12**: 589–600.

46. Petsche, H., Stumpf, C., and Gogolák, G., The significance of the rabbit's septum as a relay station between midbrain and hippocampus. I. The control of hippocampus arousal activity by septum cells. Electroenceph. clin. Neurophysiol., 1962, **14**: 202–211.

47. Prince, D. A., and Wilder, B. J., Control mechanisms in cortical epileptogenic foci. "Surround" inhibition. Arch. Neurol., 1967, **16**: 194–202.

48. Purpura, D. P., McMurthy, J. G., Leonard, C. F., and Mailiani, A., Evidence for dendritic origin of spikes without depolarizing prepotentials in hippocampal neurons during and after seizure. J. Neurophysiol., 1966, **29**: 954.

49. Rose, M., Cytoarchitektonischer Atlas der Grosshirnrinde des Kaninchens. J. Physiol. Neurol. (Leipzig), 1931, **43**: 353–440.

50. Scheibel, M. E., and Scheibel, A. B., Organization of spinal motoneuron dendrites in bundles. Exp. Neurol., 1970, **28**: 106–112.

51. Skoglund, C. R., Transsynaptic and direct stimulation of postfibers in the artificial synapse formed by severed mammalian nerve. J. Neurophysiol., 1945, **8**: 365–376.

52. Sotelo, C., and Taxi, J., Ultrastructural aspects of electrotonic junctions in the spinal cord of the frog. Brain Res., 1970, **17**: 137–141.

53. Stensaas, L. J., and Stensaas, S. S., Light and electron microscopy in the amphibian spinal cord. Brain Res., 1971, **31**: 67–84.

54. Strumwasser, F., and Rosenthal, S., Prolonged and patterned direct extracellular stimulation of single neurons. Am. J. Physiol., 1960, **198**: 405–413.

55. Szentágothai, J., Architecture of the cerebral cortex. In: *Basic Mechanisms of the Epilepsies* (H. H. Jasper *et al.*, Eds.). Little, Brown, Boston, 1969: 13–40.

56. Terzuolo, C. A., and Bullock, T. H., Measurement of imposed voltage gradient adequate to modulate neuronal firing. *Proc. Natl. Acad. Sci. VSA* 1956, **42:** 687–694.

57. Tömböl, T., A Golgi analysis of the sensori-motor cortex in the rabbit. In: *Synchronization of EEG Activity in Epilepsies* (H. Petsche and M. A. B. Brazier, Eds.). Springer-Verlag, Berlin and New York, 1972: 25–36.

58. Walker, A. E., The generalization of a seizure from a focal discharge. In: *The Physiopathogenesis of the Epilepsies* (H. Gastaut *et al.*, Eds.). Thomas, Springfield, Illinois, 1969: 273–276.

59. Walter, D. O., Spectral analysis for electroencephalograms: Mathematical determination of neurophysiological relationships from records of limited duration. *Exp. Neurol.*, 1963, **8:** 155–181.

60. Welker, C., Microelectrode delineation of fine grain somatotopic organization and SM I cerebral neocortex in albino rat. *Anat. Rec.*, 1968, **160:** 449.

61. Woolsey, T. A., and van der Loos, H., The structural organization of layer IV in the somatosensory region (S 1) of mouse cerebral cortex. *Brain Res.*, 1970, **17:** 205–242.

ELECTRICAL SEIZURE DISCHARGES WITHIN THE HUMAN BRAIN: THE PROBLEM OF SPREAD

MARY A. B. BRAZIER*

Brain Research Institute, University of California, Los Angeles, California

The question being examined in the studies reported here is whether evidence can be found for the hypothesis that abnormal synaptic input may be the principal abnormality in the epileptic brain.

The opportunity to test this concept in man during spontaneous seizures has been provided by a program in this Institute for recording from deep structures in the epileptic brain.

As described by Crandall elsewhere in this volume, the goal of implanting electrodes in the depths of the brain in epileptic patients is to lateralize and, if possible, localize the site from which the seizure is triggered. The patients in this series, which now number over 50, are mostly cases of temporal lobe epilepsy who, because control of their seizures by medication has failed, are candidates for unilateral therapeutic surgery. A smaller number are cases of partial epilepsy.

When recordings are available only from the scalp, detection of the site of origin is, of course, impossible except in those cases where the trigger zone lies in the cortical layers, for scalp electrodes record only the electrical activity of the outer mantle of the brain. One can hypothesize about a thalamic site for a disturbance at the surface from anatomical knowledge of the cortical projection areas of the various thalamic nuclei but, in the case of temporal lobe epilepsy involving the limbic system, projections to the convexity of the neocortex from suspected deep structures, such as the hippocampus, are not known, and those from the amygdala are probably restricted to the fasciculus amygdalotemporalis, identified (in man) by Klingler and Gloor (28).

In scalp electroencephalography the custom has, therefore, developed of searching in the ink record for the first sign of electrical seizure discharge. However, experience with recording from the limbic system in temporal lobe epilepsy has taught us that the arrival of the abnormal discharge at the cortex of the convexity may be the end point rather than the initiator

* The work of this investigator is supported by Career Award No. 5 K6-18608 and Grants NS 11379 and NS 09774 from the National Institute of Neurological Diseases and Stroke.

to the efferent system as a motor movement, or activates signs from the signs. The latter can only be observed when the seizure discharge spreads of the activity. A similar comment can be made in regard to the clinical sympathetic system, or is communicated verbally to the observer as a description by the patient of sensory experiences.

In recent studies within this program* at the Brain Research Institute, a search has been made for trigger zones and an attempt made to follow the route or routes of spread of the discharge throughout the brain by timing the arrival of the abnormal activity at the various loci where it can be detected. As the velocity of spread is in the order of milliseconds, this cannot be measured by eye. A computer program† has, therefore, been used to detect the site of the first appearance of abnormal frequencies and to follow the time-course of their spread to other regions of activity developing the same characteristics.

In the case of each individual patient, primary interest lies in evidence for the location of the abnormal pace-making region responsible for driving the spread of his seizure discharge. A second interest, in the general field of the study of epilepsy, is to investigate whether the spread of this abnormal activity proceeds by excessive discharge in anatomically well-known connections or whether there is a breakthrough of synapses to pathways over which traffic does not normally flow.

Some preliminary attempts to test the usefulness of this concept, namely, of the importance of the locus that drives and paces other regions into epileptic discharge, have been published (15–18) and, as these have proved promising, the method is being given in more detail below.

The procedure for tracing the spread of wave trains is very similar in concept, although different in technique, from that which Petsche and his group (24, 36–40) originated in their work in lower animals (see, also, chapter by Petsche and Rappelsberger in this volume). Their initial studies established, in the rabbit, that when monorhythmic theta rhythm was present in the septum, rhythms of similar frequency were present also in the hippocampus, hypothalamus, and thalamus, although the wave-trains were never exactly in phase; that is, they were not in true synchrony. Later work by this group showed that rhythmically occurring groups of unit discharges in certain neurons in the septal region were the pacemakers for the waves recorded by gross electrodes in these other loci, all of which lagged behind those of the septum. The periodicity of the groups of these unit discharges arriving at the hippocampus from the septum proved to be the determining factor for the frequency of the wave-trains.

* The Clinical Neurophysiology Program under the leadership of Dr. Paul H. Crandall, supported by Grant NS 02808 from the National Institute of Neurological Diseases and Stroke.

† Fast Fourier Transform. Program X92 (Biomedical Computer Programs) available from the Health Sciences Computer Facility at the University of California, Los Angeles. Supported by Grant FR-3 from the National Institutes of Health of the U.S. Public Health Service.

In the work just described, by Petsche and his colleagues, the wave-trains studied were the normal ones of the rabbit when aroused. In the case of our patients, we have no data from man's normal brain and have had to use, as controls for the epileptic patients, the recordings from a few non-epileptic patients with intractable psychoses studied by colleagues in the Department of Psychiatry at the Neuropsychiatric Institute of this medical school. The only other form of control available to us is the interictal record of our epileptic patients and, in the case of entirely lateralized discharge, of the opposite uninvolved hemisphere, each patient serving as his own control.

As the information being sought is the spread of the unprovoked seizure discharge as compared with normal transmission in the interictal state, it is clear that artificial means of evoking either a seizure or an after-discharge by electrical stimulation must be avoided, for this procedure has the effect of synchronizing all discharge from the stimulus site. The result is the sudden impingement of an abnormally concentrated barrage of impulses at the next synapses—a barrage condensed in temporal terms and excessive in intensity. Such a barrage may open trans-synaptic connections not normally traversed and give false evidence for the relationships operating in the interictal state. One of the questions being asked about the ictal stage is whether or not a breakthrough of this kind might be responsible for the spread in some cases, for abnormal synaptic input may be the major abnormality in epileptic brain tissue.

METHOD

Recording Procedure

Recordings are made simultaneously from very many pairs of electrodes linked to give information from deep sites as well as from surface electrodes on the dura, the exact number in each case being decided by the clinical problem but usually amounting to about twenty-four. Such a large number of electrodes imposes a series of such recordings in order to obtain information from the many possible combinations. The stereotactic placement of the implanted electrodes is determined by the surgeon, Dr. Paul Crandall, solely according to the clinical need for diagnostic and localizing information in each particular patient. It follows that the tracing of discharges within the brain is restricted in every case to the electrode sites required by the clinical problem.

The electroencephalograms (EEGs) are recorded simultaneously on an ink-writing oscillograph and on analog FM tape with one channel reserved for the code that signals eventual instructions to the computer indicating which section of the tape is to be analyzed. A preliminary editing of the tape is made on a PDP12 computer in this laboratory, chosen samples being submitted later to the IBM 360/91 computer in the Health Sciences Computing Facility. Calibrations (by sine waves) of the amplitude settings are made for every channel of the tape, and this information is given to the computer for a scaling program so that the output in the form of the auto-spectra is comparable for all leads in terms of μV^2 per cm (although amplification may have been unequal in the original recording).

The information needed for determination of routes of spread is a record of a spontaneously occurring seizure. For patients who have not had a seizure while in the laboratory, use has been made of their telemetered tape recordings. As mentioned above, the question of whether spread during seizures in epilepsy is achieved through abnormal synaptic inputs or only via normal anatomical connections rules out the technique of electrical stimulation and the search for after-discharges, for this procedure itself begs the question of possible breakthrough of pathways by the electric stimulus.

Quantification of the Spread of Discharge

The investigator has the choice of length of epoch to be analyzed (as well as the number of epochs) and of the width of the individual frequency bands in terms of cycles per second, and of total extent of the spectrum. The values chosen will determine the degrees of freedom and, hence, the level of significance necessary for the analysis of a single epoch. Consistent values from epoch to epoch, of course, increase the significance.

The first step in the analysis is the calculation by the computer of coherence. This is independent of individual amplitudes, because the purpose of this measurement is solely to make a comparison of the frequencies present in any pair (and all pairs) among the recording sites. The coherence program detects the frequency of wave-trains common to any pair, calculates the percentage of this activity in the given epoch, and the phase difference between them; that is: the degree by which one wave train leads or lags behind another wave train of similar frequency in some other channel. Should there be any ambiguity introduced by the polarity in which the plug containing the recording electrodes was inserted, study of the ink record (both for ictal and interictal periods) will usually indicate whether the phase should be calculated as displacement from $0°$ or from $180°$.

The phase difference in degrees can be converted into time differences in milliseconds for the specific frequency under study. A frequent finding is that, as the frequency of discharge changes with the developing seizure, the phase also changes, but when converted into milliseconds remains approximately the same.

Useful references for more detail about these forms of computer analysis can be found in Davenport and Root (21), Blackman and Tukey (8), Walter (47), Koopmans (30), Cooley and Tukey (20), and Bendat and Piersol (6).

Examples of Results Obtained by this Procedure

(1) AN EXAMPLE WHICH RAISES THE QUESTION OF EFFERENT
HIPPOCAMPAL CONNECTIONS TO IPSILATERAL HIPPOCAMPAL
GYRUS AND INVOLVEMENT OF CENTRE MÉDIAN

Figure 1A illustrates a seizure episode in an 18-year-old girl with a severe convulsive disorder of 8 years' duration and a history of a partial topectomy 2 years previously. Her seizures had continued and were mixed in sign, some being similar to temporal lobe epilepsy but with occasional grand mal convulsions; some signs of mental deterioration were also present.

During the recording of the EEG she fell asleep and, while sleeping, had a brief seizure episode (Figure 1A) which awakened her and of which she was aware. The discharge was far from monorhythmic, but when the coherences had been computed a striking emergence of high coherences was found in frequencies peaking essentially at 24 c/sec. This increase in coherence is illustrated in Figure 2 for the 24 c/sec activity for several pairs of electrodes.

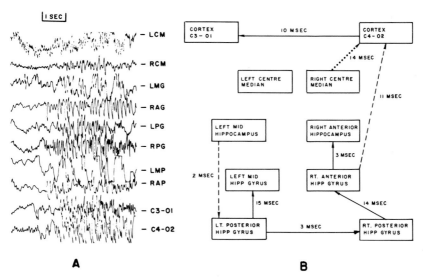

Figure 1. (A) A burst of electrical seizure activity in an epileptic patient, involving both hemispheres (Case 1). (B) Chart of analysis of phase for the electroencephalogram shown in A and summarized in Table 1. Note that the direction of the arrows indicates phase lead and not anatomical tracts. Broken lines denote routes not established anatomically. LCM, left centre médian; RCM right centre médian; LMG, left mid-hippocampal gyrus; RAG—right anterior hippocampal gyrus; LPG, left posterior hippocampal gyrus; RPG, right posterior hippocampal gyrus; LMP, left mid-hippocampus; RAP, right anterior hippocampus; C3-01 and C4-02, surface leads (international placements).

EMERGENCE OF COHERENCES DURING BURST OF SEIZURE DISCHARGES (24 cps)

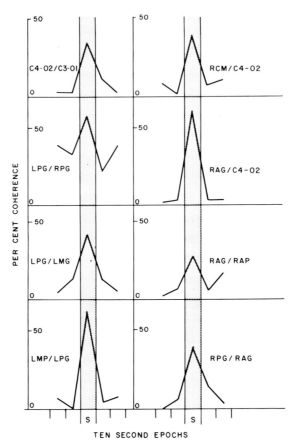

Figure 2. Results of analysis of coherence in the electroencephalogram shown in Figure 1A. The emerging most common frequency was 24 c/sec, and this chart gives the values for coherence at this frequency for several pairs of loci. S = the 10-second period of the discharge. Plotted also are the coherence values 20 and 10 seconds before and after the episode.

In this case, as can be seen from the values for phase relations given in Table 1, the activity appeared to be driven from the left hippocampus (LMP) to the posterior hippocampal gyrus (LPG) and from there to the mid-hippocampal gyrus (LMG) (see also Figure 1B). In this schematic chart, it should be emphasized that the arrows represent *phase lead* and not anatomical pathways. The crossing, in the anterior commissure, from LPG to the hippocampal gyrus of the opposite hemisphere (RPG) is ana-tomically known in lower animals, as is the route to the hippocampus of the same side (9, 35). Unknown to us from our restricted electrode place-ments is the way by which the right centre médian and the centro-occipital linkage on the surface became involved (broken lines (Figure 1B). The

TABLE 1

Epileptic Discharge with a Dominant Frequency of 24 c/sec

Pairs of sites[a]	% Coherence	Phase difference	Equivalent in milliseconds
LMP → LPG	57	19°	2
LPG → LMG	41	129°	15
LPG → RPG (crossing)	57	26°	3
RPG → RAG	39	123°	14
RAG → RAP	27	22°	3
C4-02 → C3-01 (crossing)	34	83°	10
(RAG → C4-02)	60	94°	11
(RCM → C4-02)	36	124°	14

[a] Key to abbreviations: LMP = left mid-hippocampus; LMG = left mid-hippocampal gyrus; LPG = left posterior hippocampal gyrus; RAG = right anterior hippocampal gyrus; RPG = right posterior hippocampal gyrus; RAP = right anterior hippocampus; RCM = right centre médian; C4-02 = surface leads, right central to occipital; C3-01 = surface leads, left central to occipital (international placements).

crossing at the cortical level is presumably via the corpus callosum. The left centre médian (CM), although its activity was disturbed, did not share this frequency or cohere with any other site from which our electrodes were recording.

A fiber inflow from the hippocampus to the ipsilateral hippocampal gyrus is controversial among the anatomists and is, therefore, shown by a broken line in the schematic chart in this figure. Yet the evocation of short latency responses in the gyrus as well as after-discharges by stimulation of the hippocampus is well known to electrophysiologists [for example, Ajmone Marsan and Stoll (2) and Green and Adey (25) in the cat; Brazier (11) in man]. If the consensus is that these electrical stimuli forced an unusual breakthrough, one may perhaps consider the action of the seizure discharge to be analogous.

The connections of the CM, both afferent and efferent, apart from striatal endings, are still controversial. Quite possibly some of the confusion is due to species differences. Totibadze and Moniava (45), in degeneration studies in the cat, found evidence for direct connections from the CM which terminated diffusely in layers V and VI of the cortex. Less diffuse connections ended in the layers III and IV of some gyri only, mainly the ectosylvian, suprasylvian, and coronal gyri. Some evidence from preterminal degeneration in the deepest layers of the cortex of the superior frontal gyrus in the monkey has been reported by Bowsher (10).

Electrophysiological evidence for long-sought projections from the CM to the neocortex is more readily available [e.g., Albe-Fessard and Rougeul (5) and Albe-Fessard and co-workers (3) in the cat]. Several workers have found short latency responses in the premotor cortex from electrical stimulation in the CM in the cat, some so short (2–4 msec) as to suggest monosynaptic transmission. Once again it may be noted that the artificial stimuli of electric shocks were used and, in some cases, the facilitating effect of chloralose. More direct evidence has been provided by the microelectrode studies of Albe-Fessard and her colleagues in the cat (4), but studies, neither by anatomical methods nor by electrophysiological stimulation have yet given any clues to involvement with limbic system structures. Our results reveal such long phase lags that only some involved polysynaptic route would be possible.

(2) AN EXAMPLE WHICH RAISES THE QUESTION OF AMYGDALO-
CORTICAL RELATIONS AND EFFERENT HIPPOCAMPAL CONNECTIONS

The second example is an 18-year-old man who experienced seizures starting 4 years previously and increasing in frequency and complexity, varying from brief episodes of staring to occasional full grand mal seizures. The EEG of one of the brief seizure bursts is shown in Figure 3A. When analyzed by the method described above, the ruling frequency was found to be 12 c/sec, and the coherence values found at this frequency are listed in Table 2.

According to the phase differences found, the driving locus appeared to be the right anterior hippocampus (RAP) from which the activity spread rapidly to the ipsilateral anterior hippocampal gyrus (RAG). After longer delay this activity appeared in the mid part of the same gyrus (RMG) from which it rapidly reached the amygdala (RAm) and also crossed to

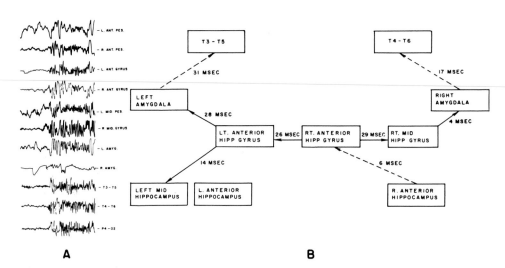

Figure 3. (A) Electroencephalogram (EEG) of wide-spread seizure discharge (Case 2). (B) Chart of analysis of phase for the EEG shown in A and summarized in Table 2. T4-T6 and T3-T5, surface leads (international placements).

TABLE 2

EPILEPTIC DISCHARGE WITH A DOMINANT FREQUENCY OF 12 C/SEC

Pairs of sites[a]	% Coherence	Phase difference	Equivalent in milliseconds
RAP → RAG	63	25°	6
RAG → RMG	63	123°	29
RMG → RAm	63	16°	4
RAm → T4-T6	53	74°	17
RAG → LAG	34	113°	26
LAG → LMP	34	61°	14
LAG → LAm	48	122°	28
LAm → T3-T5	18	132°	31
LAP → LMP	(Insignificant coherence)	—	—
LAG → LAP	(Insignificant coherence)	—	—

[a] Key to abbreviations: RAP = right anterior hippocampus; RAG = right anterior hippocampal gyrus; RAm = right amygdala; RMG = right mid-hippocampal gyrus; LAP = left anterior hippocampus; LMP = left mid-hippocampus; LAG = left anterior hippocampus gyrus; LAm = left amygdala; T3-T5 = left temporal dural leads; T4-T6 = right temporal dural leads (international placements).

the opposite hemisphere, presumably via the anterior commissure. In both hemispheres the amygdala became involved, and, after some delay, the temporal cortex on both sides (Figure 3B).

Several points relevant to known anatomical routes are raised by this example, as well as some controversial ones, namely, the connections of the hippocampus with the hippocampal gyrus, the hippocampal gyrus with the amygdala, and those of the amygdala with the neocortex.

The known data on hippocampal–gyrus relations have already been discussed above in the findings in the first case. Connections between the basolateral amygdala and the hippocampal gyrus receive recognition from anatomists (19, 27, 42). But the amygdalo-neocortical relationships are more complex.

The amygdaloid composite of nuclear groups has quite restricted afferent connections from the neocortex, and, in the case of our patients whose temporal lobes carry surface electrodes solely on the convexity, there is no placement on the dura that has direct fiber projections to the amygdala. There is, however, good evidence that fiber connections run from the anterior orbital area to the amygdala. Koikegami (29), working in the cat, found these to be restricted to the lateral part of the amygdala, but Valverde (46), in the same animal, found projections from the orbital gyrus to all the nuclei of the ipsilateral amygdala except the central nucleus.

There are, no doubt, some species differences (44) for, in the monkey, Whitlock and Nauta (48) followed connections from the inferior temporal region to the central as well as the basolateral amygdaloid nucleus. This finding was confirmed Lammers (31) and by Lammers and Lohman (32) in the same animal. However, in the rat, these connections although searched for, have not been found according to Powell and co-workers (41) and to Leonard (33). Of special interest to us who work in man is the finding of Klingler and Gloor (28) that fibers from the cingulum pass not only to the hippocampal gyrus but also to the amygdala. There would seem to be a species difference (22) here, for in lower animals no afferent fibers from the cingulum to the amygdala have been found (1).

Again in the case of efferents from the amygdaloid complex, there are differences in findings—possibly owing to species differences (22). The connections with the hypothalamus and olfactory bulb will not be discussed here, because they are irrelevant to our work in these patients.

Valverde (46), in his book, reports that in the rat he was able to trace fibers, originating in the periamygdaloid region, to the preoptic area (as well as to the hypothalamus), although axons from the amygdaloid nuclei themselves did not proceed that far. Similar results were obtained by Leonard and Scott (34). Of relevant interest to our work in patients are the connections found in man, and here we again find the most intensive studies in the work of Klingler and Gloor (28) with their evidence for a bundle of fibers (the fasciculus amygdalotemporalis) emerging from the lateral surface of the amygdala and running uninterruptedly to the cortex of the temporal lobe.

Fiber connections between both the amygdala and the anterior temporal cortex with the medial thalamus have been traced by Klingler and Gloor (28) in man; this other tract was known by earlier anatomists as the inferior thalamic peduncle and presumably could be the pathway used in those of our patients in whom a high coherence is found between amygdala and the dorsal medial nucleus of the thalamus. The identification in the monkey, by Whitlock and Nauta (48), of fibers originating in the inferior temporal region and the second temporal convolution and reaching the thalamus could apparently be the analog of the route in man for the activity responsible for the high coherences found in some of our patients and for the responses evoked in the dorsal medial nucleus by stimulation of the temporal cortex in animals (2, 23).

(3) INVOLVEMENT OF ALL HIPPOCAMPAL SITES OF ONE HEMISPHERE ONLY, WITH BILATERAL INVASION OF CORTEX

The patient was a 25-year-old woman with a complaint of short seizures in which she began to stare, dropped objects she was holding, and fell to the floor. She had a stereotyped automatism in which she scratched herself with her right hand. These seizures (for which she had an aura) were very frequent but lasted only a few minutes or even seconds. There were no tonic-clonic movements although there was a past history of generalized convulsions.

The EEG from the available depth electrodes showed a seizure discharge in all linkages from the right hemisphere and appearing on the left only at the cortex. The erupting seizure discharge was very evident in the auto-spectra, as displayed by the computer program for compressed spatial arrays, devised by Bickford and his colleagues (7), and illustrated in Figure 4. When the coherences were computed between pairs of leads, the short

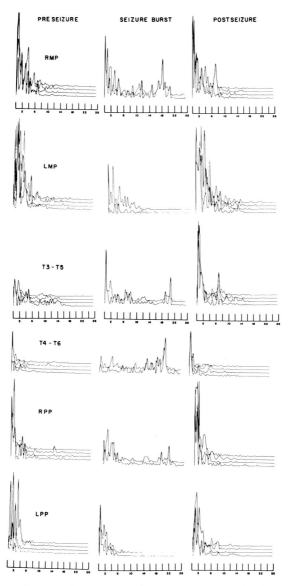

Figure 4. Compressed spectral arrays of consecutive time epochs (progressing vertically at intervals of 2.46 seconds on the ordinates) during the 20 seconds before a brief seizure burst, the 10-second period of the burst, and the 20 seconds after it. Frequency in cycles per second on the abscissa; power in μV^2 on the ordinate. Note the eruption of activity in the fast frequencies during the brief seizure discharge (Case 3). [Program by courtesy of Dr. R. Bickford and colleagues (7).] RMP, right mid-hippocampus; LMP, left mid-hippocampus; RPP, right posterior hippocampus; LPP, left posterior hippocampus; T3-T5 and T4-T6, surface leads (international placements).

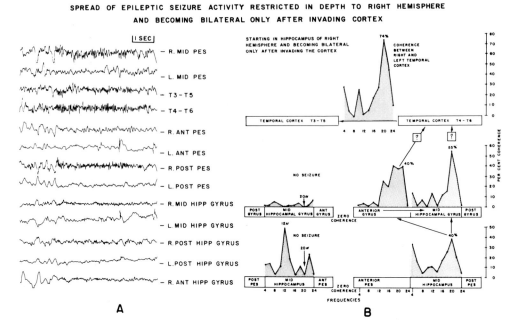

Figure 5. (A) Electroencephalogram (EEG) of the seizure discharge that yielded the spectral arrays illustrated in Figure 4 (Case 3). (B) Chart of the coherences found in the analysis of the EEG in A and listed, with their phase relations, in Table 3. T3-T5 and T4-T6, surface leads (international placements).

seizure period gave high values at 20 c/sec on the right but not on the left (Figure 5A and B).

The only significant coherence between recordings from the available electrodes on the left was the usual one (at normal, not epileptic frequency) between the hippocampus and the gyrus. As reported elsewhere (12–14), this is a common finding interictally and in nonepileptic brains. The phase analysis is listed in Table 3 and reveals that this burst of 20 c/sec discharge was led by the right mid-hippocampus from which it spread rapidly to the ipsilateral hippocampal gyrus, reaching the cortex after longer delays and by an unknown route. Once in the cortex of the initiating hemisphere the discharge passed rapidly to the opposite cortex, presumably via the corpus callosum.

This is yet another example of activity apparently efferent from the hippocampus to the hippocampal gyrus, as discussed in the first case.

(4) SPREAD OF A SEIZURE PACED FROM THE AMYGDALA

The patient, a 37-year-old woman, had a history of seizures during the preceding 10 years. These were of two types: one lasting less than a minute and consisting of staring, and, the other, of rather longer duration, in which she lost consciousness and displayed automatisms. These seizures were resistant to a variety of anticonvulsant drugs.

TABLE 3

EPILEPTIC DISCHARGE WITH A DOMINANT FREQUENCY OF 12 C/SEC

Pairs of sites[a]	% Coherence[b]	Phase difference	Equivalent in milliseconds
RMP → RMG	40	94°	13
RMP → RAG	55	55°	8
RAG → T4-T6	40	171°	24
RMG → T4-T6	55	149°	21
T4-T6 → T3-T5	74	67°	9
RAP/LAP	Nil	—	—
RMP/LMP	Nil	—	—
RPP/LPP	Nil	—	—
RMG/LMG	Nil	—	—
RPG/LPG	Nil	—	—

[a] Key to abbreviations:

RAP = right anterior hippocampus
RMP = right mid-hippocampus
RPP = right posterior hippocampus
RAG = right anterior hippocampal gyrus
RMG = right mid-hippocampal gyrus
RPG = right posterior hippocampal gyrus
T4-T6 = right temporal dural leads

LAP = left anterior hippocampus
LMP = left mid-hippocampus
LPP = left posterior hippocampus
LMG = left mid-hippocampal gyrus
LPG = left posterior hippocampal gyrus
T3-T5 = left temporal dural leads

[b] Level of significant coherence = 31%.

One of these seizures recorded in the laboratory gave the EEG of which a section is seen in Figure 6; the data are listed in Table 4. On tracing the spread of the prominent discharge at a frequency of 2 per second by analysis of coherence and phase, this striking abnormality was found to be paced from the amygdala as shown in the chart. This EEG is a good example of the well-known tendency of the hippocampus to react to abnormality with spike discharges.

The chart displays an arrow indicating passage to the hippocampus from the amygdala, a connection which is still controversial among anatomists, although plentiful evidence exists that electrical stimulation of the amygdala in man evokes responses, and even recruitment, in the hippocampus (11, 15). The anatomical evidence for connections between the amygdala and the CM is also scanty, although once again results have been described that indicate that electrical stimulation in the amygdala changes the firing pattern of units in the CM in the cat (43). A schematic diagram of such a connection in man has been published by Jasper (26).

COMMENTS

Spread of Electrical Seizure Discharge to the Opposite Hemisphere

The three main routes pertinent to temporal lobe epilepsy, each of which has been searched for in the analyses of our patients' seizure activities are the anterior commissure, the psalterium, and the corpus callosum.

SPREAD OF A SEIZURE PACED FROM THE AMYGDALA

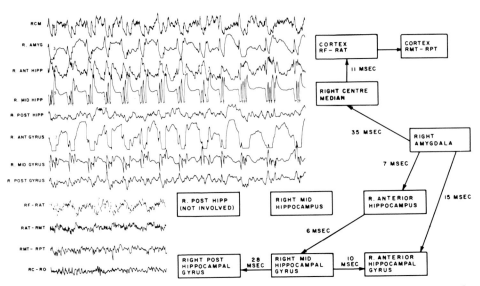

Figure 6. Electroencephalogram of a seizure and chart of spread, as indicated by the phase analyses and summarized in Table 4 (Case 4). RCM, right centre médian.

For crossings in the anterior commissure in the brain of man, Klingler and Gloor (28) found a strongly developed posterior limb carrying the interhemispheric connection of the amygdala and the temporal neocortex; some regions of the hippocampal gyri have also been found to have inter-hemispheric connections in this commissure.

The main interhemispheric crossing from the hippocampus is in the psalterium, but evidence for crossing of the seizure discharge by this route has been rare in our patients as found by this type of analysis. How strong

TABLE 4

Epileptic Discharge with a Dominant Frequency of 2 c/sec

Pairs of sites[a]	% Coherence	Phase difference	Equivalent in milliseconds
R.Cing → RAm	30	29°	4
R.Am → RMG	(16)	143°	18
RAP → RMG	77	111°	14
RMG → C4-P4	33	67°	9
C4-P4 → F8-T4	48	37°	5
F8-T4 → F4-C4	33	14°	2
RVA	No coherence with any other site	—	—

[a] Key to abbreviations: R.Cing = right anterior cingulate gyrus; R.Am = right amygdala; RAP = right anterior hippocampus; RMG = right mid-hippocampal gyrus; C4-P4, F8-T4, F4-C4 = dural leads (international placements); RVA = ventralis anterior thalami.

this hippocampal commissure is in man is a question that has been raised before; in earlier work (11), the search for responses in the hippocampus evoked by electrical stimuli in the contralateral hippocampus gave only negative results.

It should be remarked that, in as yet unpublished studies, it has proved extremely difficult to follow any route for the spread of discharge if the seizure had been induced by chemical activation. In such cases the thresholds for discharge of very many brain sites are affected by the systemic invasion of the neuronal milieu in a way that defies any explanation of spread depending on synaptic pathways.

Summary

In an attempt to examine the proposal that a crucial element in the dysfunction of the epileptic brain may be abnormal synaptic input, a method has been developed to detect the source that drives the spread of abnormal discharges with the brain. As the speed of spread is too rapid for the eye to follow, a computer program has been used that can make these measurements in milliseconds.

In the examples of seizure bursts in 4 patients whose results are presented [and in others previously published (6)], spread was found to follow not only anatomically known connections, but several pathways that have been identified only electrophysiologically. The fact that passage of impulses in these routes have been previously indicated by electrical stimulation lends probability to the suggestion that both the epileptic discharge and the artificial bombardment by an electrical stimulus are sending impulses by pathways mediated by abnormal synaptic inputs. It is of interest that no case has been found yet that gave a conduction time of zero as would be indicated were the spread to have been by volume conduction.

REFERENCES

1. Adey, W. R., and Meyer, M., An experimental study of hippocampal afferent pathways from prefrontal and cingulate areas in the monkey. *J. Anat.*, 1956, **86**: 58–74.
2. Ajmone Marsan, C., and Stoll, J., Subcortical connections of the temporal pole in relation to temporal lobe seizures. *Arch. Neurol. Psychiat.*, 1951, **66**: 669–686.
3. Albe-Fessard, D., Levante, A., and Rokyta, R., Cortical projections of cat medial thalamic cells. *Int. J. Neurosci.*, 1971, **1**: 327–338.
4. Albe-Fessard, D., Rocha-Miranda, C., and Oswaldo-Cruz, E., Activités d'origine somesthésique évoquées, au niveau du cortex nonspécifique et du centre médian du thalamus chez le singe anesthésié au chloralose. *Electroenceph. clin. Neurophysiol.*, 1951, **11**: 777–787.
5. Albe-Fessard, D., and Rougeul, A., Activités d'origine somesthésique évoquées

sur le cortex non-spécifique du chat anesthésié au chloralose: Rôle du centre médian du thalamus. *Electroenceph. clin. Neurophysiol.,* **10:** 131–152.

6. Bendat, J. S., and Piersol, A. G., *Measurement and Analysis of Random Data.* Wiley, New York, 1966.

7. Bickford, R. G., Billinger, T. W., Flemming, N. I., and Stewart, L., The compressed spectral array (CSA)—a pictorial EEG. *Proc. San Diego Biomed. Symp.,* 1972, **2:** 365–370.

8. Blackman, R. B., and Tukey, J. W., *The Measurement of Power Spectra.* Dover, New York, 1958.

9. Blackstad, T., On the termination of some afferents to the hippocampus and fascia dentata. *Acta Anat. (Basel),* 1958, **35:** 202–214.

10. Bowsher, D., Some afferent and efferent connections of the parafascicular—center median complex. In: *The Thalamus* (D. P. Purpura and M. D. Yahr, eds.). Columbia Univ. Press, New York, 1966: 99–108.

11. Brazier, M. A. B., Evoked responses from the depths of the human brain. *Ann. N.Y. Acad. Sci.,* 1964, **112:** 33–59.

12. Brazier, M. A. B., Studies of the EEG activity of limbic structures in man. *Electroenceph. clin. Neurophysiol.,* 1968, **25:** 309–318.

13. Brazier, M. A. B., Electrical activity recorded simultaneously from the scalp and deep structures of the human brain. A computer study of their relationships. *J. Nerv. Ment. Dis.,* 1968, **147:** 31–39.

14. Brazier, M. A. B., Regional activities within the human hippocampus and hippocampal gyrus. *Expl. Neurol.,* 1970, **26:** 354–368.

15. Brazier, M. A. B., The human amygdala: Electrophysiological studies. In: *The Neurobiology of the Amygdala* (B. E. Eleftheriou, ed.). Plenum, New York, 1972: 397–420.

16. Brazier, M. A. B., Spread of seizure discharges in epilepsy: Anatomical and electrophysiological correlates. *Expl. Neurol.,* 1972, **36:** 263–272.

17. Brazier, M. A. B., Interactions of deep structures during seizures in man. In: *Mechanisms of Synchronization in Epileptic Seizures* (H. Petsche and M. A. B. Brazier, eds.). Springer-Verlag, Vienna, Berlin, and New York, 1972: 409–424.

18. Brazier, M. A. B., Direct recordings from within the human brain using long-indwelling electrodes. In: *Neurophysiology Studied in Man* (G. Somjen and D. Albe-Fessard, eds.). Excerpta Med., Amsterdam, 1972: 3–13.

19. Brodal, A., The hippocampus and the sense of smell. A review. *Brain,* 1947, **70:** 179–224.

20. Cooley, J. W., and Tukey, J. W., An algorithm for the machine calculation of complex Fourier series. *Math. Comput.,* 1965, **19:** 297–301.

21. Davenport, W. B., and Root, W. L., *An Introduction to the Theory of Random Signals and Noise.* McGraw-Hill, New York, 1958.

22. De Olmos, J. S., The amygdaloid projection field in the rat as studied with the cupric-silver method. In: *The Neurobiology of the Amygdala* (B. E. Eleftheriou, ed.). Plenum, New York, 1972: 145–204.

23. Gloor, P., Electrophysiological studies on the connections of the amygdaloid

nucleus in the cat. Part I. The neuronal organization of the amygdaloid projection system. *Electroenceph. clin. Neurophysiol.*, 1955, 7: 223–242.

24. Gogolák, G., Stumpf, C., Petsche, H., and Sterč, J., The firing pattern of septal neurons and the form of the hippocampal theta wave. *Brain Res.*, 7: 201–207.

25. Green, J. D., and Adey, W. R., Electrophysiological studies of hippocampal connections and excitability. *Electroenceph. clin. Neurophysiol.*, 1956, 8: 245–262.

26. Jasper, H. H., Functional subdivisions of the temporal region. In: *Temporal Lobe Epilepsy* (M. Baldwin and P. Bailey, eds.). Thomas, Springfield, Illinois, 1958: 40–51.

27. Kahn, E. A., Bassett, R. C., Schneider, R. C., and Crosby, E. C., *Correlative Neurosurgery*. Thomas, Springfield, Illinois, 1955.

28. Klingler, J., and Gloor, P., The connections of the amygdala and of the anterior temporal cortex in the human brain. *J. Comp. Neurol.*, 1960, 115: 333–369.

29. Koikegami, H., Amygdala and other related limbic structures; experimental studies on the anatomy and function. I. Anatomical researches with some neurophysiological observations. *Acta Med. Biol.* (*Niigata*), 1963, 10: 161–277.

30. Koopmans, L. H., On the coefficient of coherence for weakly stationary stochastic processes. *Ann. Math. Stat.*, 1964, 35: 532–549.

31. Lammers, H. J., The neural connections of the amygdaloid complex in mammals. In: *The Neurobiology of the Amygdala* (B. E. Eleftheriou, ed.). Plenum, New York, 1972: 123–144.

32. Lammers, H. J., and Lohman, A. H. M., Experimental anatomisch onderzoek naar de verbindingen van piriforme cortex en amygdalakernen bij de kat. *Ned. Tijdschr. Geneeskd.*, 1957, 101: 1–2.

33. Leonard, C. M., Origin of the amygdalofugal pathways in the rat. *Anat. Rec.*, 1970, 166: 337.

34. Leonard. C. M., and Scott, J. W., Origin and distribution of the amygdalofugal pathways in the rat: An experimental neuroanatomical study. *J. Comp. Neurol.*, 1971, 144: 313–330.

35. Lorente de Nó, R., Studies on the structure of the cerebral cortex. II. Continuation of the study of the ammonic system. *J. Psychol. Neurol.* (*Leipzig*), 1934, 46: 113–167.

36. Petsche, H., The quantitative analysis of EEG data. *Progr. Brain Res.*, 1970, 33: 63–86.

37. Petsche, H., Gogolák, G., and Stumpf, C., Die Projektion der Zellen das Schrittmachers für den Thetarhythmus auf den Kaninchenhippocampus. *J. Hirnforsch.*, 1966, 8: 129–136.

38. Petsche, H., Gogolák, G., and Van Zwieten, P. A., Rhythmicity of septal cell discharges at various levels of reticular excitation. *Electroenceph. clin. Neurophysiol.*, 1965, 19: 25–33.

39. Petsche, H., and Stumpf, C., Topographic and toposcopic study of origin and spread of the regular synchronized arousal pattern in the rabbit. *Electroenceph. clin. Neurophysiol.*, 1960, 12: 589–600.

40. Petsche, H., Stumpf, C., and Gogolák, G., Significance of the rabbit's septum as a relay station between the mid brain and the hippocampus. *Electroenceph. clin. Neurophysiol.*, 1962, **14**: 202–211.

41. Powell, T. P. S., Cowan, W. M., and Raisman, G., The central olfactory connexions. *J. Anat.*, 1965, **99**: 791–813.

42. Schneider, R. C., Crosby, E. C., and Kahn, E. A., Certain afferent cortical connections of rhinencephalon. *Progr. Brain Res.*, 1963, **3**: 191–217.

43. Sommer-Smith, J. A., Powarzynski, J., Stirner, A., and Grümberg, V., Décharges cellulaires du noyau centre-médian du thalamus induites par la stimulation amygdalienne et septale. *Acta Neurol. Lat. Am.*, 1965, **11**: 360–367.

44. Stoll, J., Ajmone Marsan, C., and Jasper, H. H., Electrophysiological studies of subcortical connections of anterior temporal region in cat. *J. Neurophysiol.*, 1951, **14**: 305–316.

45. Totibadze, N. K., and Moniava, E. S., On the direct cortical connections of the nucleus centrum medianum thalami. *J. Comp. Neurol.*, 1969, **137**: 347–360.

46. Valverde, F., *Studies on the Piriform Lobe*. Harvard Univ. Press, Cambridge, 1965.

47. Walter, D. O., Spectral analysis for electroencephalograms: Mathematical determination of neurophysiological relationships from records of limited duration. *Expl. Neurol.*, 1963, **8**: 155–181.

48. Whitlock, D. G., and Nauta, W. J. H., Subcortical projections from temporal neocortex in Macaca mulatta. *J. Comp. Neurol.*, 1956, **106**: 183–212.

BEHAVIORAL CORRELATES OF GENERALIZED SPIKE-WAVE DISCHARGE IN THE ELECTROENCEPHALOGRAM

J. KIFFIN PENRY

National Institute of Neurological Diseases and Stroke, Bethesda, Maryland

Hughlings Jackson (23) provided an accurate and complete description of focal seizure activity which has been unsurpassed. Although Jackson pointed out that the hand was essentially paralyzed and could not subserve voluntary function when a march was in progress, he did not become preoccupied with the positive and negative manifestations of seizure discharge—notwithstanding their importance. With the advent of electroencephalography, investigators had no difficulty in correlating the interictal (14, 28, 40) and ictal (13, 24) electroencephalogram (EEG) with Jacksonian seizures.

However, many investigators have described the epileptic personality and the behavior of epileptic patients with far less success than Jackson (19). Although many important studies (7, 8, 33, 34, 54, 55) have statistically related intelligence and performance to various types of epilepsy or EEG abnormalities, the correlations have been of limited value for the interpretation of simultaneous behavioral and EEG abnormalities. Because human behavior, even when considered from one or two fundamental aspects, cannot be described completely, the behavioral correlates will be defined here in very general, sketchy terms. Furthermore, the fundamental aspects of generalized spike-wave discharge will not be described; a good account is given in the excellent Symposium on the Spike-and-Wave Discharge presented by Daly (6), Gastaut (11), Chatrian's group (5), Mirsky and Tecce (35), Pollen (44), Marcus and co-workers (31), and Gloor (16).

This discussion is arbitrarily confined to human behavior that may occur during a period when generalized spike-wave discharge is recorded in the EEG from scalp electrodes. First, spontaneous behavior observed during generalized spike-wave discharge will be reviewed briefly. This will be followed by a review of behavioral capacity or ability based on specific test situations, including the presentation of specific stimuli. Finally, behavioral features common to both spontaneous and tested capacity will be summarized and discussed.

SPONTANEOUS BEHAVIOR

Behavior characterized by interruption of activity, a blank stare, and unresponsiveness to ordinary environmental stimuli was probably first described by Poupart (56) in 1705 when he wrote, "If she has begun to talk and an attack interrupts her, she takes it up at precisely the point at which she stopped and she believes she has talked continuously." Such seizure activity or behavior was first related to spike-wave discharge by Gibbs, Davis, and Lennox (15) in 1935 when they stated:

> Electro-encephalograms from twelve patients with characteristic petit mal epilepsy show in all cases during the seizure an outburst of waves of great amplitude, amounting to from 100 to 300 microvolts at a frequency of 3 per second. These waves may be very smooth and approximately sinusoidal in shape but usually include a sharp negative spike breaking into the record near the positive crest of the main wave. The large 3 per second wave is invariably present. The spike is more variable in amplitude and may occasionally be absent during part of the seizure.

But the authors did not stop there, because nature does not yield its secrets so easily without putting forth a few enigmas. The authors went on to describe:

> The electro-encephalograms of these epileptic patients made between seizures are essentially normal, except that scattered here and there are brief groups of waves of pattern similar to those seen at the beginning of a seizure. . . . These we have called "larval" seizures, because they so closely resemble the beginnnig of a fully developed characteristic seizure but fade out again instead of developing the characteristic picture.

At first recognition, then, behavioral correlates of generalized spike-wave discharge encompassed two extremes: apparently normal behavior, and gross impairment of consciousness with interruption of activity. The conformation of the generalized spike-wave discharge associated with these two conditions has been apparently the same, varying only in *duration* of the spike-wave discharge.

Spontaneous behavior during generalized spike-wave discharge has attracted attention, but the published accounts of this interesting phenomenon are generally limited to a two-page case report or a two-paragraph note in a society proceedings, with emphasis on diagnostic or therapeutic significance, rather than on clinical neurophysiology. Indeed, with the latter point of view in mind, a study of these accounts yields very little valuable information, but raises many questions. In these reports a variety of terminology appears, including: "petit mal epilepsy occurring in status," "status epilepticus in petit mal," "petit mal status epilepticus," and "spike-wave stupor." The term *absence status* in the international classification (12) satisfactorily encompasses all of the terms used.

There are at least 58 cases of absence status mentioned in these reports, with some detail given for 22 of these (see Table 1). The patients ranged in age from 4 to 61 years (mean, 24 years). All except 2 had a history of one or more grand mal seizures. Behavior during absence status was described as stuporous, confused, dazed, groggy, slow or incomplete responses, wandering, "lost," and automatism. The duration of such behavior varied from hours to several days. With the exception of a few cases, EEGs during absence status were poorly correlated with behavior and not described in detail. One patient had an EEG recorded for only 107 seconds because the patient was confused and unable to cooperate; the longest continuous recording was 4 hours.

Of the 22 patients, 13 were described as having long generalized spike-wave bursts with very brief normal intervals or slowing between bursts. The other 9 were described as having "continuous spike-wave," but the meaning of the word "continuous" is justifiably questioned in at least half of these cases, because brief intervals of either slowing or normal EEG are obvious in many of the EEG illustrations.

Kellaway and Chao (27), in summarizing their 11 cases, stated: "The electroencephalogram during such episodes reveals almost continuous spike and wave activity with only occasional episodes of very brief duration of relative normality."

One of the patients reported by Thompson and Greenhouse (57) was described, during generalized spike-wave discharge, as oblivious to his environment and seemingly in a catatonic state. At that time, there was *continuous* generalized spike-wave discharge. When the patient became more alert, the generalized spike-wave discharge became *intermittent*. The EEG showed "very brief stretches, never exceeding 2 to 3 sec., with 6 to 7 c/s waves."

The case of Assael (2), reported more recently in a society proceedings, is entitled "Petit Mal Status Without Impairment of Consciousness." Yet the abstract states that the patient was referred because of peculiarities in her behavior. This report illustrates the confusion that exists in the descriptive language.

Other reported cases (1, 22, 29, 37, 39, 51) have presented interesting clinical features of diagnosis and treatment but have failed to provide data to enhance our understanding of electroclinical relationships.

Finally, nearly half the authors comment that a strong or repeated stimulus will elicit a response during paroxysmal discharge when none result from a weaker or single stimulus. Furthermore, as described by Jung (26), these stimuli often alter or temporarily normalize the EEG. Is it any wonder that the observer may be puzzled? How many of these variables can be controlled? Enough to make any consistent observations?

TABLE 1
ABSENCE STATUS

Investigator	Age of patient	Sex	Age at onset	History of grand mal	Behavior during absence status	EEG during absence status[a]
Tucker and Forster, 1950 (60)	43	F	11	Yes	Confused, groggy	Long burst generalized S-W
	4	M		Yes	Slow, incomplete responses	Long runs with short normal intervals
Vizioli and Magliocco, 1953 (61)	20	M	11	Yes	Confused, slow responses, wandering	Generalized S-W in long bursts
Schwab, 1953 (50)	28	F	13	Yes	Peculiar state of mind, dazed, could not do all of housework	Long burst generalized S-W with 1–2 seconds between, during 4 hours recording
Mann, 1954 (30)	4	F	1	Yes	Blank spells, limpness, continuous stupor	Continuous generalized S-W; almost continuous generalized S-W
	31	M	5	Yes	Blank spells and automatism	Almost continuous generalized S-W
Kellaway and Chao, 1955 (27)	?	?	?	?	(Eleven cases in children reported in abstract; not individually described)	
Zappoli, 1955 (62)	5	?	?	Yes	Stupor with slow, awkward responses	Continuous generalized S-W for 107 seconds
Friedlander and Feinstein, 1956 (10)	34	F	?	Yes	Stupor, slow responses	Continuous generalized S-W
	30	F	16	No	Confused, dazed	Continuous generalized S-W; almost continuous S-W
Bornstein et al., 1956 (3)	19	F	13	No	Incoherent, confused, disoriented, hazy	Almost continuous generalized S-W
Merlis, 1960 (32)	12	F	10	Yes	Stuporous, confused, slow responses	Continuous generalized S-W
Shev, 1964 (52)	?	?	?	Yes	(Two cases reported in abstract; not individually described)	

Reference	Age	Sex		EEG	Behavior	S-W description
Niedermeyer and Khalifeh, 1965 (38)	22	F	6	Yes	Stupor	Almost continuous generalized S-W
	28	F	?	Yes	Mental confusion	Almost continuous generalized S-W, atypical
	27	F	?	Yes	Dull, stuporous	Almost continuous generalized S-W
	15	M	?	Yes	Stupor	Almost continuous generalized S-W
	18	M	9	Yes	Stupor	Generalized S-W throughout record
	7	F	?	Yes	Dazed, lethargic	Continuous generalized S-W, with intervals of high-voltage slowing
Gumnit et al., 1965 (20)	22	F	6	Yes	(Same case reported by Niedermeyer and Khalifeh, 1965)	
Charlton and Hoefer, 1965 (4)	?	?	?	?	(Six cases reported in abstract; not individually described)	
Thompson and Greenhouse, 1968 (57)	34	M	19	Yes	Stupor, poor responses	Continuous generalized S-W
	61	F	?	Yes	Poorly responsive	Continuous generalized S-W
	42	M	?20	Yes	Stupor	Continuous generalized S-W
	41	M	?25	Yes	Confused	Long burst generalized S-W
Assael, 1969 (2)	17	F	?	?	Peculiarities in behavior	Paroxysmal outburst generalized S-W (reported in abstract)

[a] EEG—electroencephalagram; S-W—spike and wave.

Experimental Behavior

Schwab (47) made the first measurement of behavior during generalized spike-wave discharge and reported his results to the Boston Society of Psychiatry and Neurology on May 19, 1938. He designed a test situation to record the patient's EEG and manual response to a visual stimulus (150-W tungsten light) delivered after the onset of generalized spike-wave discharge. His measurement represented the patient's reaction time to a visual stimulus. He stated: "I have found that in some cases consciousness is never lost. In others it is always lost. In some it is lost during some of the attacks and preserved in others. The longer attacks seem generally to be associated with loss of consciousness."

Schwab refined his routine measurements by substituting a neon lamp for the tungsten light, but he also became fascinated by the effects of the stimulus on the EEG. He added an auditory stimulus (air whistle) and entitled his next report "The Influence of Visual and Auditory Stimuli on the Electroencephalographic Tracing of Petit Mal" (48). A diagram illustrating how he was able to measure reaction time is shown in Figure 1.

Figure 2 shows a plot of Schwab's data. For paroxysms lasting less than 2 seconds, there is a normal reaction time. If an averaging line were drawn through this scatter graph, it could be seen that reaction time increases with the duration of the attack. It cannot be concluded, however, that the reaction time is directly proportional to the duration of the spike-wave

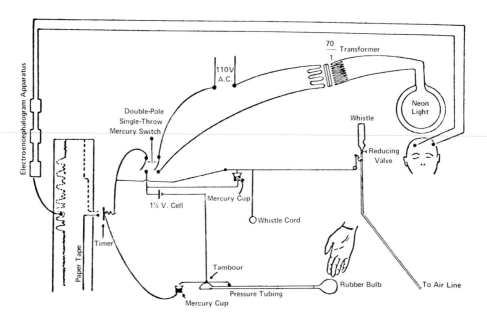

Figure 1. Diagrammatic plan of the light and whistle reaction time apparatus attached to the electroencephalograph. (Reprinted from Schwab, *Am. J. Psychiatry*, 1941, 97: 1301–1312.)

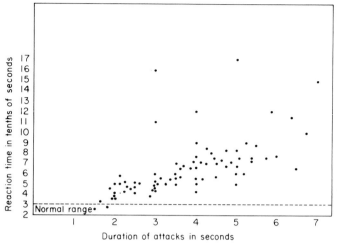

Figure 2. Relation of the neon light reaction time to duration of attack in petit mal. (Reprinted from Schwab, *Am. J. Psychiatry*, 1941, **97**: 1301–1312.)

paroxysm, because the stimulus remained until the patient reacted. Because the intensity of the stimulus in Schwab's measurements was rigidly controlled, it seems likely that the scatter graph represents different levels of attention in the same patient at the time of the stimulus. Schwab concluded from his data that six degrees of petit mal seizures exist:

1. Very short spells (1–3 seconds) with nearly normal reaction times
2. Moderately short spells (3–6 seconds) with impairment of reaction time
3. Moderately short spells that become even shorter with the light stimulus (termination by stimulus)
4. Longer spells (8–20 seconds) that fail to respond to light stimulus (transient unconsciousness)
5. Similar attacks that break up with a loud whistle (termination by stimulus)
6. Severe attacks that respond to neither form of stimulus (severe degree of unconsciousness)

It can be seen from the arrangement of the experiment and from Schwab's data that his experiment was not designed to test reaction time by presenting a stimulus at the various points within the time duration of a paroxysm. The methods and data were not extended in a subsequent report (49).

Shimazono and his colleagues (53) presented various verbal stimuli during generalized spike-wave discharge in the EEG and observed verbal responses (such as answering simple questions or doing mental calculations) or performance of a simple motor task (such as counting on the fingers). In Figure 3, their schematic diagram of what happens to consciousness during generalized spike-wave discharge reveals two slopes and a broken

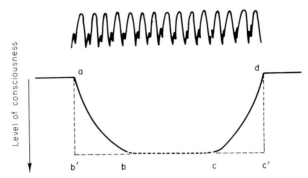

Figure 3. Schematic representation of the disturbance of consciousness in petit mal seizures. Seizure begins at *a* and ends at *d*. Curved lines *ab* and *cd* represent transition to and from impaired consciousness, respectively. Broken line *bc* indicates fluctuation in level of impaired consciousness. [From Shimazono and co-workers (53).]

line to account for their experimental findings. They could not confirm Schwab's views that attacks of long duration are associated with a more severe degree of unconsciousness. They concluded that various degrees of alteration of consciousness graded from almost no loss of consciousness to complete lapse of consciousness during generalized spike-wave discharge. They stated further that during a given petit mal seizure, the degree of disturbance of consciousness is not constant but is altered in various ways spontaneously or following various stimuli. In their opinion, this could be confirmed by applying various stimuli during the seizure.

Goldie and Green (17), utilizing questions and answers, found that the initial 3 seconds and final 1.5 seconds in any paroxysmal generalized spike-wave discharge are characterized by less impairment of consciousness than in the intervening period.

Tizard and Margerison (58) utilized the "tape test" (46) and the "5-lights test" to measure reaction time and the number of errors in response to auditory and visual stimuli in 2 patients. By evaluating their data statistically, they found response time to be the most sensitive behavioral correlate of generalized spike-wave discharge. Response time slowed significantly even for discharges of 0.5 to 1.5 seconds, even though there was no increase in errors of omission during the short discharges.

Tizard and Margerison (59) continued their studies on 6 additional patients and added additional tests to measure simple and choice reaction to visual, auditory, and tactile stimuli, and to verbal commands and questions. They corroborated their initial findings but commented that the distribution of responses during generalized spike-wave discharge did not follow the "troughlike" course often described (17, 53).

Mirsky and Van Buren (36) tested behavior in 18 patients with centrencephalic epilepsy. Their tests included the continuous performance test, the delayed identification tests, and the simple motor response test. They were concerned about the polyspikes contained in the generalized paroxysmal spike-wave discharge but found, in agreement with Fischgold (9) and Hauser (21), that the "spike" was not more likely to be associated with errors than the "wave." Evaluating the results of the continuous performance test statistically by pooling all their data (1094 "correct" stimuli recorded during 588 bursts), they found a strong tendency for errors to occur during the spike-wave burst, although some performance was preserved. The percentage of correct responses during the burst averaged 24.1, whereas the average percentage correct in absence of the burst was 84.8. The difference was highly significant. In consideration of the time course of impairment, they found that correct responses usually occurred later within the spike-wave burst than did errors.

Figure 4 is based on the continuous performance test of Mirsky and Van Buren (36). They concluded that behavioral alterations become manifest before the burst itself is evident in the EEG and that they dissipate somewhat earlier than the EEG abnormality. Notwithstanding their findings preceding the EEG abnormality, the troughlike pattern as well as the variability and breakup at the bottom of the trough can be noted when the diagram is observed from the points of the beginning to the end of the burst. The similarity to the concept put forth by Shimazono and his colleagues is striking.

Recent Investigations

The effects of generalized spike-wave discharge on pursuit rotor performance have been studied by the author in collaboration with Goode and Dreifuss (18). With respect to errors in performance occurring during those

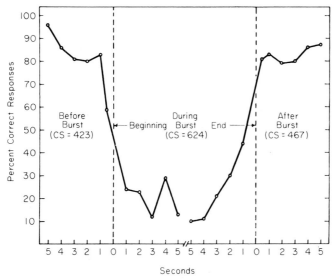

Figure 4. Relation between level of performance on the continuous performance test and the onset, development, and termination of the electrographic burst. CS refers to number of correct stimuli. [From Mirsky and Van Buren (36).]

generalized spike-wave paroxysms that lasted longer than 3 seconds, we found either a troughlike pattern of dysfunction (error) or fluctuating performance (errors mixed with correct pursuit).

In pursuit rotor performance, the error begins well after the onset of generalized spike-wave discharge and ends well before the end of the EEG abnormality (Figure 5). This pattern of error performance in relation to duration of spike-wave burst is essentially the same as that found by other investigators utilizing different techniques (17, 36, 53). Moreover, errors in pursuit rotor performance illustrate the "broken" or fluctuating level of consciousness (performance) during generalized spike-wave discharge (Figure 6).

In a different series of studies performed in collaboration with Dreifuss (41), one of the patients illustrated the complexities of behavior that can be observed during generalized spike-wave discharge. This patient had a period of confusion or stupor but could follow simple commands which often had to be repeated. All movements were slow. Speech consisted of simple responses such as "yes" or "no." The patient's behavior during absence status was intensively analyzed from a replay of the video tapes of the split screen. The patient took a cup of soft drink into her right hand when it was offered to her during generalized spike-wave discharge. The generalized spike-wave discharge fluctuated with her activity. A few moments later, she transferred the cup to her left hand and drank from it. When the generalized spike-wave discharge ceased (indicated by arrow), she touched the cup to her lips (Figure 7). A few seconds later, she removed the cup from her lips, and generalized spike-wave discharge returned.

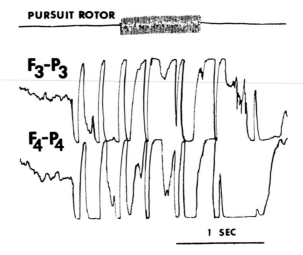

Figure 5. Electroencephalogram during pursuit rotor performance. Upper trace shows 0.8-second pursuit rotor error which occurs in the middle of generalized spike-wave burst. F₃-P₃ and F₄-P₄—electrodes.

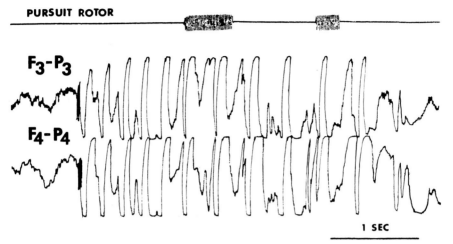

Figure 6. Electroencephalogram during pursuit rotor performance. Upper trace shows 0.5 and 0.3-second pursuit rotor errors occurring during generalized spike-wave discharge. F₃-P₃ and F₄-P₄—electrodes.

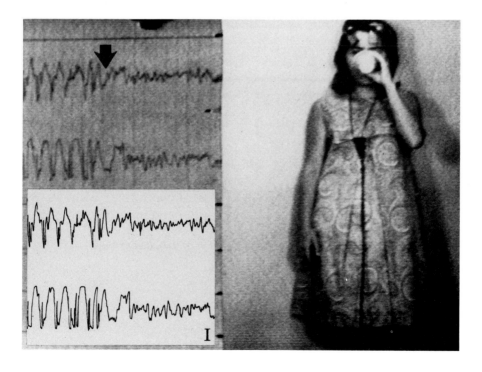

Figure 7. Patient drinking from cup held in her left hand. Arrow on (EEG) electroencephalogram indicates moment the cup touched her lips. (Photographed from split screen during video tape replay. Two channels of telemetered EEG are shown.) Insert montage labeled I is a photograph of telemetered spike-wave discharge from EEG.

An analysis of the video tape of this patient during the 16-minute period revealed seventy-seven paroxysms, lasting a total time of 11 minutes and 34 seconds. These ranged in duration from 0.4 to 39.6 seconds (mean, 9.1 seconds). The total duration of the normal intervals was 4 minutes and 26 seconds. The seventy-six normal intervals ranged from 0.6 to 16.1 seconds (mean, 3.6 seconds).

In a study using a paroxysm-triggered method for measuring reaction time at specific time points during spike-wave discharge, reaction time was delayed at the exact onset of the burst in more than half of the paroxysms (45). Could the trough effect result from those normal reaction times at the onset? This seems to be the best explanation. Of even greater importance, however, is the question of why some of these reaction times are normal. Nearly half the spike-wave bursts, on detailed observation, were not fully generalized at the onset, that is, the slow waves frequently did not reach full voltage until the second or third wave (0.3 to 1.0 second). It appears, therefore, that a delayed reaction time (impaired performance) occurs only when high-voltage slow waves are generalized and synchronous. Quantitative measurements to test this hypothesis are now being carried out.

Impaired performance during generalized spike-wave bursts can be demonstrated by special laboratory techniques. But what is the limit of clinical observation? While developing techniques to measure the efficacy of drugs for control of absence seizures, untreated hospitalized patients underwent observation during four 2-hour periods (42, 43). A 12-hour telemetered EEG was recorded continuously. The number of observed seizures was compared to the number and duration of spike-wave bursts recorded during an 8-hour period (see Table 2). The ratio of the number of observed seizures to spike-wave bursts was plotted as a function of the average duration of the spike-wave bursts (Figure 8). From this illustration, it can be seen that the limit of clinical observation is significantly related to the duration of the burst. Spike-wave bursts of less than 3 seconds in duration were generally unidentified by intensive clinical observation, unless the patient was speaking, writing, or engaged in fine movements of the upper extremities. Behavioral alterations generally were not clinically observed during spike-wave bursts lasting less than 1 second.

Discussion

From a review of reported cases of absence status, it may be concluded that details of behavioral alterations have been inadequately correlated with details of generalized spike-wave discharge in the EEG. It is apparent from recent studies that behavior is altered during continuous spike-wave discharge in the EEG and must be considered as a *dynamic spectrum of abnormal behavior*. This spectrum is characterized at one end by an increase in reaction time to environmental stimuli and stupor at the other;

TABLE 2

Comparison of Clinical Seizures and Spike-Wave Bursts

| Patients | Seizures seen by trained observer (8 hr) | Spike-wave bursts (8-hr telemetered EEG[a]) | | Ratio of observed seizures to number of spike-wave bursts |
		No.	Average duration (sec)	
T. D.	9	19	5.9	0.474
M. S.	64	137	7.5	0.467
L. S.	14	43	9.7	0.326
H. F.	1	1,613	1.7	0.001
J. J.	3	33	1.9	0.091
E. C.	0	5	1.3	0.000
L. D.	44	113	2.5	0.389
V. W.	19	23	19.2	0.826
S. D.	28	51	14.5	0.546
D. W.	2	26	4.1	0.077
L. F.	3	9	29.5	0.333
G. L.	28	140	3.9	0.200
A. R.	11	23	10.8	0.478
J. H.	25	39	16.5	0.641
S. R.	0	199	2.3	0.000
W. W.	38	73	3.0	0.521
H. P.	2	20	7.0	0.100
L. W.	9	65	1.3	0.138

[a] EEG—electroencephalogram.

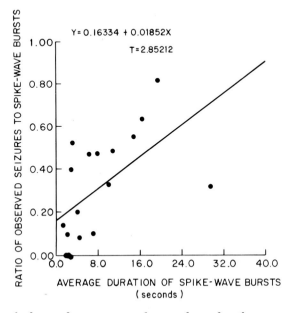

Figure 8. Ratio of observed seizures to the number of spike-wave bursts is plotted as a function of average duration of spike-wave bursts over an 8-hour period for 8 patients (see Table 2). A linear regression line reveals a significant relationship ($p < 0.05$). Therefore, the probability of observing a clinical absence attack during a spike-wave burst increases with the increasing duration of the burst.

the latter being further characterized by loss of response to stimuli in all modalities of sensation, except painful stimuli (withdrawal) and maintenance of posture. In clinical terms, this range in behavior would vary from mild lethargy to deep stupor. Intermingled with this spectrum of behavior would also be found the well-known stereotyped fundamental correlates of generalized spike-wave discharge. These are the blank stare; mild clonic twitches about the eyes, face, or extremities; mild increase or decrease in postural tone; automatisms which are environmentally influenced (41); and autonomic phenomena (36), such as flushing of the face or borborygmi. This spectrum of altered behavior becomes dynamic when each phase of behavioral response changes its rate and character according to the intensity of the stimulus. This dynamic spectrum, then, encompasses the behavioral correlates of generalized spike-wave discharge.

The split screen video tape technique combined with the telemetered EEG (41) is a valuable method for further EEG–behavior correlation studies. Although this technique does not control any of the numerous variables just described, it does make possible the identification and thorough study of them. The question may be asked, Why study the relationship of behavior and the scalp-recorded EEG? These two crude parameters have not been studied simultaneously in adequate detail. It is recognized that electrical events deep in the cerebral structures are frequently not apparent in the EEG recorded from the scalp or cortex, but this fact serves only to point up the limitations of the scalp-recorded EEG. Even during experimentally produced seizures, a clinical event does not always accompany an electrical discharge. Nevertheless, such experimental models are valid for studying the epileptic process (25).

The EEG–behavior correlation studies are of more than academic importance. Observation alone is too often an unreliable indicator of seizure frequency to serve as a guide in medical treatment. Moreover, it is not satisfactory for the scientific appraisal of new drugs in the case of absence seizures. Advances in our understanding of the relationship of spike-wave bursts to behavior have permitted the use of electrical events that have been reliably detected and measured (42, 43, 45).

CONCLUDING REMARKS

Further attempts to define and measure behavioral events and electroencephalographic events and to study their relationship are warranted because of the widely held concept that EEG events are either ictal or interictal. Unless measurements of similar reliability and precision are made simultaneously, assumptions cannot be made about the relationships. Knowledge about the relationship of behavior to the EEG is not only important physiologically but is of value to prove the efficacy of antiepileptic drugs and in the treatment of patients with epilepsy.

REFERENCES

1. Andermann, F., and Robb, J. P., Absence status: A reappraisal following review of thirty-eight patients. *Epilepsia*, 1972, **13**: 177–187.
2. Assael, M. I., Petit mal status without impairment of consciousness. *Electroenceph. clin. Neurophysiol.*, 1969, **27**: 218.
3. Bornstein, M., Coddon, D., and Song, S., Prolonged alterations in behavior associated with a continuous electroencephalographic (spike and dome) abnormality. *Neurology (Minneap.)*, 1956, **6**: 444–448.
4. Charlton, M. H., and Hoefer, P. F. A., Petit mal status epilepticus. *Electroenceph. clin. Neurophysiol.*, 1965, **19**: 535.
5. Chatrian, G. E., Somasundaram, M., and Tassinari, C. A., DC changes recorded transcranially during "typical" three per second spike and wave discharges in man. *Epilepsia*, 1968, **9**: 185–209.
6. Daly, D. D., Reflections on the concept of petit mal. *Epilepsia*, 1968, **9**: 175–178.
7. Dongier, S., Statistical study of clinical and electroencephalographic manifestations of 536 psychotic episodes occurring in 516 epileptics between clinical seizures. *Epilepsia*, 1959–1960, **1**: 117–142.
8. Ervin, F., Epstein, A. W., and King, H. E., Behavior of epileptic and nonepileptic patients with "temporal spikes." *Arch. Neurol. Psychiatry*, 1955, **74**: 488–497.
9. Fischgold, H., La conscience et ses modifications. Systèmes de references en EEG clinique. *Congr. Int. Sci. Neurol.*, 1957, 181–208.
10. Friedlander, W. J., and Feinstein, G. H., Petit mal status. Epilepsia minoris continua. *Neurology (Minneap.)*, 1956, **6**: 357–362.
11. Gastaut, H., Clinical and electroencephalographic correlates of generalized spike and wave bursts occurring spontaneously in man. *Epilepsia*, 1968, **9**: 179–184.
12. Gastaut, H., Clinical and electroencephalographical classification of epileptic seizures. *Epilepsia*, 1970, **11**: 102–113.
13. Gastaut, H., and Dell, M. B., Etude électro-encéphalographique des foyers epileptiques corticaux. *Encéphale*, 1949, **38**: 97–107.
14. Gibbs, E. L., Merritt, H. H., and Gibbs, F. A., Electroencephalographic foci associated with epilepsy. *Arch. Neurol. Psychiatry*, 1943, **49**: 793–801.
15. Gibbs, F. A., Davis, H., and Lennox, W. G., The electro-encephalogram in epilepsy and in conditions of impaired consciousness. *Arch. Neurol. Psychiatry*, 1935, **34**: 1133–1148.
16. Gloor, P., Generalized cortico-reticular epilepsies. Some considerations on the pathophysiology of generalized bilaterally synchronous spike and wave discharge. *Epilepsia*, 1968, **9**: 249–263.
17. Goldie, L., and Green, J. M., Spike and wave discharges and alterations of conscious awareness. *Nature (Lond.)*, 1961, **191**: 200–201.
18. Goode, D. J., Penry, J. K., and Dreifuss, F. E., Effects of paroxysmal spike-wave on continuous visual-motor performance. *Epilepsia*, 1970, **11**: 241–254.
19. Guerrant, J., Anderson, W. W., Fischer, A., Weinstein, M. R., Jaros, R. M.,

and Deskins, A., *Personality in Epilepsy.* Thomas, Springfield, Illinois, 1962.

20. Gumnit, R. J., Niedermeyer, E., and Spreen, O., Seizure activity uniquely inhibited by patterned vision. *Arch. Neurol.,* 1965, **13**: 363–368.

21. Hauser, F., *Perception et réponses motrices au cours des paroxysmes de pointes-ondes.* Foulon, Paris, 1960.

22. Hosokawa, K., Booker, H. E., Okumura, N., Ikeda, H., and Kumashiro, H., Spike-wave stupor. *Folia Psychiatr. Neurol. Jap.,* 1970, **24**: 37–47.

23. Jackson, J. H., In: *Selected Writings of John Hughlings Jackson.* (J. Taylor, ed.). Hodder & Stoughton, London, 1931: Vol. 1.

24. Jasper, H. H., Electroencephalography. In: *Epilepsy and Cerebral Localization* (W. Penfield and T. C. Erickson, eds.). Thomas, Springfield, Illinois, 1941: 380–453.

25. Jasper, H. H., Application of experimental models to human epilepsy. In: *Experimental Models of Epilepsy—A Manual for the Laboratory Worker* (D. P. Purpura *et al.,* eds.). Raven Press, New York, 1972: 585–601.

26. Jung, R., Blocking of petit-mal attacks by sensory arousal and inhibition of attacks by an active change in attention during the epileptic aura. *Epilepsia,* 1962, **3**: 435–437.

27. Kellaway, P., and Chao, D., Prolonged status epilepticus in petit mal. *Electroenceph. clin. Neurophysiol.,* 1955, **7**: 145.

28. Kornmüller, A. E., and Janzen, R., Uber lokalisierte hirnbioelektrische Erscheinungen bei Kranken, ins besondere Epileptikern. *Z. ges. Neurol. Psychiatr.,* 1939, **165**: 372–374.

29. Lipman, I. J., Isaacs, E. R., and Suter, C. G., Petit mal status epilepticus. *Electroenceph. clin. Neurophysiol.,* 1971, **30**: 159–162.

30. Mann, L. B., Jr., Status epilepticus occurring in petit mal. *Los Angeles Neurol. Soc. Bull.,* 1954, **19**: 96–104.

31. Marcus, E. M., Watson, C. W., and Simon, S. A., An experimental model of some varieties of petit mal epilepsy. Electrical-behavioral correlations of acute bilateral epileptogenic foci in cerebral cortex. *Epilepsia,* 1968, **9**: 233–248.

32. Merlis, S., Status epilepticus in petit mal. *Pediatrics,* 1960, **26**: 654–656.

33. Milstein, V., and Stevens, J. R., Verbal and conditioned avoidance learning during abnormal EEG discharge. *J. Nerv. Ment. Dis.,* 1961, **132**: 50–60.

34. Mirsky, A. F., Primac, D. W., Ajmone Marsan, C., Rosvold, H. E., and Stevens, J. R., A comparison of the psychological test performance of patients with focal and nonfocal epilepsy. *Expl. Neurol.,* 1960, **2**: 75–89.

35. Mirsky, A. F., and Tecce, J. J., The analysis of visual evoked potentials during spike and wave EEG activity. *Epilepsia,* 1968, **9**: 211–220.

36. Mirsky, A. F., and Van Buren, J. M., On the nature of the "absence" in centrencephalic epilepsy: A study of some behavioral, electroencephalographic and antonomic factors. *Electroenceph. clin. Neurophysiol.,* 1965, **18**: 334–348.

37. Moe, P. G., Spike-wave stupor: Petit mal status. *Am. J. Dis. Child,* 1971, **121**: 307–313.

38. Niedermeyer, E., and Khalifeh, R., Petit mal status ("spike-wave stupor"). An electroclinical appraisal. *Epilepsia,* 1965, **6**: 250–262.

39. Novak, J., Corke, P., and Fairley, N., "Petit mal status" in adults. *Dis. Nerv. Syst.*, 1971, **32**: 245–248.

40. O'Leary, J. L., and Fields, W. S., Focal disorder of brain activity as it relates to the character of convulsive seizures: Electroencephalogram in focal seizures. *Arch. Neurol. Psychiatry*, 1949, **62**: 590–609.

41. Penry, J. K., and Dreifuss, F. E., Automatisms associated with the absence of petit mal epilepsy. *Arch. Neurol.*, 1969, **21**: 142–149.

42. Penry, J. K., Porter, R. J., and Dreifuss, F. E., Quantitation of paroxysmal abnormal discharge in the EEGs of patients with absence (petit mal) seizures for evaluation of antiepileptic drugs. *Epilepsia*, 1971, **12**: 277–278.

43. Penry, J. K., Porter, R. J., and Dreifuss, F. E., Ethosuximide: Relation of plasma levels to clinical control. In: *Antiepileptic Drugs* (D. M. Woodbury, J. K. Penry, and R. P. Schmidt, eds.). Raven Press, New York, 1972: 431–441.

44. Pollen, D. A., Experimental spike and wave responses and petit mal epilepsy. *Epilepsia*, 1968, **9**: 221–232.

45. Porter, R. J., Penry, J. K., and Dreifuss, F. E., Responsiveness at the onset of spike-wave bursts. *Electroenceph. clin. Neurophysiol.*, 1973, **34**: 239–245.

46. Rosvold, H. E., Mirsky, A. F., Sarason, I., Bransome, E. B., Jr., and Beck, L. H., A continuous performance test of brain damage. *J. Consult. Psychol.*, 1956, **20**: 343–350.

47. Schwab, R. S., Method of measuring consciousness in attacks of petit mal epilepsy. *Arch. Neurol. Psychiatry*, 1939, **41**: 215–217.

48. Schwab, R. S., The influence of visual and auditory stimuli on the electroencephalographic tracing of petit mal. *Am. J. Psychiatry*, 1941, **97**: 1301–1312.

49. Schwab, R. S., Reaction time in petit mal epilepsy. *Res. Publ. Assoc. Res. Nerv. Ment. Dis.*, 1947, **26**: 339–341.

50. Schwab, R. S., A case of status epilepticus in petit mal. *Electroenceph. clin. Neurophysiol.*, 1953, **5**: 441

51. Schwartz, M. S., and Scott, D. F., Isolated petit-mal status presenting de novo in middle age. *Lancet*, 1971, **2**: 1399–1401.

52. Shev, E. E., Syndrome of status petit mal in the adult. *Electroenceph. clin. Neurophysiol.*, 1964, **17**: 466.

53. Shimazono, Y., Hirai, T., Okuma, T., Fukuda, T., and Yamamasu, E., Disturbance of consciousness in petit mal epilepsy. *Epilepsia*, 1953, **2**: 49–55.

54. Small, J. G., Milstein, V., and Stevens, J. R., Are psychomotor epileptics different? *Arch. Neurol.*, 1962, **7**: 187–194.

55. Stevens, J. R., Sachdev, K., and Milstein, V., Behavior disorders of childhood and the electroencephalogram. *Arch. Neurol.*, 1968, **18**: 160–177.

56. Temkin, O., *The Falling Sickness*. Johns Hopkins Press, Baltimore, Maryland, 1945.

57. Thompson, S. W., and Greenhouse, A. H., Petit mal status in adults. *Ann. Intern. Med.*, 1968, **68**: 1271–1279.

58. Tizard, B., and Margerison, J. H., The relationship between generalized paroxysmal EEG discharges and various test situations in two epileptic patients. *J. Neurol. Neurosurg. Psychiatry*, 1963, **26**: 308–313.

59. Tizard, B., and Margerison, J. H., Psychological functions during wave spike discharge. *Br. J. Soc. Clin. Psychol.*, 1963, **3:** 6–15.

60. Tucker, W. M., and Forster, F. M., Petit mal epilepsy occurring in status. *Arch. Neurol. Psychiatry*, 1950, **64:** 823–827.

61. Vizioli, R., and Magliocco, E. B., A case of prolonged petit mal seizures. *Electroenceph. clin. Neurophysiol.*, 1953, **5:** 439–440.

62. Zappoli, R., Two cases of prolonged epileptic twilight state with almost continuous "wave-spikes." *Electroenceph. clin. Neurophysiol.*, 1955, **7:** 421–423.

PSYCHOMOTOR EPILEPSY AND SCHIZOPHRENIA:
A COMMON ANATOMY? *

JANICE R. STEVENS

University of Oregon School of Medicine, Portland, Oregon

Epilepsy and mental disorders were considered to be closely related until the last century. More recently a specific relationship between psychomotor epilepsy and schizophrenia has been alleged, denied, described, or decried in an increasingly voluminous literature. Anecdotal evidence of the coincidence of the two disorders abounds. Similarities between the clinical syndromes are numerous and indubitable, but controlled studies have regularly failed to provide convincing evidence that the incidence of schizophrenia is higher among patients with psychomotor epilepsy than in individuals with other forms of epilepsy or, indeed, other chronic brain disorders (2, 20, 66, 80, 87).

However, the sharing of numerous symptoms, the occasional alternation or reciprocity between schizophreniform and temporal lobe epileptic attacks, and the frequency of spikes or other abnormalities in the electroencephalogram (EEG) over the temporal regions of the scalp in both disorders are powerful arguments in favor of at least a common anatomical substrate. Introduction of neuroleptic agents that act by blocking postsynaptic catecholamine receptor sites has opened new avenues of investigation for neurology as well as psychiatry. A number of the drugs that are potent antipsychotic agents lower the threshold for convulsive discharge (86, 89), a fact of some interest when it is recalled that the original reason for introduction of convulsive treatment for the major psychoses was Meduna's now dubious observation that epilepsy was so unusual in patients with schizophrenia that a biological antagonism between these disorders was probable (63). Subsequently, a series of reports indicating a coincidence of epilepsy and schizophrenia, calling attention to the frequency of similar EEG abnormality, clinical parallels, and temporal relationships have led to the opposite contention, that is, that the two disorders are closely related (26, 27, 74, 79). The evidence for and against this relationship has been reviewed

* Supported in part by Grant No. 18055-03, National Institute of Mental Health and the Epilepsy Foundation of America. From the Department of Psychiatry, Massachusetts General Hospital, and the Erich Lindemann Mental Health Center, Boston, Massachusetts.

The author expresses gratitude to Dr. Walla Nauta, who launched many of the ideas in this report but who is not responsible for the flaws in their development.

elsewhere and will not be reconsidered here (5, 80, 84, 87). Data emerging from recent studies of psychopharmacological and histochemical properties of antipsychotic agents which suggest possible new interpretations of the relationships between epilepsy and schizophrenia are the subject of this communication.

CLINICAL STUDIES

Recent examination of the coincidence of schizophrenia and epilepsy in a state mental hospital of 1400 patients yielded 25 individuals with a diagnosis of schizophrenia who have some kind of "seizures" (Table 1). Careful review of each of these cases indicated that only 9 patients had distinct evidence of recurrent epileptic seizures in the absence of gross cerebral pathology or disorders of the senium. If 3 cases of "childhood" schizophrenia are excluded [for, in contrast to adults, some 40% of children diagnosed schizophrenic develop seizures (76)], the incidence of epilepsy among other schizophrenic patients is around 0.6% or slightly in excess of the 0.5% reported for the general population. Similar statistics are reported from more extensive and detailed surveys (5).

Acute Schizophrenia

Numerous investigators and clinicians have pointed out similarities between clinical features of psychomotor epilepsy and schizophrenia (Table 2) (14, 47). Among the most interesting of these to a neurologist are the "absence like" episodes characterized by psychomotor blocking and episodic sensory inundation experienced by schizophrenic patients. The former is a curious state of "sticking" of thought process and motor behavior in which the individual becomes mute or motionless, often displaying reaction times lasting 30 seconds or more. Occasionally chewing, smacking and swallowing accompany such arrests. In contrast to psychomotor

TABLE 1

COINCIDENCE OF EPILEPSY AND SCHIZOPHRENIA AMONG 1400
STATE HOSPITAL PATIENTS[a]

Diagnosis	No. of patients
Epilepsy followed by schizophrenia	2 (1 childhood epilepsy only)
Schizophrenia followed by epilepsy	6 (3 child. schizophrenia)
Simultaneous onset epilepsy and schizophrenia	1
Postlobotomy	2
Focal lesion—? tumor	1
Onset of seizures over age 65	5
Postencephalitic	1
Atypical seizures or psychotic impulsions?	7
Total	26

[a] From Rydjewski and Stevens (77).

TABLE 2

CLINICAL COMPARISON OF SCHIZOPHRENIC AND EPILEPTIC DISTURBANCES OF CONSCIOUSNESS[a]

Clinical features	Psychomotor	Schizophrenia
Onset	Abrupt	Abrupt
Sensory or affective precipitants	Infrequent	Very frequent
Approximate duration of attack	0.5–5 minutes	Seconds to days
Subjective experiences:		
Aura	Frequent	Absent
Disturbance of body image	Infrequent and mild	Present and severe
Ideokinetic dyspraxia	Absent	Present
Echopractic impulses	Absent	Present
Inability to screen out irrelevant stimuli	Slight	Severe
Effect of distraction on short-term memory	Mild	Severe
Disturbance of sensory perception	Mild, occasional	Severe and generalized
Impairment of identity	Mild (mental diplopia)	Severe
Hallucinations	Rare	Frequent
Anxiety, fear	Frequent, epigastric	Severe pervasive
Dysphasia	Frequent	Present
Intrusion or crowding of thoughts, percepts	Occasional	Frequent
Observable changes during attack:		
Fixed gaze and blank expression	Frequent	Present
Immobility	Frequent	Present
Incoherence of speech	Frequent	Present
Incontinence	Infrequent, usually urination	Rare, both urine and feces
Self-injury	Usually absent	Occasional
Injury to others	Very rare, only if restrained	Unpredictable, unprovoked often in response to hallucinated auditory commands
Disturbance of consciousness	Severe	Questionable, brief, mild, clouding
Amnesia	Complete for automatism	Can recall much of attack
Cessation of attack	Gradual, independent of external stimuli	Abrupt, often in response to external stimuli
Symptoms or signs following attack	Headache, confusion, dysarthria not rare	Absent

[a] Adapted after Chapman (14).

epilepsy, however, such spells are usually accompanied by bizarre ideas, crowding of thoughts or images, and a *distraction* of consciousness rather than the total amnesia typically associated with psychomotor automatisms. Furthermore, in patients with schizophrenia such attacks are most often precipitated in situations of heightened affective input and can be promptly aborted by a number of different sensory stimuli. The *paroxysmal sensory inundation* which may accompany these attacks is a more extreme instance of perhaps related etiology during which there is a sudden intensification of sensory or ideational experience. During such attacks patients may start violently, jump from a chair, or throw themselves over a wall or through a window. When asked to describe the subjective state accompanying such responses, replies are typically vague: "I'm burning up," "Everything jumped at me in the third dimension," "Lights got too bright, like a police station," "The voices made me do it."

Some clinical examples may be useful in illustrating these phenomena.

CASE 1

A 17-year-old boy with an excellent school record became indolent and inattentive during his junior year of high school. He became preoccupied with the Bible, took copious notes day and night, slept increasingly less, and finally became agitated, hallucinated, obsessed with his own crucifixion, suspicious and combative when restrained. Admitted to the hospital, he seemed dazed and intensely hypervigilant, stood in the middle of the ward transfixed, eyes unwinking, staring ahead, arms extended to the side, pupils widely dilated, with episodic, marked lateral deviation of the eyes to either side followed by strong head turning as though he heard or saw someone behind him. Consciousness was not lost—he could nearly always reply when coaxed and then denied that anything unusual was happening to him. Lying stiffly on the examining table he held his head rigidly off the mattress, seemed bewildered by a series of peculiar sensations, clutched at his heart, his genitals, stared at the ceiling fearfully; suddenly his eyes swerved to the ground and he reached for his shoe as though it were a pet and stroked it, muttering "What's that? Right! Right!" "Keep it in. Keep it in. Stick it in. Shut up!" There were brief twitches of muscles in the hands and arms followed by snapping of the fingers. Perseverated, stereotyped opening and closing of his trousers, and repeated tucking in of his shirt persisted for many minutes after which he shouted, "Jacob! Yes, yes," nodded, followed by a sudden myoclonic jerk of the entire body. He then stood in a rigid listening posture followed by a prolonged period of spontaneous hyperventilation during which his attention could not be obtained. After several days' treatment with large doses of phenothiazines, he became alert, friendly, and able to describe some of the experiences of the previous day although memory was incomplete. He recalled electrical and tactile sensations over his body and genitalia, a foul stench in his room, and above all the intense interest, importance, and reality of the experience. Questions made him anxious and bewildered and he again became mute, glanced sharply and suspiciously about, and did not wish to continue the interrogation.

During the height of the hallucinatory episode the EEG demonstrated low-voltage fast activity from all regions of the head. The patient could not or would not voluntarily keep his eyes closed but when they were held shut, spindled 20-c/sec activity appeared anteriorly, and bilateral theta was obtained over the temporal regions. Photic stimulation induced strong myoclonic jerks followed by spindled "ringing" phenomena at 14 c/sec Rhythmic flash elicited high-voltage driving responses from frontal regions and rhythmic jerks of the body. The patient smiled and laughed aloud during stimulation at 14 flashes per second, reporting vivid images. Finally, he stuck his handkerchief in his mouth to help him to stop laughing. Auditory stimulation induced sharp myoclonic jerks without significant EEG change.

COMMENT

This patient was seemingly at the mercy of polysensory, ideational, and affective perceptions which dominated consciousness with a continuous stream of bewildering intensely preoccupying experiences, many of which are strikingly reminiscent of the fragmentary perceptions characteristic of psychomotor–temporal lobe epilepsy auras. As the episode concluded following several days of neuroleptic medication at high dosage, the patient became hyperdocile, withdrawn, had little volition, and appeared to have suffered mild loss of intellectual incisiveness as well as moderate affective blunting. In sharp contrast to the postictal interpretation of patients with psychomotor automatisms, he remembered many aspects of his acute illness, including his own actions and beliefs, and, most important, was still not certain that the bizarre experiences were not really true. Seemingly, the perceptual and ideational inundation, the sense of panic, the absorption of interest are so totally convincing that they supersede the importance of external reality and thus lead to a search for meaning and significance, often satisfied by the invocation of external forces.

The early manifestations of an acute schizophrenic illness are dominated by sensory bewilderment, compelling preoccupations with internal somatic stimuli, and remembered or imagined ideational experience. Hallucinations and delusions of bodily functions as well as auditory, visual, tactile, olfactory, and gustatory sense, but above all the excessive rumination over stereotyped and often meaningless ideas preempt the paths to both awareness and bodily action, leading to unusual behavior. The coincident motor automatisms may represent responses to the sensory alterations or often seem to be due to inappropriate appearance or perseveration of habitual primitive behaviors or speech fragments. Thoughts and ideas are confused with memories of real experiences and the affective significance of sensory perceptions is unaccountably heightened and altered.

EXAMPLES

A patient who repeatedly rises from his chair and stands immobile and rigid for a few seconds explained that "someone put a machine under me." Another chronic schizophrenic, a former University honor student of history, after latencies of 40 to 50 seconds, solemnly replies with profoundly irrelevant banalities and clichés of academia in response to quite unrelated questions. Although occasionally reminiscent of the automatisms of psycho-motor epilepsy, such behaviors differ in that there may be altered but not lost consciousness and the veracity and the reality of the experience is indisputable for the schizophrenic patient. In contrast, the many similar experiences reported by patients with psychomotor epilepsy are nearly always viewed in retrospect with some detachment and are rarely incorporated into a delusory belief.

Repeated opportunities to record the scalp EEG during episodes of acute hallucinosis and agitation, including several 24–48 hour telemetered recordings during catatonic episodes, reveal no ictal pattern at the scalp, but only transient disappearance of background rhythms coincident with episodes of rapid eye movement, blinking, acute hallucinosis, or impulsive behavior (Figure 1). Monophasic sharp waves in the occipital region dur-

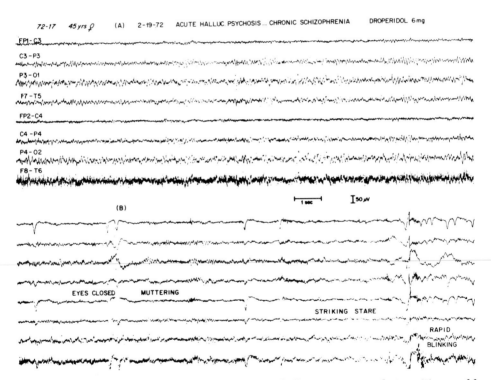

Figure 1. Scalp electroencephalogram during acute hallucinatory episode in a 45-year-old housewife with chronic schizophrenia. (A) Patient is quiet with eyes closed. Many sharp waves are superimposed on background of alpha activity from parieto-occipital regions. (B) "Paroxysmal sensory inundation" and auditory hallucinations. Alpha activity suddenly disappears, then patient opens her eyes, cannot or will not close them, mutters in agitated fashion as though replying to members of her family. Suddenly, her eyes become fixed, bulging, staring fearfully, followed by a paroxysm of rapid blinking during which she fails to respond.

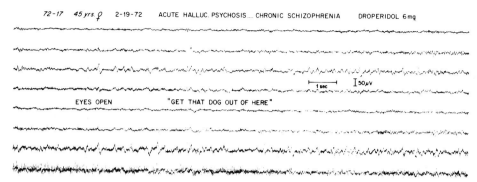

72-17 45 yrs. ♀ 2-19-72   ACUTE HALLUC. PSYCHOSIS.... CHRONIC SCHIZOPHRENIA   DROPERIDOL 6 mg

EYES OPEN   "GET THAT DOG OUT OF HERE"

Figure 2. Visual hallucinations Same patient and montage as in Figure 1, a few seconds later. Patient sits up suddenly and stares at corner of room where she apparently sees an imaginary animal. Note sharp irregular 50–60 μV potentials from parieto-occipital regions bilaterally, which in contrast to Figure 1A, when eyes were closed, now appear without background alpha.

ing such episodes resemble the "PGO spikes" recorded from pons, geniculate, and occipital regions during rapid eye movement (REM) sleep of the cat (Figure 2). During the hallucinatory episode these waves momentarily disappeared as the gaze became fixed (Figure 1B).

Electroencephalographic Studies

Photic stimulation may precipitate a paroxysmal EEG discharge during acute exacerbations of schizophrenia (Figure 3). Decline of photometrazol threshold for convulsive discharge to zero during catatonic states was described by Corriol and Bert in 1950 (17), and a review of the early literature indicates that catatonic episodes were reportedly not infrequently accompanied by, or terminated by, epileptic seizures (51). The case histories which we have examined suggest that many such attacks labeled seizures were not frank convulsions but rather episodes of intense psychomotor excitement, blocking, or immobility. The EEGs we have recorded from the scalp in many similar episodes are very different from those of epilepsy. The spikes over the temporal regions, in up to 25% of EEGs from patients with schizophrenia observed by Hill (42) and others, or from deep structures (39, 40) are consistent with an underlying abnormality of neuronal activity but need not necessarily be identified with an epileptic process.

Chronic Schizophrenia

Schizophrenias of insidious onset or chronic course display less florid but highly distinctive evidence of loss of integration of sensory and associative patterns characteristic of excitation or ablation of limbic structures. The pervasiveness of intrusive obligatory sexual ruminations, hallucinations, and delusions of genital manipulation suggest an ideational hypersexuality consistent with the experimental evidence of genital sensation evoked during electrical or cholinergic stimulation of septal areas in monkey and man

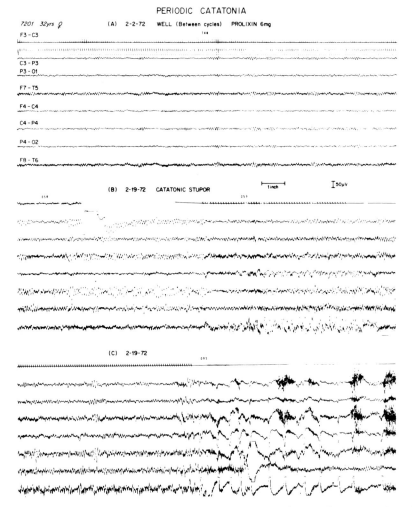

Figure 3. Case 2. Thirty-two-year-old former secretary with periodic catatonic episodes and chronic progressive schizophrenia. (A) Response to rhythmic photic stimulation (12 flashes/second, top line) is unremarkable during usual state between catatonic exacerbations. (B) Catatonic stupor, medication unchanged. Patient appears preoccupied, walks and obeys automatically, replies monosyllabically, displays waxy flexibility, catatonic postures, poor eye contact. Twelve per second flash (top line) now precipitates paroxysmal hypersynchrony of theta frequencies over right temporal region (electrodes F8-T6). (C) Continuation of B. As rhythmic 12 per second flash is sustained, a burst of irregular theta and sharp waves appears from all scalp leads, continues briefly as flash is terminated, and is followed by paroxysmal blinking and chewing. The electroencephalogram following such episodes displays no postictal features. Patient unable to describe what happened.

(40, 59). Symptoms reminiscent of postamygdalotomy hypersexuality, apathy, psychic blindness, as well as attention and phagic disturbances described by Kluver and Bucy (52) and by Schreiner and Kling (78) are represented in the following patient.

CASE 2

Patient P.P. is a thirty-four-year-old ex-secretary, first admitted to a psychiatric hospital at age 21 following progressive social withdrawal, loss of will, increasing fearfulness, and sexual preoccupation. During the subsequent 12 years in hospital, she gradually regressed to an indifferent, apathetic state of idleness punctuated by episodic stereotyped pacing, rocking, and chewing. During the long course of her illness, her chronic affective devastation has been relieved for short periods following electroconvulsive therapy or change in antipsychotic medication. For a few days or weeks, she is then able to type copy accurately and quickly, to participate in drama groups and other ward activities, run errands, etc. Every 3 to 4 weeks, however, often just prior to her menses, she begins to regress, becomes mute, avoids social contacts, appears restless and preoccupied, paces the halls, loses interest in or eye contact with others, is indifferent to smoke in her eyes or burns of her skin from cigarettes, eats prodigiously and indiscriminately both edibles and inedibles, and unless reminded, soils and wets herself and is indifferent to dirty, disheveled, often bizarre, dress. For 4 to 8 days, she demonstrates episodic momentary psychomotor blocking, during which she seems out of contact, chews, swallows, and fails to reply unless forcibly encouraged or tempted by food. Waxy flexibility, automatic obedience, and echolalia alternate with extremes of affection during which she indiscriminately hugs and kisses friends and strangers alike. Her typing of copy, usually precise, accurate and speedy, is now accomplished without regard to margins, with repetition of words, and occasionally by intrusion of material from her own thoughts. During all these evidences of polysensory agnosia, consciousness is "clear" in that structured questions devoid of emotional importance can be readily answered. Neurological examination during her well periods is unremarkable except for blunted affect, hyperdocility, loss of ability to keep her mind to a steady idea such as the continuity of a story, and unusual difficulty in map-reading and construction. During the acute catatonic exacerbations, bilateral grasp and palmomental reflexes are obtained. Radiological and routine laboratory studies are unremarkable except for a flat glucose tolerance test during the catatonic period. After several months of treatment with high doses of thyroid hormone [as recommended by Gjessing (33) in periodic catatonia], she became hostile, combative, and required full restraints. An incessant stream of stereotyped repetitive phrases during this period was concerned with references to sexual activity and fears of death. Waking EEGs made during relatively well periods are entirely normal and demonstrate no unusual susceptibility to photic stimulation. Sleep tracings reveal a few small sharp spikes over the temporal regions. During the catatonic stuporous phase the background EEG is relatively unchanged but photic stimulation precipitates high-voltage paroxysmal discharges over either temporal region (Figure 3). Such episodes are often followed by smacking and chewing behavior and distracted consciousness from which she is easily diverted. Similar oral activity occurs frequently in the absence of EEG paroxysms or photic stimulation.

Addition of anticonvulsant drugs to the neuroleptic regimen of these patients with blocking, chewing, or blinking automatisms has not decreased the occurrence of the latter nor in any way alleviated the subjective and objective signs and symptoms of their schizophrenia, whereas the antipsychotic neuroleptics usually have had a dramatic ameliorative effect. This fact, coupled with the markedly different EEG from that recorded during psychomotor seizures, the readiness with which exacerbations and remissions of symptoms can be induced by environmental factors, and the loss of reality orientation in the schizophrenic interpretation of experiences, sharply separate the epileptic and schizophrenic disorders. Although the psychomotor blocking episodes with chewing and swallowing resemble epileptic automatisms of temporal lobe epilepsy, the differences noted above seem to require the use of similar anatomical structures but to invoke quite different physiological mechanisms in the two processes.

EXPERIMENTAL STUDIES

Transient disturbances in behavior and affect following prolonged electrical stimulation of limbic structures or protracted generalized convulsions are well known. In 1963, Grossman reported permanent behavioral alteration in cats following recovery from prolonged severe generalized seizures produced by instillation of minute amounts of carbachol in amygdala bilaterally (36). Such animals behaved relatively normally unless they were approached by other animals or by man, when they attacked viciously. There is abundant evidence that marked change in electrical properties and even histology may occur in regions "downstream" from or contralateral to a primary epileptic focus or when certain regions, such as amygdala are subjected to repeated electrical stimulation (19, 35, 67). Among the most interesting of these studies is the work of Guzman-Flores (37) who recently described changes in unit activity in hypothalamus and contralateral amygdala following generalized seizures induced by penicillin instillation of amygdala nucleus unilaterally. Following recovery from such seizures, cats received parenteral progesterone for several days, after which they became permanently "psychotic," appeared to hallucinate, displayed excessive fear, and attacked viciously if approached by other animals or by man. Only cats in which sustained seizures had occurred displayed such behavior following the steroid. Extracellular unit activity recorded from chronically implanted microelectrodes demonstrated bursts of high-frequency activity in both amygdala and other limbic structures during the epileptic seizures in association with characteristic high-voltage spike-and-wave activity recorded by gross EEG electrodes. In contrast, during the chronic, postictal, hyperirritable psychotic state, the surface EEG displayed only a moderate increase in fast activity and the extracellular microelectrodes demonstrated a steady increase in the rate of unit discharge without bursting quality (Figure 4).

During either the epileptic or hyperirritable state, there was also a distinct change in the rate of firing from units in the reticular formation of the brainstem, suggesting a possible substrate for altered "consciousness" and disturbance in regulatory function. Guzman-Flores' studies have important implications for many unexplained cyclic phenomena characteristic of both schizophrenia and epilepsy. Evidently excessive neuronal discharge, although universally present in epilepsy, is by no means pathognomonic

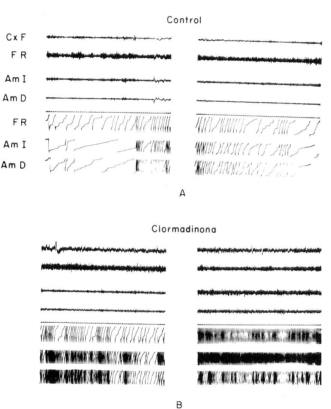

Figure 4. Samples of typical activity found in cortical and subcortical electroencephalogram (EEG) and extracellular microelectrodes in cat following recovery from seizures induced by penicillin in right amygdala. (A) Control recordings prior to administration of a synthetic progesterone compound (Clormadinoma). Top four lines of each section represent conventional EEG; fifth line is time in seconds; bottom four lines record integrated multiunit activity. CxF, frontal cortex; FR, reticular formation; AMI, left amygdala; Am D = right amygdala. (B) Two samples of EEG and unit activity from implanted electrodes in same postictal animal following administration of Clormadinona, 10 mg/kg. Cat appears hypervigilant, hallucinated, and attacks if approached. Note modest increase in fast activity in EEG but striking increase in rate of unit discharge. (Courtesy of Dr. Carlos Guzman-Flores, Mexico City, Mexico.)

of epilepsy, that is, it is a necessary but not sufficient cause. When excessive discharge was confined to subcortical structures and was steady rather than bursting, neither the gross EEG spike nor spontaneous disturbance in behavior was observed. However, use of the system involved, for example, induced by external stimuli, provoked marked affective and behavioral anomalies, which, as we have noted in previous studies, may be associated with abnormal EEG events (82, 84). Clinical and electrical parallels to acute and chronic psychotic disturbances in man are compelling. Recent demonstrations of altered unit firing patterns in limbic structures in response to local hormone effects in normal animals (32, 57) raise the question as to whether the unusual electrical and behavioral changes induced by hormones following seizures represent examples of deafferentation supersensitivity to local hormone and transmitter effects or relate to the temporal association of endocrine changes and occurrence of seizure phenomena and psychoses.

PHARMACOLOGICAL STUDIES

One of the most striking events in the search for cause and treatment of schizophrenia has been the development over the past 20 years of a series of antipsychotic drugs, the efficacy of which is in general proportional to, although not necessarily dependent on, their tendency to induce a variety of motor disturbances long known to be associated with Parkinsonism and other disorders of the basal ganglia. Many of these agents also have a tendency to lower the threshold to epileptic discharge but this epileptogenic effect seems much less closely related to therapeutic efficacy against the psychoses than is the case for the extrapyramidal effects. Indeed, examination of the relative potency of the various neuroleptics in relation to antipsychotic and epileptogenic properties and relative blocking effect on norepinephrine (NE) and dopamine (DA), respectively [as measured by acid metabolite and histochemical studies (4, 12, 25, 30, 60, 72, 73)], indicates that in general the antipsychotic drugs with maximum anti-NE effect (promazine, chlorpromazine) are less potent antipsychotics but more epileptogenic than agents with principally DA blocking and extrapyramidal effects (86, 89).

The demonstration by Hornykiewicz (43) that paralysis agitans is associated with a significantly decreased DA content in caudate nucleus, secondary to degeneration of axon terminals of a DA pathway originating in substantia nigra, raised the distinct possibility that certain psychoses, including schizophrenia, the early symptoms of which are often dramatically alleviated by agents that maximally block DA receptors, may be closely related to a disturbance of DA (or derivative NE) production, inactivation, or receptor sensitivity. Support for such a hypothesis is strengthened by the precipitation of frank hallucinatory, paranoid, or schizophreniform psychoses in a significant proportion of individuals receiving L-dopa therapy and amphetamines (9, 13, 56). Experimental evidence of pharmacological reciprocity which may relate to competition for receptor sites or metabolic routes by DA and 5-hydroxytryptamine (5-HT) is supported by the amelioration of L-dopa-induced psychoses by L-tryptophan, the precursor of serotonin (7) and the exacerbation of extrapyramidal signs by the same agent (15). The psychotogenic effect of amphetamines, which potentiate NE and especially DA at central synapses (31), and the hallucinogenic effect of serotonin-blocking agents such as D-lysergic acid diethylamide (LSD) (1) contrast with the general decrease in convulsive threshold induced by agents that deplete catecholamines or augment serotonin (5-HT) (55, 93). On the other hand, diphenylhydantoin is reported to potentiate NE in cerebral cortex (38).

Kety and co-workers (50) demonstrated that one effect of convulsive therapies is an increased turnover of catecholamines, a role also served by the neuroleptic antipsychotic agents that block central catecholamine receptor sites (18). A similar function may be served by endogenous epilepsies. These observations arouse new interest in the relationship between catecholamines, schizophrenia, epilepsy, and disorders of the basal ganglia.

ANATOMICAL AND HISTOCHEMICAL STUDIES

Introduction of histofluorescence methods for demonstration of intraneuronal catechol- and indoleamines in the central nervous system by Carlsson and his collaborators (11) has demonstrated a distinctive anatomic distribution of NE-, DA- and 5-HT-containing neurons. Arising from specific nuclear groups almost entirely restricted to the brain stem (with the notable exception of the dopaminergic hypophyseal–infundibular pathway and specific cells of retina and olfactory bulb), the NE and 5-HT axons descend to the spinal cord (where DA terminals have not been described) and terminate on cell bodies in lateral columns and anterior and dorsal horns (88). There are two major ascending norepinephrine systems arising in locus coeruleus and medial reticular formation, respectively, and proceeding rostrally within the medial forebrain bundle to hypothalamus, median eminence, amygdala, on the one hand, and the entire neocortex on the other (Figure 5).

Two major ascending pathways from cell bodies of origin in brain stem have also been identified for the dopamine system: (a) the well-known nigrostriatal tract originating in fluorescent cells of *substantia nigra*, the axons of which ascend principally, if not exclusively, to terminate on small interneurons of *caudate nucleus* and *putamen* (94) and (b) a second major dopaminergic pathway that originates from cells of the *ventral tegmental nucleus* of *Tsai*, medial and rostral to *substantia nigra* and from which axons ascend uncrossed in the medial forebrain bundle in close proximity to the nigrostriatal tract, terminating in a rich network of DA endings in the *olfactory tubercle,* in the *nucleus accumbens septi,* and in the *bed*

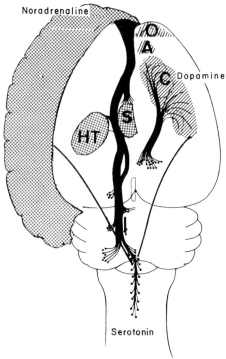

Figure 5. Diagrammatic representation contrasting termination of principal *noradrenergic* pathways in cortex, septum (S), and hypothalamus (HT) with *dopaminergic* terminals in caudate–putamen (C), accumbens–bed nucleus of stria terminalis (A), and olfactory tubercle (O). Serotonergic fluorescence is reported at all these sites. [Adapted from Ungerstedt (88).]

nucleus of the stria terminalis (3, 22, 88). Whereas histofluorescence techniques demonstrate little NE in basal ganglia, DA fluorescence is similarly absent in neocortex, allocortex, hippocampus, and amygdala (with the exception of central nucleus of amygdala which is architecturally and ontogenetically striatal in origin and, significantly, does receive dopaminergic terminals).

In contrast, serotonergic fibers originate further caudally in the median raphé of the pons, descend in spinal cord to innervate the same area in which NE axons have been identified, and ascend from the more rostral raphé in the medial forebrain bundle after passing through interpeduncular nucleus, to terminate on both striatal and cortical sites as well as throughout the limbic and hypothalamic regions. As Dahlstrom (21) has pointed out, monoamine-containing neurons belong to phylogenetically ancient systems, including most invertebrates, as attested to by their localization and arborization in lower brain stem of mammals as well as their role in modulating such basic adaptive processes as arousal, sleep, locomotion, thermal regulation, defense, and reproduction.

Although the necessity for extremely fresh material for accurate use of the histofluorescence method presents formidable problems for the investigation of the disposition of central amines in the human brain, Constantinidis and co-workers (16) confirmed that the characteristic green fluorescence in human material is distributed similarly to that found in the rat and drew attention to the DA fluorescence in infundibulum, caudate-putamen, and particularly in *nucleus accumbens septi.*

Demonstration of these three ascending monoaminergic systems and the rapid development of increasingly potent and specific psychopharmacological blocking agents, potentiators, and precursors have revolutionized many concepts of cerebral anatomy, physiology, and clinical neuropsychiatry. With respect to the possible relationship between temporal lobe epilepsy and psychosis, the relevant anatomical and neurophysiological data suggest that the second ascending dopaminergic pathway, arising in ventral tegmental nucleus among the fibers of the medial forebrain bundle and terminating in limbic striatum may be of particular importance in the regulation of limbic system function and, thus, be of special interest in analysis of possible relationships between these clinical syndromes.

Mesolimbic (Tegmento–Accumbens) Dopamine System

Nauta (70) has called attention to several striking parallels between the nigrostriatal and tegmento–accumbens systems. In addition to the common dopamine fluorescence (essentially unique with the exception of the hypothalamic hypophyseal pathway), both systems originate among the melanin-containing cells in midbrain tegmentum and terminate on small interneurons of neo- and limbic striatum, which, in turn, project to architecturally similar DA-free outflow systems. Histologically, the three DA-receiving structures at the anterior pole of the caudate nucleus, comprising the limbic striatum or olfactory striatum, share with the neostriatum a histological structure characterized by a great number of small, short-axoned, Golgi Type 2 cells with spiny dendrites upon which converge afferents from cortex and thalamus and DA axons from brain stem. The cortically derived axons tend to travel perpendicular to dendrites of striatal interneurons, contacting many cells by synapses as they pass. Projecting out of the nucleus are large spindle-shaped neurons with smooth dendrites which comprise 1–2% of the total neuron population of striatum (29, 48).

The accumbens complex, located at a crossroad of olfactory tract, septum, pyriform cortex, and amygdala, poses a functional dilemma to anatomists. First described by Meynert (65) who considered the region to be the anterior polar area of caudate nucleus, Ziehen (95) gave the name *nucleus accumbens septi* because the nuclear group appeared to be "leaning against" the septum. Histologically and histochemically two parts are discernible: an outer, less cellular region that merges with caudate nucleus and contains DA terminals and a denser inner region confluent with septum which is noradrenergic (3). Stimulation of the latter causes ovulation in the rabbit, and cells in the adjacent islands of Calleja have recently been claimed to project to hypothalamic centers responsible for control of gonadotropic-releasing factors and specifically and avidly take up radioactive estrogen granules following parenteral injection (53). Although traditionally assimilated into the taxonomy of the olfactory brain, there is little evidence that an olfactory function is subserved by limbic striatum in higher mammals, a conjecture supported by the persistence of these structures in anolfactory cetaceans (70).

Topographic Projections on Accumbens–Caudate Crescent

Kemp and Powell (49) have recently confirmed earlier evidence (23, 24, 91) of an orderly topographic projection of nearly the entire cerebral mantle to the caudate–putamen complex, such that premotor and motor areas project to the head of the caudate whereas parietal and occipital areas project to ventral and posterior regions of the complex, a topography in which "only the projections from the temporal lobe remain unclear." This orderly topographic relationship between neocortex and caudoputamen is maintained in the projection of striatum to globus pallidus, the lateral segment of which projects to subthalamic nucleus and the medial segment to the thalamic nuclei ventrolateralis, centrum medianum, and to the midbrain tegmentum (71). In rather striking parallel, the "nucleus capitis caudati," that is, the olfactory tubercle–accumbens–bed nucleus complex, receives projections from the primitive olfactory cortex of the pyriform lobe, from subcallosal regions of the cingulate gyrus, from septum, intralaminar, and anterior thalamic nuclei, and from amygdala and hippocampus, both of which are at least in part derivatives of the limbic cortex (62). Thus, the amygdala projects to the bed nucleus via the stria terminalis, the hippocampus projects to accumbens via fornix, and the pyriform cortex to olfactory tubercle and septum (68–71, 92).

The entire system of neo- and limbic striatal structures comprised by accumbens complex, caudate, and their contributory afferents may be visualized as two open fans, the folds of one of which represents fibers converging from the wide neocortical mantle onto the caudoputamen, whereas those of the other, an anteroventrolateral fan, converge upon the *accumbens, tubercle,* and *bed nucleus* of *stria terminalis* from allocortical structures and from the amygdala. After entering the caudate–accumbens crescent, the cortical and thalamic afferents traverse a grid of hyperpolarized dendrites, apparently synapsing on spines of the same neurons that receive dopamine afferents from brain stem. To carry the "fan" analogy a little further, the confluent folds collect into two "handles," one emerging from the globus pallidus as the ansa lenticularis, whereas the other, from the "ventral fan" of limbic structures, emerges from the tubercle–accumbens complex via substantia innominata to course toward hypothalamus and frontal lobe (Figure 6.)

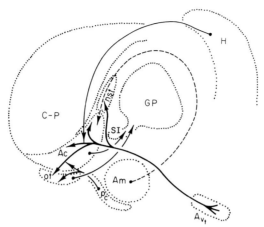

Figure 6. Dopaminergic input from ventral tegmental area of Tsai (Avt) to accumbens (Ac), olfactory tubercle (ot), and bed nucleus of stria terminalis (nst) "mesolimbic system"), which, in turn, receive afferents from pyriform cortex (pc), hippocampus (H), and amygdala (Am). Efferents from accumbens complex pass through an anteroventral extension of globus pallidus (GP), the substantia innominata (SI), en route to hypothalamus and frontal lobe. CP = caudate–putamen. [Diagram by Nauta (70).]

PHYSIOLOGICAL STUDIES

The ascending fibers of the nigrostriatal tract, arising from a few thousand dopaminergic cells in ventral midbrain and widely distributed to dendrites of striatum, have been shown by Buchwald *et al.* (8, 45) to exercise a specific effect on membrane potential and duration of postsynaptic potentials of caudate cells which respond to cortical and thalamic afferents. The UCLA investigators have shown that neurons of caudate nucleus fire infrequently, are strongly hyperpolarized during the resting state, and are further hyperpolarized by cortical stimulation. Extracellular recordings from nucleus accumbens by Matthysse and Schnaas (61) also indicate sparse firing, the pattern of which is altered by stimulation of ventral tegmental area. Altered cortical potentials to peripheral stimuli were recorded following caudate stimulation by Krauthamer and Albe-Fessard (54). Cholinergic and electrical stimulation of caudate nucleus in waking animals induces circling movements, drowsing, or sleep spindles and inhibition of spontaneous and cortically induced movement (8, 64, 81). According to Koikegami (53), electrical stimulation of nucleus accumbens is followed by increased respiration, mydriasis, defecation, and ovulation. Dopamine placed directly in caudate nucleus of freely moving cats causes bizarre stereotyped behavior; NE was without similar effect (75). Catecholamine (DA, NE, epinephrine) instillation in accumbens and septum of man had little effect according to Heath, in contrast to cholinergic or electrical stimulation, which reportedly induced intensely pleasureable orgastic effect (40). Injection of L-dopa, potentiation of dopaminergic effect by amphetamines, or by DA receptor sensitization with apomorphine induces a remarkable series of stereotyped behaviors in rodents and other animals, including continuous sniffing, compulsive gnawing, and bizarre forms of social interaction. Rats so treated react to sound by running around in their cage until they meet another rat, then the pair stand on hind legs with noses in close contact making rhythmic synchronous movements with their front legs and hissing. This behavior can be blocked by low doses of the potent neuroleptic, haloperidol (75).

Caudate–Accumbens: A Central Gating Mechanism for Neo- and Paleocortex?

The crescentic nuclear mass comprised by limbic and neostriata, a second, inner limbus within the limbic arch, strategically interposed between cortical and thalamic suprastructures and final common paths to brain stem, hypothalamus, and frontal lobe, poses a mystery to clinicians and physiologists for whom the striking developments in neuropharmacology and histochemistry of the past two decades are beginning to provide new answers and are raising numerous new questions. The presence of a second dopaminergic pathway to an area contiguous with the head of the caudate nucleus and which so resembles neostriatum architecturally, permits the hypothesis that olfactory tubercle–accumbens–bed nucleus form a unit functionally parallel for the limbic cortex, including amygdala and hippocampus, to caudate–putamen for neocortex, the inputs and outputs providing the essential difference. The unique anatomical interposition of caudate–accumbens between cortex and brain stem–hypothalamus and the orderly topographic projection thereon of afferents from motor, sensory, association, and visceral afferents suggest that the striata may act as a giant sieve or filter through which the wide input from neocortex and limbic cortex funnel for special "processing" by amine-mediated interneurons, for which serotonin and dopamine systems reciprocally set membrane threshold.

The ascending brain stem monoaminergic, strionigral and mesolimbic axons and their probable recurrent branches or return loops to cells of origin in brain stem could thus function as self-regulating servosystems in which the DA and 5-HT terminals in striatum exert a "push–pull" biasing effect on discharge threshold of interneurons which, in turn, receive the multiplicity of signals converging on caudate–accumbens complex from wide areas of neocortex and limbic cortex and from amygdala and thalamus.

The inhibitory and regulatory role assigned to caudate–putamen on the basis of physiological, ablative, and clinical studies has traditionally emphasized motor function but, more recently, has been extended to include the processing of information received from visual and associative cortex (24, 49). The anatomic and neurophysiological parallels emphasized in the preceding paragraphs lead to the suggestion that the accumbens complex may exert a gating or filtering function over affective, ideational, and visceral perceptions and species-specific automatisms funneled from limbic structures en route to final paths in hypothalamus and frontal lobe. The normally hyperpolarized cells of caudate–putamen–accumbens complex, whose threshold may be influenced by the reciprocal action of DA and 5-HT terminals synapsing upon interneurones that receive axons from neocortex and limbic cortex, could thus affect the selection of endogenous and exogenous stimuli for access to attention and behavior.

If the hypothesized neostriatal gate normally limits inundation by general sensory and motor afferents via caudate–putamen interneurons, the limbic striatal structures may be expected to serve a similar function with respect to the access to consciousness and action of peculiarly temporal lobe mechanisms, such as auditory and visual memories and species-specific survival automatisms.

Epilepsy and Schizophrenia: Phenomenological Considerations

Intrusion of endogenous percepts and behavioral automatisms in psychomotor epilepsy secondary to "excessive neuronal discharge" of cortical structures seems one step removed from the similar sensory deceptions of psychosis, which more often represent an enhancement or distortion of various aspects of perceived experience. The evidence presented suggests that an explanation for the disturbance in selection and amplification of various aspects of endogenous and exogenous percepts in these disorders may lie in the overactivity of the cortex in seizures, and in defective regulation "downstream" from the cortex in psychosis.

Clinical support for a dopamine-biased limbic striatal "gate" between limbic inputs and perception–behavior outputs emerges with particular clarity in the study of schizophrenia. As noted above, the "dopamine hypothesis" for this disorder originated principally from the observation that neuroleptic agents most effective against the acute symptoms of schizophrenia were those that had generally the highest incidence and severity of extrapyramidal side effects. [European psychopharmacologists have emphasized an even stronger relationship between antipsychotic potency and antagonism to DA-induced stereotyped or cataleptic behavior in experimental animals (31, 46).]

In contrast, the epileptogenic effect of neuroleptic agents appears to be maximum in the weakest antipsychotic neuroleptics, which also have least extrapyramidal side effect or anti-DA action, suggesting important physiological and chemical distinctions between schizophrenia and epilepsy. Although most patients with seizures appear to be protected against the chronic perceptual, affective, and ideational deceptions which compromise the sense of reality in schizophrenia, data have been presented which indicate that repeated or prolonged seizures may be followed by permanent alterations in distant structures. Electrical stimulation and hormone effects as well as the striking changes in brainstem amines during maturation and sleep also influence the onset of disturbances in amine-modulated systems (58, 83).

Although approximately half of the patients with psychomotor epilepsy who come to surgery or autopsy demonstrate some pathology of the temporal lobe (28), for most of the idiopathic epilepsies, no etiology has been demonstrated. There is, however, circumstantial evidence that a deficiency in the brain stem arousal system is also a factor in permitting bilaterally synchronous high-voltage activity from cortex associated with "essential" or genetic epilepsy. Thus, paroxysmal and convulsive responses in the EEG to rhythmic photic stimulation, characteristic of approximately one-third of patients with generalized epilepsy, are potentiated by depressants delivered to brain stem via vertebral artery (6, 34), and experimental lesions of midbrain tegmentum confer susceptibility to photically induced spike-wave in animals (44, 85).

Clinical observations led Mettler in 1955 (64) to propose that there was an important relationship between schizophrenia and disturbed function of corpus striatum. Psychopharmacological, histochemical, and electroencephalographic data assembled in this report support such a hypothesis but suggest that the disturbance is primarily in the most anterior part of striatum which receives afferent input from limbic structures. It must be admitted that direct evidence in support of this hypothesis is sparse. Although several relatively recent studies report unusually formed small cells in substantia innominata of patients with schizophrenia (10, 90), pathological abnormalities have been described by various observers from so many different regions of the brain in this disorder that skepticism must prevail until further evidence is forthcoming. From the electroencephalographer's standpoint, it is of interest that Heath (40) and, more recently, Hanley and co-workers from the University of California, Los Angeles (39), reported spikes in schizophrenic patients uniquely from chronic electrodes in the so-called septum but actually located 2–4 millimeters from the midline in the nucleus accumbens (41).

In conclusion, although both psychomotor seizures and schizophrenia share a similar clinical phenomenology of altered affect, distorted percepts, and stereotyped behaviors which may originate in or be interpreted through limbic and temporal structures, the two maladies appear to be derangements of separate anatomical and biochemical systems. One is primarily cortical and, thus, more influenced by brain stem NE-5-HT modulation; the other is predominantly limbic striatal, and in receipt of DA and 5-HT terminals from brain stem fluorescent nuclei. Clinical and experimental studies indicate important interactions between these systems.

SUMMARY

The evidence for a relationship between schizophrenia and psychomotor epilepsy is considered in the light of clinical and EEG similarities and recent developments in psychopharmacology and histochemistry. The contrasting distribution of dopamine and norepinephrine terminals to striatum and cortex, respectively, and the relative influence of neuroleptic agents on these monoamines, on psychotic symptoms, and on convulsive threshold has led to a hypothesis that the limbic striatum, which receives input from limbic cortex, amygdala, and hippocampus serves a "gating" function for impulses arising in these structures similar to that which may obtain for caudate–putamen for pathways converging thereon from neocortex. Disturbance in this function related to faulty production of, sensitivity to, or inactivation of local monamines in limbic striatum may influence the threshold for transmission of peculiarly limbic affective, interpretative, and behavioral patterns transmitted by predominantly cholinergic pathways from cortical structures to final common paths in consciousness and behavior.

REFERENCES

1. Aghajanian, G. K., Foote, W. E., and Sheard, M. H., Lysergic acid diethylamide: Sensitive neuronal units in the midbrain raphe. *Science*, 1968, **161:** 706–708.
2. Alström, C. H., A study of epilepsy in its chemical, social and genetic aspects. *Acta Psychiatr. Scand., Suppl.*, 1950, **63:** 1–284.
3. Andén, N. E., Dahlström, A., Fuxe, K., and Larsson, K., Mapping out of catecholamine and 5-hydroxy-tryptamine neurons innervating the telencephalon and diencephalon. *Life Sci.*, 1965, 4: 1275–1279.
4. Andén, N. E., Roos, B. E. and Werdinius, B., Effects of chlorpromazine, haloperidol and reserpine on the levels of phenolic acids in rabbit corpus striatum. *Life Sci.*, 1964, **3:** 149–158.
5. Bartlet, J. E. A., Chronic psychosis following epilepsy. *Am. J. Psychiatry*, 1957, **114:** 338–343.
6. Bennett, F. E., Intracarotid and intra vertebral metrazol in petit mal epilepsy. *Neurology (Minneap.)*, 1953, **3:** 668–673.
7. Birkmayer, W., Personal communication.
8. Buchwald, N. A., Hull, C. D., Vernon, L. M., and Barnardi, G. A., physiological and psychological aspects of basal ganglia functions. In: *Psychotropic Drugs and Dysfunctions of the Basal Ganglia* (G. Crane and R. Gardner, Jr., Eds.). U.S. Govt. Printing Office, Washington, D.C., 1969: Publ. Health Serv. Publ. No. 1938: 82–91.
9. Bunney, W. E., Present status of psychological reaction to L-dopa. *Am. J. Psychiatry*, 1970, **127:** 361–362.
10. Buttlar-Brentano, K. von, Pathohistologische Feststellungen am basalkern Schizophrener. *J. Nerv. Ment. Dis.*, 1952, **116:** 646–653.
11. Carlsson, A., Falck, B., Hillarp, N. R., Torp, A., Histochemical localization at the cellular level of hypothalamic noradrenalin. *Acta Physiol. Scand.*, 1962, **54:** 385–386.
12. Carlsson, A., and Lindqvist, M., Effect of chlorpromazine or haloperidol on formation of 3-methoxytyramine and normetanephrine in mouse brain. *Acta Pharmacol. Toxicol.*, 1963, **20:** 140–144.

13. Celesia, G. G., and Varr, A. N., Psychosis and other psychiatric manifesta-
    tions of levodopa therapy. *Arch. Neurol.*, 1970, **23**: 193–200.
14. Chapman, J., The early symptoms of schizophrenia. *Br. J. Psychiatry*, 1966,
    112: 225–251.
15. Chase, T. N., Ng, L. K. Y., and Watanabe, A. M., Parkinson's Disease:
    Modifications by 5-hydroxytryptophane. *Neurology* (*Minneap.*), 1972,
    22: 479–484.
16. Constantinidis, J., Tissot, R., de la Torre, J. C., and Geissbuhler, F., Essai
    de localisation des monoamines dans l'hypothalamus humain. *Pathol.
    Biol.* (*Paris*) 1969, **17**: 361–363.
17. Corriol, J., and Bert, J., Electroencéphalographie et schizophrénie. Etude
    des seuils convulsivants. *Ann. Med. Psychol.* (*Paris*), 1950, **108**: 588–597.
18. Corrodi, H., Fuxe, K., and Hökfelt, T., The effect of neuroleptics on the
    activity of central catecholamine neurones. *Life Sci.*, 1967, **6**: 767–774.
19. Crowell, R. M., Wyss, F. T., Fankhauser, H., and Akert, K., Spontaneous
    cure of limbic system epilepsy in the cat. *Epilepsia*, 1968, **9**: 291–301.
20. Currie, S., Heathfield, K. W. G., Henson, R. A., and Scott, D. F., Clinical
    course and prognosis of temporal lobe epilepsy. A survey of 666 patients.
    Brain, 1970, **94**: 173–190.
21. Dahlström, A., Fluorescence histochemistry of monoamines in the ceneral
    nervous system. Discussion. In: *Basic Mechanisms of the Epilepsies*
    (H. H. Jasper, A. A. Ward, and A. Pope, Eds.). Churchill, London, and
    Little, Brown, Boston, 1969: 212–214.
22. Dahlstrom, A., Fuxe, K., Olson, L., and Ungerstedt, U., Ascending systems
    of catecholamine neurons from the lower brainstem. *Acta Physiol.
    Scand.*, 1964, **62**: 485–486.
23. Daitz, H. M., and Powell, T. P. S., Studies of the connexions of the fornix
    system. *J. Neurol. Neurosurg. Psychiatry*, 1954, **17**: 75–82.
24. Denny-Brown, D., *The Basal Ganglia and Their Relation to Disorders of
    Movement.* Oxford, London, and New York, 1962.
25. Ernst, A. M., and Smelik, P. G., Site of action of dopamine and apomorphine
    in compulsive gnawing behavior in rats. *Experientia*, 1966, **22**: 837–838.
26. Ervin, F., Epstein, A. W., and King, H. E., Behavior of epileptic and non-
    epileptic patients with temporal spikes. *Arch. Neurol. Psychiatry*, 1955,
    74: 488–497.
27. Flor-Henry, P., Psychosis and temporal lobe epilepsy. *Epilepsia*, 1969, **10**:
    363–395.
28. Falconer, M. A., and Cavanagh, J. B., Clinico-pathological considerations
    of temporal lobe epilepsy due to small focal lesions. *Brain*, 1959, **82**:
    483–504.
29. Fox, C. A., Hillman, D. E., Siegsmund, K. A., and Sether, L. A., The primate
    globus pallidus and its feline and avian homologues, a Golgi and elec-
    tron microscopic study. In: *Evolution of the Forebrain* (R. Hassler
    and H. Stephan, Eds.). Thieme, Stuttgart, 1966: 237–248.
30. Fuxe, K., Discussion: Histological and molecular biochemistry. In: *Modern
    Problems of Pharmacopsychiatry* (D. P. Bobon, P. A. J. Janssen and
    J. Bobon, Eds.). Karger, Basel, 1970: Vol. 5: 6–8, 121–124.
31. Fuxe, K., and Ungerstedt, U., Histochemical, biochemical and functional

studies on central monoamine neurons after acute and chronic amphetamine administration. In: *International Symposium on Amphetamines and Related Compounds* (E. Costa and S. Garattini, Eds.). Raven Press, New York, 1970: 257.

32. Gerlach, J. L., and McEwen, B. S., Rat brain binds adrenal steroid hormone: Radioautography of hippocampus with corticosterone. *Science*, 1972, **175**: 1133–1136.

33. Gjessing, R., Disturbances of somatic functions in catatonia with periodic course and their compensation. *J. Ment. Sci.* 1938, **84**: 608–621.

34. Gloor, P. Generalized cortico-reticular epilepsies. *Epilepsia*, 1968, **9**: 249–263.

35. Goddard, G. V., McIntyre, D. C., and Leech, C. K., A permanent change in brain function resulting from daily electrical stimulation *Exp. Neurol.*, 1969, **25**: 295–330.

36. Grossman, S. P., Chemically induced epileptiform seizures in the cat. *Science*, 1963, **142**: 409–411.

37. Guzman-Flores, C., Progesterone-induced chronic behaviour disorders following amygdala seizures in the cat. *5th Natl. Congr. Physiol. Sci., 1970*, Tepic, Mexico.

38. Hadfield, M. G., Uptake and binding of catecholamines. *Arch. Neurol.*, 1972, **26**: 78–84.

39. Hanley, J., Berkhout, J., Crandall, P., Rickles, W. R., and Walter, R. D., Spectral characteristics of EEG activity accompanying deep spiking in a patient with schizophrenia. *Electroenceph. clin. Neurophysiol.*, 1970, **28**: 90.

40. Heath, R. G., *Studies in Schizophrenia*. Harvard Univ. Press, Cambridge, 1959.

41. Heath, R. G., Personal communications, 1972.

42. Hill, D., EEG in episodic psychotic and psychopathic behavior. *Electroenceph. clin. Neurophysiol.*, 1952, **4**: 419–442.

43. Hornykiewicz, O., Die topische Localisation das verhalten von Noradrenalin un Dopamin (3-hydroxytyramin) in der Substantia nigra des normalen und Parkinsonkranken Menschen. *Wien. Klin. Wochenschr.*, 1963, **75**: 309–312.

44. Hubel, D. H., and Nauta, W. J. H., Electrocorticograms of cats with chronic lesions of rostral mesencephalic tegmentum, *Fed. Proc.*, 1960, **19**: 287.

45. Hull, C. D., Bernardi, G., and Buchwald, N. A., Intracellular responses of caudate neurons to brainstem stimulation. *Brain Res.*, 1970, **22**: 163–179.

46. Janssen, P. A. J., Chemical and pharmacological classification of neuroleptics. In: *The Neuroleptics* (D. P. Bobon, P. J. Janssen, and J. Bobon, Eds.). Karger, Basel, 1970, 33–36.

47. Karagulla, S., and Robertson, E., Psychic phenomena in temporal lobe epilepsy and the psychoses. *Br. Med. J.*, 1955, **1**: 748–752.

48. Kemp, J. M., An electron microscopic study of the termination of afferent fibers in the caudate nucleus. *Brain Res.*, 1968, **11**: 464–467.

49. Kemp, J. M., and Powell, T. P. The corticostriate projection in the monkey. *Brain*, 1970, **93**: 525–546.

50. Kety, S. S., Javoy, F., Thierry, A. M., Julou, L., and Glowinksi, J., A sustained effect of electroconvulsive shock on the turnover of norepineprhine in

the central nervous system of the rat. *Proc. Natl. Acad. Sci. USA*, 1967, **58**: 1249–1254.

51. Kleist, K., Schizophrenic symptoms and cerebral pathology, *J. Ment. Sci.*, 1960, **106**: 246–255.

52. Klüver, H., and Bucy, P. C., Preliminary analysis of the functions of temporal lobes in monkeys. *Arch. Neurol. Psychiatry*, 1939, **42**: 979–1000.

53. Koikegami, H., Hirata, Y., and Oguma, J., Studies on the paralimbic brain structures. I. Definition and delimitation of the paralimbic brain structures and some experiments on the nucleus accumbens. *Folia Psychiatr. Neurol. Jap.*, 1967, **21**: 151–179.

54. Krauthamer, G., and Albe-Fessard, D., Electrophysiologic studies of the basal ganglia and striopallidal inhibition of non-specific afferent activity. *Neuropsychologia*, 1964, **2**: 73–77.

55. Lambert, P. A., Perrin, J., Revol, L., Achaintre, A., Balzet, P., Beaujard, M., Berthier, C., Brousolle, P., and Requet, A., Essai de classification des neuroleptiques d'après leurs activités psychopharmacologiques et cliniques. In: *Neuropsychopharmacology* (P. B. Bradley, P. Deniker, and C. Radouco-Thomas, Eds.). Elsevier, Amsterdam, 1958: 613–624.

56. Langrall, H. M., and Joseph, C., Evaluation of safety and efficacy of levodopa in Parkinson's disease and syndrome, results of a collaborative study. *Neurology* (*Minneap.*), **22**: No. 5, 1972 Part 21 Suppl. 3–16.

57. Lisk, R. D., Sexual behaviour: Hormonal control. In: *Neuroendocrinology* (L. Martini and W. F. Ganong, Eds.). Academic Press, New York, 1967: Vol. 2: 197–239.

58. Loup, M., and Cadilhac, J., Le développement des neurones à monoamines du cerveau chez le chaton. *C. R. Soc. Biol.* (*Paris*), 1970, **164**: 1582–1587.

59. Maclean, P. D., New findings relevant to the evolution of psychosexual functions of the brain. *J. Nerv. Ment. Dis.*, 1962, **135**: 289–301.

60. Matthysse, S., Antipsychotic drug actions: A clue to the neuropathology of schizophrenia. *Fed. Proc.*, 1973, **32**: 200–205.

61. Matthysse, S., and Schnaas, F., Unpublished observations.

62. McLardy, T., Some cell and fiber peculiarities of uncal hippocampus. *Progr. Brain Res.*, 1963, **3**: 71–88.

63. Meduna, L. von., *Die Konvulsionstherapie der Schizophrenie.* Halle, Marburg, 1937.

64. Mettler, F. A., Perceptual capacity, functions of the corpus striatum and schizophrenia. *Psychiatr. Q.*, 1955, **29**: 89–111.

65. Meynert, T., Von Gehirne der Saugetiere. In: *Handbuch der Lehre von den Geweben des Menschen und der Tiere* (S. Stricker, Ed.). Engelmann, Leipzig, 1817: Vol. II: 694–808.

66. Mignone, R. J., Donnelly, E. F., and Sadowsky, D., Psychological and neurological comparisons of psychomotor and non-psychmotor epileptic patients. *Epilepsia*, 1970, **11**: 345–359.

67. Morrell, F., Secondary epileptogenic lesions. *Epilepsia*, 1960, **1**: 538–560.

68. Nauta, W. J. H., Hippocampal projections and related neural pathways to the midbrain in the cat. *Brain*, 1958, **81**: 319–340.

69. Nauta, W. J. H., The problem of the frontal lobe: A reinterpretation. *J. Psychiatr. Res.*, 1971, **8**: 167–187.

70. Nauta, W. J. H., Personal communications, 1972.
71. Nauta, W. J. H., and Mehler, W. R., Projections of the lentiform nucleus in the monkey. *Brain Res.*, 1966, 1: 3–42.
72. Nybäck, H., Borzecki, Z., and Sedvall, G., Accumulation and disappearance of catecholamines formed from tyrosine-14C in mouse brain; the effect of some psychotropic drugs. *Eur. J. Pharmacol.*, 1968, 4: 395–403.
73. Pletscher, A., Pharmacological changes of the dopamine metabolism in the basal ganglia. In: *Psychotropic* Drugs and Dysfunctions of the Basal Ganglia (G. Crane and R. Gardner, Jr., Eds.). US Govt. Printing Office, Washington, D.C., 1969: Public Health Serv. Publ. No. 1938: 82–91.
74. Rodin, E., Pesarg, R. N., Waggoner, R. W., and Baggchi, B. K., Relationship between certain forms of psychomotor epilepsy and schizophrenia. *Arch. Neurol. Psychiatry*, 1957, 77: 449–463.
75. Rossum, J. M., The significance of dopamine receptor blockade for the action of neuroleptic drugs. In: *Neuropsychopharmacology* (H. Brill, J. O. Cole, and P. B. Bradley, Eds.). Excepta Med., Amsterdam, 1967: 321–329.
76. Rutter, M., and Lockyer, L., A five to fifteen year follow-up study of infantile psychosis. *Br. J. Psychiatry*, 1967, 113: 1169–1199.
77. Rydjewski, J., and Stevens, J. R., Unpublished observations, 1972.
78. Schreiner, L., and Kling, A., Behavioral changes following rhinencephalic injury in cat. *J. Neurophysiol.*, 1953, 16: 643–659.
79. Slater, E., Beard, A. W., and Glithero, E., The schizophrenia-like psychoses of epilepsy. *Br. J. Psychiatry*, 1963, 109: 95–150.
80. Stevens, J. R., Psychiatric implications of psychomotor epilepsy. *Arch. Gen. Psychiatry*, 1966, 14: 461–471.
81. Stevens, J. R., Kim, C., and Maclean, P. D., Stimulation of caudate nucleus: Behavioral effects of chemical and electrical excitation. *Arch. Neurol.*, 1961, 4: 47–54.
82. Stevens, J. R., Lonsbury, B., and Goel, S., Electroencephalographic spectra and reaction time in disorders of higher nervous function. *Science*, 1972, 176: 1346–1349.
83. Stevens, J. R., Lonsbury, B. L., and Goel, S. L., Seizure occurrence and interspike interval. *Arch. Neurol.*, 1972, 26: 409–419.
84. Stevens, J. R., Milstein, V. M., and Goldstein, S., Psychometric test performance in psychomotor epilepsy. *Arch. Gen. Psychiatry*, 1972, 26: 532–538.
85. Stevens, J. R., Nakamura, Y., Milstein, V., Okuma, P., and Llinas, R., Central and peripheral factors in epileptic discharge. Part II. Experimental studies in the cat. *Arch. Neurol.*, 1964, 11: 463–476.
86. Tedeschi, D. H., Benigni, J. P., Elder, C. J., Yeager, J. C., and Flanigan, J. V., Effects of various phenothiazines on minimal electroshock seizure threshold and spontaneous motor activity of mice. *J. Pharmacol. Exp. Ther.*, 1958, 123: 35–42.
87. Tizard, B., The personality of epileptics: A discussion of the evidence. *Psychol. Bull.*, 1962, 59: 196–210.
88. Ungerstedt, U., Stereotaxic mapping of the monoamine pathways of the rat brain. *Acta Physiol. Scand., Suppl.*, 1971, 367: 1–122.
89. Verdeaux, G., Verdeaux, J., and Sakelaridis, N., Les modifications paroxy-

stiques de l'EEG sous l'influence des neuroleptiques. *Rev. Neurol.* (*Paris*), 1960, **102:** 344.

90. Weinstein, M. R. Histopathological changes in the brain in schizophrenia. A critical review. *Arch. Neurol. Psychiatry,* 1954, **71:** 539–553.

91. Whitlock, D. G., and Nauta, W. J. H., Subcortical projections from temporal neocortex in macaca mulatta. *J. Comp. Anat.,* 1956, **106:** 183–212.

92. Wilson, R. D., The neural associations of nucleus accumbens septi in the albino rat. Masters Thesis, Dept. of Psychology, Massachusetts Institute of Technology, Cambridge, Massachusetts, 1972.

93. Woolley, D. W., *The Biochemical Basis of Psychoses.* Wiley, New York, 1962: 195–198.

94. York, D. H., Dopamine receptor blockade—a central action of chlorpromazine on striatal neurones. *Brain Res.,* 1972, **37:** 91–100.

95. Ziehen, T., *Das central nerven System der Monotremen und Marsupilier.* Fischer, Jena, 1904.

CIRCADIAN CYCLES AND SEIZURES

DAVID D. DALY

University of Texas, Southwestern Medical School, Dallas, Texas

Since ancient times physicians have recognized an association between seizures and sleep. In discussing sleeping and waking, Aristotle remarked "sleep is similar to epilepsy and in some way, sleep is epilepsy" (56). He also observed that in some persons the disease originated in sleep and never attacked them while awake. Posidonius, a fourth century physician, remarked "what epileptics suffer in their attacks when awake, sufferers from incubus undergo in their sleep." In the nineteenth century, Hughlings Jackson studied focal seizures as a strategem for unraveling the problems of cerebral localization. His contemporary Gowers focused his attention primarily on the causes of seizures, their symptoms, and treatment. These interests have carried forward in this century in a series of classifications of types of seizures and their underlying causes. In terms of pathophysiology, efforts have focused on the mechanisms of neuronal hyperexcitability, processes underlying the propagation of epileptic discharge, experimental models that simulate the naturally occurring disorder, and studies of the modifying effects of ontogeny and phylogeny. Less often have authors studied the relationship between time of occurrence of seizures and the circadian cycle.

The observation by Aserinsky and Kleitman (2) that sleep was not a homogeneous continuum but, rather, consisted of two strikingly distinct phases has generated a continuously increasing volume of research into the physiology and pathology of sleep, which has formed the basis for several comprehensive monographs (31). Briefly, sleep consists of an initial period of slow regular respirations, reduced muscle tone, and slow disconjugate eye movements; during this time the electroencephalogram (EEG) shows synchronized slow activity, spindles of 12 to 14 c/sec rhythms, surface negative transients at the vertex and K complexes. This stage has been variously termed synchronized sleep, slow wave sleep, or non-rapid-eye-movement (NREM) sleep. This stage is succeeded by a second phase characterized by an even greater loss of muscle tone upon which are superimposed small twitching movements of the face and limbs, rapid conjugate, usually horizontal, eye movements which resemble normal waking eye movements, and irregular heart and respiratory rates. The EEG at this time shows a striking reduction in voltage and increase in frequency to a pattern resembling drowsiness. This phase has been variously termed paradoxical sleep, activated sleep, low-voltage fast sleep, D sleep, or rapid eye movement (REM) sleep. Recent studies have shown that these two dramatically different states are controlled by anatomically distinct mono-aminergic systems (30). Serotonin-containing neurons in the midline ponto-medullary raphé nuclei initiate NREM sleep, whereas norepinephrine-containing neurons in the locus ceruleus modulate REM sleep.

The discovery of the complex nature of sleep has inevitably awakened interest in the interaction of this process with epileptic mechanisms. In this article, the evidence is reviewed on the time of occurrence of seizures in the sleep–waking cycle, on the modifications in interictal EEG discharges by wakefulness and both phases of sleep, on the effects of sleep deprivation and photic stimulation on the epileptic process, and, finally, on the inverse effects of the epileptic process on normal sleep cycles. For various reasons this review has proven difficult and I have made no attempt at citation of all articles. For example, some articles were available only in abstract form because of their original language, e.g., Japanese; various authors have used diverse terminology for sleep stages; some report anecdotal observations, and finally the lack of a unifying theory makes the data difficult to organize.

TIME OF OCCURRENCE OF SEIZURES

Gowers (26) studied 840 patients and noted that seizures occurred exclusively, "or almost only," at night in 21%, diurnally in 43%, and throughout the circadian period in 37%. He concluded that if the first seizure occurred during the day, seizures would most likely continue to do so and would not occur at night. The converse observation also seemed to hold. Stimulated by this, Langdon-Down and Brain (36) extended these observations. They studied 66 institutionalized epileptics who suffered a total of 2524 seizures in 6 months. They proposed a classification of diurnal, nocturnal, and "diffused" seizures, the latter category referring to those occurring with equal frequency by day and night. The diurnal group constituted the largest number of patients who, nevertheless, suffered fewer seizures. When data on time of occurrence were pooled for all patients, several peak times of occurrence emerged (Figure 1). Patients with nocturnal seizures showed two peaks, one occurring in the second hour after retirement and another approximately 6 hours later between 5 and 6 in the morning. In contrast, the diurnal group showed a dramatic peaking in the first hour after awakening, a second peak in midafternoon approximately 9 hours after awakening, and a third less marked peak some 4 hours later in the early evening. In contrast, patients in the diffused group "show no special

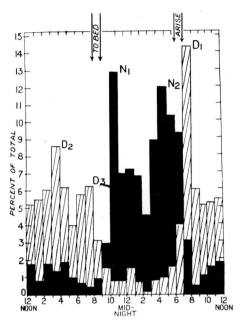

Figure 1. Circadian distribution of 2524 seizures occurring over a 6-month period in 66 patients. The fits of the nocturnal group are represented in black, those of diurnal group in cross-hatching. [Reproduced from Langdon-Down and Brain (36).]

time incidence in their attacks. . . . " The authors also noted a greater disposition for nocturnal or diurnal cycling in those patients having a shorter duration of illness although, even after seizures had persisted for over 20 years, the majority of patients still showed a "clear-cut diurnal or nocturnal type."

Patry (44) has reported strikingly similar observations on 31 adult institutionalized epileptics experiencing a total of 1013 convulsions during a 1-year period. All studies show a remarkably similar distribution in the three groups (Table 1). In further confirmation of Langdon-Down and Brain's observations, Patry noted that diurnal seizures occurred with greatest frequency in patients with seizures of less than 10 years duration, but

TABLE 1

Comparison of Data on Time of Occurrence of Seizures from Three Different Investigations

Seizure time	Percent of total		
	Gowers	Langdon-Down and Brain	Patry
Diurnal	43	43	45
Nocturnal	21	24	19
Diffused	37	33	36

he also showed that the majority of patients (67%) continued to show a clear division into nocturnal and diurnal types even after persistence of attacks for 20 years. Patry confirmed the existence of peak times of incidence for both nocturnal and diurnal seizures although distinguishing a greater number than the previous study. He, too, noted that seizures tended to occur either in the first 2 or 3 hours after retirement or in the early morning hours prior to awakening. Diurnal seizures showed a marked increase shortly after awakening and another midafternoon rise.

Janz (29) has conducted the most extensive study, reporting on 2110 patients selected from an outpatient clinic by the sole criterion that they had suffered convulsions with or without minor seizures. He classified the seizures as follows.

1. "Epilepsies on awakening (A), that is, attacks chiefly after waking and during the period of relaxation after work. . . . This closely resembles Langdon-Down and Brain's diurnal group with its D_1 and D_2 peaks.

2. "Sleep epilepsies (S)," noting that such patients tended to have attacks mainly after falling asleep "usually from about 9–11 p.m.," or in the early morning hours before awakening, "usually between 3 and 5 a.m." These are identical with the N_1 and N_2 periods of Langdon-Down and Brain.

3. "Diffuse epilepsies."

Although these categories conform essentially to those of the previous authors, Janz noted a difference in incidence of the types, with sleep epilepsies being most frequent (45%), diffuse epilepsies least frequent (21%), and diurnal or A epilepsies being intermediate (34%). He attributed this in part to the difference in patient populations between ambulatory and institutionalized patients.

Janz found that the A type generally began between ages 10 and 25 years and had a demonstrable cause in only 10% but a familial history of seizures in 12.5%. When associated with minor seizures, "they are mostly linked with the petit mal triad." The diffuse epilepsies were the reverse, being predominantly symptomatic (54%) with a hereditary factor in only 3.8% and an onset without predilection for age. They were associated with partial seizures of either simple (focal seizures) or complex symptomatology (psychomotor seizures). The S epilepsies fell in between: 23% were symptomatic in origin with familial seizures in 7.7% and, like the diffuse epilepsies, showed no predilection for age of onset. If partial seizures occurred, they were predominantly of complex symptomatology (psychomotor seizures).

Janz has remarked on the constancy of these types throughout the disease. "Diffuse epilepsies never change permanently to one of the two connected manifestations. Sleep epilepsies never change to an awakening epilepsy, but 20% may take on a pseudo-diffuse course in the course of time." A minority of A types may change, usually into the S type. The S epilepsies occur at "regular intervals which the patients can often predict." In contrast, the A and D epilepsies occur at completely irregular intervals.

Janz's observations had begun prior to the recognition of NREM and REM sleep, and his study, therefore, has given no information on the relation of the two nocturnal peaks to REM sleep.

In an independent study of 120 patients with epilepsy upon awakening, Beyer and Jovanovic (7) have confirmed Janz's observations, noting that 95% of convulsions occurred from 10 minutes to 2 hours after awakening and that onset of seizures was between 11 and 15 years of age.

Recently the introduction of night-long polygraphic recordings and of radiotelemetry has made possible the correlation of clinical seizures, interictal and ictal discharge in the EEG, and the behavioral stages of wakefulness and sleep.

Janz has associated A epilepsies with the petit mal triad (tonic-clonic convulsions generalized from onset, absences, and myoclonic seizures). This supports the common clinical observation that myoclonic seizures commonly occur after awakening, the myoclonic jerks often causing the child to drop silverware and dishes at breakfast and books when leaving for school. Meier-Ewert and Broughton (38) have shown that myoclonus diminishes with the onset of NREM sleep, accompanied by a paradoxical increase in generalized spike-wave discharges, which will be discussed in greater detail later. During REM periods myoclonus virtually disappeared. The response to arousal differed dramatically in the two phases of sleep. Arousal from REM produced a return of myoclonic jerks in mild degree associated with generalized spike-wave discharges. In contrast, arousal from NREM produced prolonged and intense myoclonus lasting up to 40 minutes but, surprisingly, not terminating in a convulsion. During the myoclonic jerks patients retained consciousness despite almost continuous polyspike and polyspike-wave discharges.

Few authors have reported on the effects of sleep on absence attacks, possibly because of the difficulties in recognizing such attacks during sleep. Niedermeyer (39) has reported "fluttering of the eyelids" during spike-wave bursts in NREM sleep. In contrast, Ross et al. (49) have observed no behavioral effects during bursts of spike-wave discharge in NREM. Gastaut et al. (19) have reported on 4 patients suffering "petit mal status." In 3, this consisted of confusional states whereas the fourth was of a "type myoclonique." In all subjects, clinical and electrical manifestations of status disappeared in sleep with a prompt recurrence upon arousal. In another patient suffering petit mal status, EEG abnormality persisted in both NREM and REM sleep but apparently without clinical accompaniment. Gastaut and colleagues have proposed as a general rule that status epilepticus differs from isolated seizures, tending to ameliorate or disappear during sleep.

Stevens and her co-workers (54) have used continuous radiotelemetry to study clinical ictus as well as ictal and interictal EEG discharges. In one 20-year-old male with absence and generalized convulsions, they noted that "clinical petit mal attacks occurred in clusters at intervals of or multiples of 1 and $\frac{1}{2}$ hours." No absence occurred during sleep. In a second patient, withdrawing of diphenylhydantoin resulted in sixteen "brief tonic seizures" during sleep which occurred in three clusters approximately 90 minutes apart. Their precise observations merit detailed quotation:

> Each brief tonic seizure was preceded by a marked increase in the irregularity of the interictal spike rate and a tendency for spikes to increase in frequency until seven to ten seconds prior to the onset of clinical ictus. At this time, interictal spikes abruptly and totally arrested, and REMs appeared on the ocular channel, after which there was a sudden burst of rhythmic, high voltage spike-wave activity accompanied by a tonic generalized seizure. Following each attack, interictal spikes disappeared entirely for two to six minutes, then resumed the previous waxing and waning oscillation around a mean of circa 20 spikes per minute. Sinusoidal bursts of REMs were apparent in the electro-oculogram (EOG) for five to ten seconds preceding and following each tonic fit.

The first cluster of seizures lasted 35 minutes and was followed by a period of slow wave sleep. After 90 minutes, an identical episode, consisting of three seizures in 12 minutes, recurred and was also succeeded by a period of slow wave sleep for 80 minutes. A third episode of REM associated with two tonic seizures was terminated by intravenous injection of a barbiturate.

Several reports dealing with seizures associated with diffuse encephalopathies, including myoclonus associated with Hunt's syndrome or dyssynergia cerebellaris myoclonica (6) and Unverricht-Lundborg's myoclonus epilepsy (18), constitute a special group. Most authors agree that in these patients a marked increase in myoclonic jerking develops in the early stages (I-II) of NREM followed by a gradual decrease in stage III and almost total disappearance in stage IV (6, 18, 42, 55). Both Bergamasco and colleagues (6) and Gambi and co-workers (18) have described a total absence of REM sleep in their patients. In contrast, Passouant and Cadilhac (42) have reported observing REM stages with a modification in the myoclonus. They have seen a disappearance of generalized myoclonus with a persistence of focal or unilateral spikes often accompanied by small localized twitchings on the opposite side.

Bergamasco's group (6) have described in considerable detail two types of seizures occurring in 1 patient with dyssynergia cerebellaris myoclonica. The first type consisted of generalized myoclonic jerkings during NREM sleep, being most marked in the deeper levels. The seizures, which varied in duration from 2 to 35 minutes, were accompanied by generalized polyspike-wave discharges. Surprisingly, the patient did not awaken. "The longest lasting seizures were followed by a period of slow, disorganized, low voltage EEG activity lasting 4–6 minutes with simultaneous appearance of rapid eye movements in the EOG." These episodes occurred at the end of periods of NREM of variable duration, and one is tempted to conclude they preceded the onset of REM sleep. The second type of seizure consisted of tonic extension of the upper limbs and tachycardia without arousal. Electroencephalographic desynchronization accompanied these attacks which typically occurred in the "first stages of sleep, in varying number per night and not every night. . . ."

In the so-called Lennox syndrome or "childhood epileptic encephalopathy" (22), tonic seizures have been reported in large numbers during slow wave sleep (20). During REM sleep, slow spike-wave discharges persist but without motor manifestations (42).

Partial seizures of complex symptomatology (psychomotor seizures) have been reported in slow wave sleep (20). Kikuchi (33) described polygraphic studies of 20 patients with seizures of temporal lobe origin in which 7 patients experienced 9 seizures. Seven seizures occurred in slow wave sleep, usually in the deeper levels, and two occurred during REM sleep. The patients usually did not awaken after the seizure. Passouant and Cadilhac (42) have described 1 patient in whom each REM period was preceded by a clinical seizure and implied that temporal lobe seizures commonly occur at the onset of or during REM periods. In another patient, in whom recordings were made from electrodes implanted in the hippocampus, electrographic seizures began with the onset of REM periods and persisted throughout this time. Stevens' group (53) have recorded twenty-eight nocturnal seizures in a girl with "typical psychomotor seizures." They did not specify the sleep stage in which these seizures occurred but commented upon the "remarkably symmetrical distribution of both seizure duration and inter-seizure intervals, suggesting some internal 'clock' for both the generation of and resistance to seizures." A subsequent report (54) described another patient with psychomotor seizures whose EEG showed a right temporal spike focus. Six clinical seizures occurred in a 24-hour period, with the seizures separated by "intervals or multiples of intervals of one and one-half hours." They attempted to relate these to NREM/REM or basic rest–activity cycle (BRAC) (34), although curiously in this patient they state that "no distinct REM sleep was recorded. . . ."

Epstein and Hill (14) have described a patient whose EEG showed a focus of spikes in the right frontotemporal region. They observed that "rhythmic [sic] continuous spiking from the right temporal area [occurred] during all but one REM sleep period." In five such periods, they aroused the patient during the REM period with repetitive spiking: the patient reported an unpleasant dream accompanied by an epigastric sensation typical of the onset of his seizures.

INTERICTAL ELECTROENCEPHALOGRAPHIC ABNORMALITY

Because interictal discharge occurs frequently, numerous reports have described the effects of sleep on various types of abnormal EEG activity.

General agreement exists that NREM sleep activates all types of interictal discharge. In contrast, REM sleep exerts a differential effect depending on whether the discharges are generalized or localized; generalized discharges disappear during REM sleep. Schwartz and co-workers (51) have shown that in a patient whose EEG showed different types of abnormality, this differential effect of sleep persists. In their Case 3, left occipital spikes were recorded in the waking state as well as in both NREM and REM sleep; in contrast, bursts of bilateral multiple spikes appeared only in NREM and were absent in the waking and REM sleep states. Because of these differential effects, these types of abnormalities will be discussed separately.

Generalized Discharges

Since 1946 it has been recognized that NREM sleep activates the generalized 3-cps spike-wave bursts seen in patients with absences and tonic-clonic convulsions generalized from the onset (24). Gibbs and Gibbs (25) reported that spike-wave discharges occurred in 84% of waking recordings and 89% of NREM sleep recordings. Gastaut *et al.* (20) observed a lower incidence of spike-wave discharges in the waking state, in only 25% of patients. A marked activation occurred with the onset of stage I NREM with bursts appearing in 88%, rising to 90% in stage II, and declining to 70% in stage III and 60% in stage IV. Ross *et al.* (49) have reported a comprehensive study of 13 ambulatory patients suffering from absences or generalized convulsions or both. They calculated the number of discharges per minute in the various phases of the circadian cycle. During the daytime waking state, the median value for the group was 0.24 discharge/minute. This dropped in the period immediately prior to sleep to only 0.08 discharge/minute. The onset of NREM sleep showed a dramatic sixfold increase to 0.46 discharge/minute which rose steadily to reach a maximum of 1.09 discharge/minute in stage IV (Figure 2).

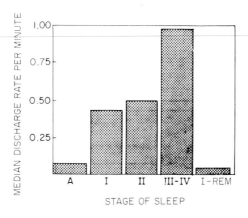

Figure 2. Incidence of spike-wave bursts during the waking state and different stages of sleep based on pooled observations on 13 patients. [Reproduced with permission from Ross *et al.* (49).]

Angeleri's group (1) have reported on 5 patients with absence attacks, 6 with absence and generalized convulsions, and 5 with only generalized convulsions associated with diffuse polyspike-wave discharges in the EEG. The patients with only absence attacks showed spike-wave activity maximally in stage IV, whereas patients with absence and generalized convulsions had peak activity in stages II and III. In patients with only generalized convulsions, great variability occurred among different patients.

Rather constant morphological changes occur with progression into deeper levels of NREM sleep (20, 32, 49). During the waking state the EEG shows well organized, relatively long bursts of generalized 2.5–3.5 cps spike-wave discharges. These persist into levels of drowsiness; however, with the onset of spindles and K complexes the bursts become more disorganized and shorter in duration. The spikes vary in amplitude, and the rhythmical slow waves become more variable in duration and in amplitude. Single spikes are replaced by polyspikes or polyspike-wave complexes. "By the time Stage IV was reached, the tracing showed an anarchic and irregular recording. . . . The EEG was grossly abnormal with a preponderance of high voltage, irregular, $\frac{1}{2}$ to 2 c/sec waves interspersed with high voltage fast and slow spikes" (49). Stevens' group (53) have shown a striking alteration in the statistical properties of bursts between the waking and sleeping states. In the waking state the bursts show a strongly unimodal distribution with a predominant seizure duration of 15 to 20 seconds. In contrast, the nocturnal attacks shortened dramatically, with the distribution of duration exhibiting an exponential character (Figure 3).

During slow wave sleep, Niedermeyer (40) has remarked on a "consistent relationship between the seizure discharges and arousal responses such as vertex waves and especially K complexes." He argues that "most patients with CGE [common generalized epilepsy] suffer from a *faulty*

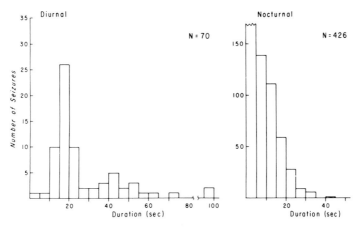

Figure 3. Alteration of duration properties of spike-wave bursts during periods of wakefulness and non-rapid-eye-movement sleep. [Reproduced with permission from Stevens *et al.* (53).]

arousal mechanism which induces both seizure discharges and clinical seizures." He has coined the term *dyshormia* to characterize this deviant arousal mechanism which he believes "might be due to a biochemical disturbance which is genetically transmitted."

In contrast with the activating effects of slow wave sleep, REM sleep is consistently associated with a diminution or total disappearance of generalized epileptiform discharges (10, 11, 13). Gastaut's group (20) have reported a complete disappearance of spike-wave discharges in 27% of patients and a reduction in 70%. Kazamatsuri (32) observed spike-wave bursts during REM in about one-half of 21 cases of petit mal epielpsy, the morphology during this stage resembling the well-organized spike-wave complexes seen in the waking state. In contrast, Ross and colleagues (49) have observed complete absence of spike-wave discharge in only 3 of 13 patients. The remaining patients showed a dramatic drop in the number of discharges per minute to a level equal to or below that seen in the waking state (Figure 2). The median value for the group was 0.07 discharge/minute in REM sleep as opposed to a maximum rate of 1.09 in NREM and 0.24 during daytime waking states. They also commented that "when rapid eye movements were present during I-REM, the discharge rate was even lower" (0.03 discharge/minute as opposed to 0.07).

In infants suffering from infantile spasms or massive myoclonus, the waking EEG shows a complex chaotic pattern of generalized slow waves and multifocal spikes which has been termed *hypsarhythmia*. With the onset of NREM sleep these discharges persist. Batini and co-workers (4) felt that usually the discharges tended to become more bisynchronous than in the waking states, although in some instances they noted a tendency toward fragmentation with the bursts being less numerous and of shorter duration. Gastaut's group (20) believed that the fragmentation increased with deepening of sleep. Both report a disappearance of all discharges in REM sleep. In the Lennox syndrome, slow spike-wave discharges persist, particularly in lighter levels of sleep (20) or may even increase in occurrence (41) but disappear completely during REM sleep. In contrast, in REM sleep, Passouant and Cadilhac (42) have reported a persistence of discharges which are, however, short in duration and without clinical accompaniment. Patry and co-workers (45) have reported on 6 children who clinically showed retardation and evidence of focal or multifocal cerebral lesions and 5 of whom suffered seizures. All children developed an electrical spike-wave status with the onset of slow wave sleep. This persisted relentlessly during this phase of sleep although without clinical accompaniment. The onset of REM sleep and arousal were associated with a dramatic reduction of paroxysmal discharges.

Focal Discharges

Fuster and the Gibbs (17) early called attention to a marked increase during slow wave sleep in the occurrence of spikes in the temporal region of patients suffering from psychomotor seizures. Delange and co-workers (13) reported 3 patients whose EEGs showed temporal spike foci; the abnormalities persisted both in NREM and REM sleep. Passouant and colleagues (43) have also reported persistence of temporal foci in NREM sleep. The rate of discharge increased with deepening NREM and increased even further during REM sleep. Gastaut's group (20) have described a striking activation during NREM sleep in patients, with temporal lobe spikes appearing in 67% of patients in stage I, 77% in stage II, 64% in stage III, and 55% in stage IV. They did note disappearance of temporal spikes in a small (7%) number of patients. During REM sleep, 7% of these patients had no abnormality in the EEG whereas, of the remaining patients, 40% showed an augmentation of discharge rate, in 40% the rate remained unchanged, and in 13% it was reduced. The majority of their patients had spike foci in the temporal, parietal, or occipital regions. During NREM sleep they also noted a change in the morphological character of the spikes which became longer in duration and higher in amplitude; in contrast, during REM sleep the spikes resembled those occurring in the waking state. In NREM the focus enlarged in size and often spike discharges appeared in the homologous area of the opposite hemisphere. In contrast, during REM sleep the focus constricted to resemble that seen in the waking state. From a study of 20 patients with temporal lobe epilepsy, Kikuchi (33) has reported somewhat divergent findings. He concurred that the incidence of temporal spikes was greatest during moderately deep sleep but observed suppression of spikes during REM sleep.

Ferroni and colleagues (16) have studied 22 patients with psychomotor seizures whose EEGs showed temporal spike foci and distinguished two types of alterations in NREM sleep. The first group show highly localized, short duration spikes which tend to cease firing in NREM; these patients have infrequent, predominantly nocturnal seizures. The second group shows longer duration spikes which tend to "propagate" and are activated during NREM; these patients have more frequent seizures which are largely diurnal. While speculating that these differences may reflect differing pathophysiological involvements of deep temporal structures, the authors could offer no definitive explanation. Passouant and Cadilhac (42) have reported that during REM sleep recordings from scalp electrodes may show no abnormalities and yet spike discharges will persist unchanged in the amygdala and hippocampus.

SLEEP DEPRIVATION

Lack of sleep has long been recognized as a precipitant of seizures. Janz (28) reported it as the third most common cause of status epilepticus. Janz (29) has also remarked that "deprivation of sleep, especially combined with consumption of alcohol, and sudden awakening can therefore be considered as specifically provocative of attacks in epilepsies on awakening." Beyer and Jovanovic (7) have reached similar conclusions. Bennett

(5) has reported the occurrence of generalized convulsions in 4 otherwise healthy young men in military service after unusual stress including sleep deprivation.

Mattson and co-workers (37) have reported on activation of the EEG following sleep deprivation of patients with known epilepsy. Approximately one-third of 89 patients with normal or borderline EEGs developed abnormalities of various types following 24 hours of sleep deprivation. In addition, sleep deprivation led to worsening of the EEG in 56% of patients showing abnormalities in routine EEGs. In contrast, 20 control subjects showed no abnormalities in the EEG after 24 hours without sleep. In a subsequent prospective study of 114 epileptic patients having normal or borderline interictal EEGs, sleep deprivation for 24 hours resulted in activation in 41% of patients (47). In 16 patients, spike-wave complexes appeared after sleep deprivation whereas in 28 other patients, focal spikes or sharp waves appeared and three patients suffered an "electrographic ictal episode." The authors have concluded that activation resulted directly from sleep deprivation in 54%. In 28% of patients the abnormality occurred in drowsiness or sleep. The authors did not indicate how many patients had sleep recordings in the predeprivation examination, stating only "spontaneous sleep or drowsiness was obtained in many patients." In another 18% activation was attributed to a "sampling" effect. The authors also noted that of all patients, 37% reported sleep loss in the 24-hour period preceding spontaneous seizures. Patients showing EEG activation had a slightly higher incidence (42%) of such seizures compared with those patients not showing activation (33%).

Sleep deprivation may exert more general effects since Welch and Stephens (58) have reported abnormalities after 24-hour sleep deprivation in the EEGs of 12 of 78 patients with neurological complaints other than seizure disorders. No available experimental evidence provides a clue as to the mechanism for the effects of sleep deprivation.

PHOTIC STIMULATION

The effect of intermittent photic stimulation (IPS) in inducing photoconvulsive and photomyoclonic responses has been long known and thoroughly investigated (8). Photoconvulsive responses and clinical ictus occur almost exclusively in generalized epilepsies. In contrast to the extensive reports on the effects of IPS in the waking state, relatively few reports describe the effects of sleep on photoconvulsive responses. In an early study of NREM sleep, Rodin's group (48) have reported that photoconvulsive responses disappeared in 9 of 26 patients, 6 of whom had clinical photoepilepsy. None of 46 patients who were insensitive to IPS in the waking state showed photosensitivity in sleep. In general, the stimuli became decreasingly potent as the sleep level increased, and relatively little response occurred in stages III and IV. The authors reported 1 patient with awakening epilepsy who exhibited light sensitivity for a brief period of time following arousal from NREM sleep. Similar observations have been reported by Meier-Ewert and Broughton (38). In contrast, Hishikawa and colleagues (27) reported on 15 patients with photosensitive epilepsy in whom IPS induced generalized discharges. They reported a marked decrease in photosensitivity during drowsiness and an inability to induce epileptiform discharges during slow wave sleep.

Both Meier-Ewert and Broughton (38) and Scollo-Lavizzari and Hess (52) have observed a disappearance of photoconvulsive responses during photic stimulation in REM sleep; in contrast, Hishikawa's group (27) report that during REM sleep discharges were "induced as promptly as in the waking state." No obvious explanation exists for these discordant observations, although the patient groups are not identical in terms of seizure types and underlying causes.

EFFECTS OF SEIZURES ON NORMAL CIRCADIAN CYCLES

In view of the strong influence of circadian cycles on seizures, one may reasonably ask the converse question as to whether seizures modify the sleep mechanisms of epileptics. Christian (12) has claimed that patients with nocturnal seizures go rapidly into deep levels of sleep remaining there until the early morning hours when the depth of sleep decreases. In contrast, patients with epilepsy on awakening experience great difficulty in falling asleep and do not sleep deeply until the early morning hours. Janz (29) has confirmed this, observing that "patients with epilepsies on awakening delay getting up for as long as possible, and when they are awakened, as necessity usually demands it, they are often drowsy for a long time afterward." In view of the striking modifications of the organization of sleep at different ages (15), one wonders whether part of this may reflect the age differences noted by Janz in the A and S epilepsies (see above).

In studies of 21 patients with absence attacks, Kazamatsuri (32) saw no evidence of alteration in the nocturnal sleep patterns. Similar observations were made by Ross and colleagues (49) who commented that "the sleep pattern of these epileptic patients was very similar to that found for other subjects during their first night of laboratory sleep."

In patients with generalized myoclonus or tonic seizures, Passouant and Cadilhac (42) have reported a reduction in the number of sleep cycles and the total duration of REM sleep. With diffuse encephalopathies, various abnormalities occur in NREM: absence of distinct stages, shortening of duration, and disappearance of sigma rhythms and K complexes. Bergamasco's group (6) have found a complete lack of REM sleep in a 13-year-old girl with dyssynergia cerebellaris myoclonica, although cycling through various levels of NREM did occur during the night. In a study of two brothers with progressive myoclonus epilepsy, Gambi and co-workers (18) have noted a marked disorganization of sleep and complete absence of REM sleep paralleling the previous observations.

In a study of 20 patients with temporal lobe epilepsy, Kikuchi (33) observed deranged nocturnal sleep in the majority of patients. Typically there was prolongation of state III and shortening of stage IV, whereas REM sleep appeared in an irregular fashion. Stevens and co-workers (53, 54) have failed to observe REM sleep in 1 patient with temporal lobe seizures but otherwise did not comment on deviations from normal circadian cycles. Passouant and Cadilhac (42) have remarked that in patients with temporal lobe seizures NREM is little disturbed but imply unspecified changes in REM.

Conclusions

This profusion of reports defies simple summarization, much less organization into a logically coherent schema. Some observations are anecdotal. At times data are incomplete or, even, contradictory. We also lack basic understanding of certain normal sleep processes; for example, in view of the differential effect on myoclonus of arousal from NREM sleep (38), do different arousal mechanisms operate in these two states? Do the biochemical-anatomical systems underlying the BRAC continue to operate in the waking state (57) and, indeed, influence the time of occurrence of diurnal seizures? Despite all these reservations, one can perhaps draw some general conclusions.

1. Patients with symptomatic seizures constitute the majority of the "diffuse" epilepsies (29). In these patients partial seizures of both simple and complex symptomatology occur intermingled with convulsions. These convulsions are secondarily generalized from a focal onset and, under these circumstances, one may postulate that derangements, both electrophysiological and biochemical, in local neuronal networks control the occurrence of ictus and remain less influenced by circadian cycles. In contrast, seizures on awakening seem associated with those epilepsies variously termed *centrencephalic, reticulocortical,* or *common generalized* (29). In these patients, hereditary factors play a much stronger role, and convulsions tend to occur in the first hour or two after arousal (7). Arousal from NREM sleep may produce prolonged myoclonus in patients not otherwise subject to such episodes (38), and electrographic signs of arousal during sleep (K complexes) often precede the abnormal discharges appearing in the EEG at this time (40). The D_2 peak of Langdon-Down and Brain (36) does occur some 9 hours after the D_1 and is, thus, a multiple of the 90-minute BRAC; however, pooled observations on many patients yield these data from which it would be rash to extrapolate that BRAC cycling does, indeed, continue during wakefulness. Clearly altered arousal processes are deeply involved in these epilepsies. The term *dyshormia* (40) adds nothing to our understanding of such processes, but it does formalize the idea that

the ultimate biochemical clue to this group of seizure disorders possibly lies in genetically dictated changes in the biochemistry of monoaminergic neuronal systems.

The N_1 and N_2 peaks described in the nocturnal or "sleep" epilepsies occur in the first 2 hours of sleep and again shortly before arousal (36) and generate the same unsupported impulse to relate them to the first and last REM cycles of the night. However, this would not explain the apparent lack of influence of the intervening REM cycles on nocturnal convulsions. Janz (29) has noted that patients with sleep epilepsies usually suffer partial seizures of complex symptomatology (psychomotor seizures) and that the incidence of seizures in the family lay intermediate between the high incidence of awakening epilepsies and the low incidence of diffuse epilepsies. In fact, this nocturnal group may be a nonhomogeneous one containing patients with seizures due to acquired causes, such as hippocampal sclerosis, and others in which the focal electrical abnormality in the temporal region may be genetically determined (9).

2. With regard to interictal abnormality, NREM sleep consistently activates epilepsies of generalized as well as localized nature. In the generalized epilepsies associated with 3-per sec spike-wave or polyspike-wave discharges, the dramatic activation in NREM sleep contrasts with a marked reduction or disappearance of such discharges during REM sleep. Pompeiano (46) has suggested that the augmentation of the recruiting response seen after stimulation of the thalamic nonspecific projection system during synchronized slow wave sleep is accompanied by a parallel unleashing of neuronal circuits generating the spike-wave discharge. Conversely, the cortical response to stimulation of this system diminishes strikingly during both REM sleep and waking (50, 59), concomitant with the disappearance or reduction of the generalized epileptic discharges in this stage of sleep as well as in the waking state.

Stevens' group (54) have suggested a reciprocal relation between interictal spikes and ictus, commenting "in our patients slow-wave sleep was associated with increased spike rate without clinical seizures. In contrast and as has been shown by others, during REM periods, the rate of interictal epileptiform bursts from the scalp is sharply altered from the inter-REM mean, apparently disposing to ictus." In this sense, the steadily recurring interictal discharges may be viewed as epiphenomena signaling the operation of an inhibitory "fail-safe" mechanism. Short-term biological cycling, in this case BRAC, would modify this process yielding a periodic or quasiperiodic appearance of seizures. "Catamenial epilepsy" (35) provides inferential evidence of longer-term fluctuations in seizure thresholds as a result of changes in biochemical, in this case hormonal, milieu.

3. Finally, the epileptic process may, in turn, modify normal circadian cycles and particularly the BRAC. At present evidence is too scanty to permit definitive conclusions. Some alterations may be incidental to the

effects of anticonvulsant drugs, for example, suppression of REM sleep by barbiturates, on normal nocturnal sleep cycles. On the other hand, alterations of normal nocturnal cycles in patients with temporal lobe epilepsy may reflect in part the influence of disordered function in limbic structures on the waking-sleeping mechanisms. Finally, in diffuse diseases which involve the brain stem itself, for example Hunt's syndrome, the basic pathological process that produces seizures may also derange the monoaminergic neuronal systems located in the brainstem.

Clearly more questions remain unanswered than answered. The complexities of all-night polygraphic recording and radiotelemetry have no doubt deterred many investigators from exploring these areas. Nevertheless, important problems remain unsolved. The solution to some of these may contain answers not only to important theoretical questions but to the practical problems of controlling clinical seizures.

REFERENCES

1. Angeleri, F., Ferroni, A., and Bergonzi, F., Studio sulla quantificazione dell' attivita epilettica punta-onda e polipunta-onda diffusa e sincrona in registrazioni poligrafiche notturne di epilettica. *Riv. Patol. Nerv. Ment.*, 1967, **88**: 413–431.
2. Aserinsky, E., and Kleitman, N., Regularly occurring periods of eye motility and concomitant phenomena during sleep. *Science*, 1953, **118**: 273.
3. Bancaud, J., Talairach, J., Bordas-Ferrer, M., Auber, J. L., and Marchand, H., Les accès épileptiques au cours du sommeil de nuit. In: *Sommeil de Nuit Normal et Pathologique*. Masson, Paris, 1965: 255–274.
4. Batini, C., Criticos, A., Fressy, J., and Gastaut, H., A propos du sommeil nocturne chez sujets présentants une épilepsie à expression EEG bisynchrone. *Rev. Neurol. (Paris)*, 1962, **106**: 221–224.
5. Bennett, D. R., Sleep deprivation and major motor convulsions. *Neurology (Minneap.)*, 1963, **13**: 953–958.
6. Bergamasco, B., Bergamini, L., and Mutani, R., Spontaneous sleep abnormalities in the case of dyssynergia cerebellaris myoclonica. *Epilepsia*, 1967, **8**: 271–281.
7. Beyer, L., and Jovanovic, U. J., Elektrencephalographische und klinische Korrelate bei Aufwachepileptikern mit besonderer Berucksichtigung der therapeutischen Probleme. *Nervenarzt*, 1966, **37**: 333–336.
8. Bickford, R. G., and Klass, D. W., Sensory precipitation and reflex mechanisms. In: *Basic Mechanisms of the Epilepsies* (H. H. Jasper, A. A. Ward, and A. Pope, Eds.). Churchill, London, and Little, Brown, Boston, 1969: 543–564.
9. Bray, P., and Wiser, W., Evidence for a genetic etiology of temporal-central abnormalities in focal epilepsy. *N. Engl. J. Med.*, 1964, **271**: 926–933.
10. Cadilhac, J., Vlahovitch, B., and Delange-Walter, M., Considérations sur les modifications des décharges épileptiques au cours de la période des

mouvements oculaires. In: *Sommeil de Nuit Normal et Pathologique.* Masson, Paris, 1965: 275–282.

11. Castellotti, V., and Pittaluca, E., Rilievi elettroencefalografici durante sonno spontaneo nell'epilessia 'morfeica'. *Riv. Neurol.,* 1965, **35**: 568–587.

12. Christian, W., Bioelektrische Charakteristik tagesperiodisch gebundener verlaufsformen epileptischer Erkrankungen. *Dtsch. Z. Nervenheilkd.,* 1960, **181**: 413–444.

13. Delange, M., Castan, P., Cadilhac, J., and Passouant, P., Etude du sommeil de nuit au cours d'épilepsies centrencéphaliques et temporales. *Rev. Neurol. (Paris),* 1962, **106**: 106–113.

14. Epstein, A. W., and Hill, W., Ictal phenomena during REM sleep of a temporal lobe epileptic. *Arch. Neurol.,* 1966, **15**: 367–375.

15. Feinberg, I., Effects of age on human sleep patterns. In: *Sleep, Physiology and Pathology* (A. Kales, Ed.). Lippincott, Philadelphia, 1969: 39–52.

16. Ferroni, A., Chirulla, C., and Signorini, E., L'attivita elettrica di focolai epilettici temporali in rapporto alla veglia e alle fasi del sonno notturno. Studio su 31 registrazioni poligrafiche. *Riv. Neurol.,* 1969, **34**: 652–657.

17. Fuster, B., Gibbs, E. L., and Gibbs, F. A., Pentothal sleep as an aid to the diagnosis and localization of seizure discharges of the psychomotor type. *Dis. Nerv. Syst.,* 1948, 9: 199–202.

18. Gambi, D., Ferro, F. M., and Mazza, S., Analysis of sleep in progressive myoclonus epilepsy. *Tur. Neurol.,* 1970, 3: 347–364.

19. Gastaut, H., Balletto, M., Rhodes, J., Batini, C., and Fressy, J., Etude du sommeil nocturne de 9 sujets présentants un état de mal épileptique generalisé ou focalisé. *Rev. Neurol. (Paris),* 1963, **108**: 173.

20. Gastaut, H., Batini, C., Fressy, J., Broughton, R., Tassinari, C. A., and Vittini, F., Etude électroencéphalographique des phénomènes épisodiques au cours du sommeil. In: *Sommeil de Nuit Normal et Pathologique.* Masson, Paris, 1965: 239–254.

21. Gastaut, H., Roger, J., Ouachi, S., Timsit, M., and Broughton, R., An electroclinical study of seizures of tonic expression. *Epilepsia,* 1963, 4: 15–44.

22. Gastaut, H., Roger, J., Soulayrol, R., Tassinari, C. A., Regis, H., Dravet, C., Bernard, R., Pinsard, N., and St. Jean, M., Childhood epileptic encephalopathy with diffuse slow spike-waves (otherwise known as "petit-mal variant" or Lennox syndrome). *Epilepsia* 1966, 7: 139–179.

23. Gastaut, H., and Tassinari, C. A., Triggering mechanisms in epilepsy: the electroclinical point of view. *Epilepsia,* 1966, 7: 85–138.

24. Gibbs, E. L., and Gibbs, F. A., Diagnostic and localizing value of electroencephalographic studies in sleep. *Res. Publ. Assoc. Res. Nerv. Ment. Dis.,* 1946, **26**: 366–376.

25. Gibbs, F. A., and Gibbs, E. L., *Atlas of Electroencephalography.* Addison-Wesley, Reading, Massachusetts, 1950: Vol. 1; 1952: Vol. 2.

26. Gowers, W. R., *Epilepsy and Other Chronic Convulsive Diseases,* 1885 (reprinted in American Academy of Neurology Reprint Series, Dover, New York, 1964).

27. Hishikawa, Y., Yamamoto, J., Furuya, E., Yamada, Y., Miyazaki, K., and Kaneko, Z., Photosensitive epilepsy: Relationships between the visual

evoked responses and the epileptiform discharges induced by intermittent photic stimulation. *Electroenceph. clin. Neurophysiol.*, 1967, **23:** 320–324.

28. Janz, D., Conditions and causes of status epilepticus. *Epilepsia*, 1960, **2:** 170–177.

29. Janz, D., The grand mal epilepsies and the sleeping-waking cycle. *Epilepsia*, 1962, **3:** 69–109.

30. Jouvet, M., Some monoaminergic mechanisms controlling sleep and waking. In: *Brain and Human Behavior* (A. G. Karczmar and J. C. Eccles, Eds.). Springer-Verlag, Berlin and New York, 1972: 131–161.

31. Kales, A. (Ed.), *Sleep, Physiology and Pathology.* Lippincott, Co. Philadelphia, 1969.

32. Kazamatsuri, C., Electroencephalographic studies of petit mal epilepsy during natural sleep. *Psychiatr. Neurol. Jap.*, 1964, **66:** 650–679 (in Japanese); *Epilepsy Abstr.*, 1947–1967: 3422.

33. Kikuchi, S., An electroencephalographic study of nocturnal sleep in temporal lobe epilepsy. *Folia Psychiatr. Neurol. Jap.*, 1969, **23:** 59–81.

34. Kleitman, N., Basic rest-activity cycle in relation to sleep and wakefulness. In: *Sleep, Physiology and Pathology* (A. Kales, Ed.). Lippincott, Philadelphia, 1969: 33–38.

35. Laidlaw, J., Catamenial epilepsy. *Lancet*, 1956, **2:** 1235–1237.

36. Langdon-Down, M., and Brain, W. R., Time of day in relation to convulsions in epilepsy. *Lancet*, 1929, **2:** 1029–1032.

37. Mattson, R. H., Pratt, K. L., and Calverley, J. R., Electroencephalograms of epileptics following sleep deprivation. *Arch. Neurol.*, 1965, **13:** 310–315.

38. Meier-Ewert, K., and Broughton, R., Photomyoclonic response of epileptic and nonepileptic subjects during wakefulness, sleep and arousal. *Electroenceph. clin. Neurophysiol.*, 1967, **23:** 142–151.

39. Niedermeyer, E., Sleep electroencephalograms in petit mal. *Arch. Neurol.*, 1965, **12:** 625–630.

40. Niedermeyer, E., *The Generalized Epilepsies.* Thomas, Springfield, Illinois, 1972.

41. Ohtahara, S., Oke, E., Ban, T., *et al.*, The Lennox syndrome. Electroencephalographic study. *Clin. Neurol.* (*Tokyo*), 1970, **10:** 617–625 (in Japanese); *Epilepsy Abstr.*, 1971, 4: 829.

42. Passouant, P., and Cadilhac, J., Décharges épileptiques et sommeil. In: *Modern Problems of Pharmacopsychiatry* (E. Niedermeyer, Ed.). Karger, Basel, 1970: Vol. 4: 87–104.

43. Passouant, P., Cadilhac, J., and Delange, M., Indications apportées par l'étude du sommeil de nuit sur la physiopathologie des épilepsies. *Int. J. Neurol.*, 1965, **5:** 207–216.

44. Patry, F. L., The relation of time of day, sleep and other factors to the incidence of epileptic seizures. *Am. J. Psychiatry*, 1931, **87:** 789–813.

45. Patry, G., Lyagoubi, S., and Tassinari, C. A., Sub-clinical "electrical status epilepticus" induced by sleep in children. *Arch. Neurol.*, 1971, **24:** 242–252.

46. Pompeiano, O., Sleep mechanisms. In: *Basic Mechanisms of the Epilepsies* (H. H. Jasper, A. A. Ward, and A. Pope, eds.). Churchill, London, and Little, Brown, Boston, 1969: 453–473.

47. Pratt, K. L., Mattson, R. H., Weikers, N. J., and Williams, R., EEG activation of epileptics following sleep deprivation: A prospective study of 114 cases. *Electroenceph. clin. Neurophysiol.*, 1968, **24**: 11–15.

48. Rodin, E. A., Daly, D. D., and Bickford, R. G., Effects of photic stimulation during sleep. *Neurology (Minneap.)*, 1955, **5**: 149–159.

49. Ross, J. J., Johnson, L. C., and Walter, R. D., Spike and wave discharges during stages of sleep. *Arch. Neurol.*, 1966, **14**: 399–407.

50. Rossi, G., Favale, E., Hara, T., Giussani, A., and Sacco, G., Researches on the nervous mechanism underlying deep sleep in the cat. *Arch. Ital. Biol.*, 1961, **99**: 270–292.

51. Schwartz, B. A., Guilbaud, G., and Fischgold, H., Single and multiple spikes in the night sleep of epileptics. *Electroenceph. clin. Neurophysiol.*, 1964, **16**: 56–67.

52. Scollo-Lavizzari, G., and Hess, R., Photic stimulation during paradoxical sleep in photo-sensitive subjects. *Neurology (Minneap.)*, 1967, **17**: 604–608.

53. Stevens, J. R., Kodama, H., Lonsbury, B. L., and Mills, L., Ultradian characteristics of spontaneous seizure discharges recorded by radiotelemetry in man. *Electroenceph. clin. Neurophysiol.*, 1971, **31**: 313–325.

54. Stevens, J. R., Lonsbury, B. L., and Goel, S. L., Seizure occurrence and interspike interval. *Arch. Neurol.*, 1972, **26**: 409–419.

55. Tassinari, C. A., Broughton, R., Poire, R., Roger, J., and Gastaut, H., Sur l'évolution de movements anormaux au cours du sommeil. In: *Sommeil de Nuit Normale et Pathologique*. Masson, Paris, 1965: 314–333.

56. Temkin, O., *The Falling Sickness* (2nd ed.). Johns Hopkins Press, Baltimore, Maryland, 1971.

57. Webb, W., Twenty-four-hour sleep cycling. In: *Sleep, Physiology and Pathology* (A. Kales, Ed.). Lippincott, Philadelphia, 1969: 53–66.

58. Welch, L. K., and Stephens, J. B., Clinical value of the electroencephalogram following sleep deprivation. *Aerosp. Med.*, 1971, **42**: 349–351.

59. Yamaguchi, N., Ling, C., and Marczynski, T., Recruiting responses observed during wakefulness and sleep in unanesthetized chronic cats. *Electroenceph. clin. Neurophysiol.*, 1964, **17**: 246–254.

CLINICAL ICTAL PATTERNS AND ELECTROGRAPHIC DATA IN CASES OF PARTIAL SEIZURES OF FRONTAL-CENTRAL-PARIETAL ORIGIN

C. AJMONE MARSAN and **L. GOLDHAMMER**[*]

National Institute of
Neurological Diseases and Stroke
Bethesda, Maryland

Georgetown University
School of Medicine
Washington, D.C.

In most textbooks of neurology, the focal motor epileptic seizure is generally identified with the Jacksonian attack. The occurrence of ictal episodes consisting of adversive movements of head and eyes and of other tonic motor phenomena is mentioned, but these less typical patterns are often considered as part of a generalized grand mal convulsion with asymmetrical (or focal) onset. It is, however, a common observation that focal epileptogenic lesions, particularly those located above the Sylvian fissure, in proximity to the sensory motor strip and in various portions of the frontal lobe, manifest themselves with a complex and variable seizure symptomatology (1, 4, 6, 7, 9, 10). The occurrence of a typical Jacksonian pattern of clonic movements with their characteristic march is rather uncommon in its pure form. More often this pattern is complicated by adversive movements and tonic postures of one or the other limb, in one or both sides of the body, interassociated in various complex sequences; in many cases such postures may be the exclusive or predominant feature of the entire ictal episode. In still other situations the seizure might include automatic and visceral phenomena rather than, or intermixed with, tonic and clonic motor signs; this, in spite of the commonly accepted notion that such phenomena are characteristic of seizures which have their origin below the Sylvian fissure in pararhinencephalic structures.

It seems reasonable to conclude that such complexity and variety of seizure patterns are either a property of epileptogenic lesions affecting the frontocentral regions or the result of a rapid, preferential spread of epileptiform activity from the primary focus to other cerebral structures. Whatever their underlying mechanism might be, the fact remains that the seizure will often present a diagnostic challenge for purposes of both localization and lateralization of the main epileptogenic process.

[*] *Acknowledgment:* The authors wish to thank Dr. J. Van Buren, Chief of the Branch of Neurological Surgery, National Institute of Neurological Diseases and Stroke, for permitting the use of his patient files. They also acknowledge with gratitude the assistance of Dr. T. C. Chen, Office of Biometry, National Institute of Neurological Diseases and Stroke, in the statistical evaluation of the data and of Mrs. M. Jackson for typing the manuscript.

In this study we have analyzed in detail the patterns of a large number of ictal episodes in a group of such patients in which there was some electrographic (and possibly also clinical and pathological) evidence to localize the epileptogenic process to a given region and hemisphere of the brain. The main purpose of the study was to correlate the various seizure patterns, and associations thereof, with the presumed site and side of the main epileptogenic lesion. It was hoped that through such a study one might gain a better understanding of the functional pathology of these regions and also be in a better position to evaluate the localizing and lateralizing reliability of each of these patterns. This should increase the usefulness of the observation and accurate description of seizure patterns in arriving at a correct diagnostic identification of the site of the underlying epileptogenic process.

PATIENT MATERIAL, METHOD, AND GENERALITIES

This study was carried out on a total of 187 patients. All had a seizure disorder and all had definite electrographic evidence of it, with epileptiform activity involving exclusively or primarily supra-Sylvian regions. Patients with typical centrencephalic (petit mal) patterns and with electroencephalographic (EEG) findings indicative of an exclusive or main involvement of temporal or pararhinencephalic structures were excluded. Patients with electrographic evidence of parieto-occipital or occipital foci were not included in the present study and will be the object of a separate investigation. The patients were selected from the files of our EEG Laboratory according to the above criteria and exclude only the few cases without clinical evidence of seizures in spite of the presence of epileptiform activity in their record(s) [see Zivin and Ajmone Marsan (11)] and those in which the records were persistently negative in spite of the occurrence of focal ictal episodes of unquestionable epileptic nature [see Ajmone Marsan and Zivin (3)]. Such exclusions were justified by the main purpose of this study, as outlined above.

Electroencephalogram Evaluation

Each of the 187 patients had a minimum of two and a maximum of over twenty EEG examinations. These were carried out with a minimum of twenty electrodes applied according to the standard 10–20 system, under various conditions which included routinely wakefulness, sleep, hyperventilation, and photic stimulation. The follow-up time varied from 1 week (in a few cases) to over 15 years. A considerable number of patients (88) eventually underwent surgical treatment. Among such cases, for those in whom the EEG remained abnormal and/or the seizures persisted after the operation, only the presurgery findings (both EEG and clinical) were analyzed and included in this study.

The EEG localization of epileptiform discharges would often present some problem, especially in those patients (the majority) in which a relatively large number of records were obtained. Whereas in certain patients the interictal paroxysmal potentials were clearly localized (and lateralized) at given electrode(s), and such localization would remain constant throughout the various examinations, even in follow-up studies extending over several years, in other patients the region involved by epileptiform abnormalities would vary, and emphasis and extent of the localization might change in different records. Because of this situation, an attempt was made to classify each patient according to the most prominent and constant EEG localizing features, without ignoring, at the same time, any evidence for additional or secondary localizations. For the final analysis and correlation of seizure patterns, the patients were eventually arranged into four groups according to the main localization of their paroxysmal discharges and also into four other overlapping groups to emphasize particular and/or additional localizations (see below). Thus, for instance, the group of frontal localizations includes not only patients with pure frontal foci but also patients with some evidence of possible secondary involvement of central or temporal areas. Similarly, the parasagittal group includes patients who are also in the main groups of frontal, frontocentral, central, and centroparietal localizations, and the same is true—in different degrees—for each of the other groups.

Regardless of their location, the EEG paroxysmal discharges were clearly and consistently lateralized to one or the other hemisphere exclusively, in all records of 134 patients. In 39 additional patients these discharges had some bilateral features but were clearly prominent on one side. In only 14 patients the epileptiform potentials were bilateral and symmetrical or shifting from side to side (in the same or in different records) without any definite predominance of lateralization. These data are summarized in Table 1.

Clinical Evaluation

All pertinent amnestic, physical and laboratory data obtained in one or multiple hospitalizations for each patient were collected from his chart. Particular emphasis was placed on the seizure descriptions which had been derived primarily from direct observations by hospital personnel or, occasionally, by relatives. A considerable number of spontaneously occurring ictal episodes (induced seizures are not included in this study) had also been witnessed by the senior author or by the technical staff of the EEG Laboratory. The extent and quality of this information were unavoidably uneven and rather variable in different patients: in a few of these, only one or two ictal episodes could be observed, whereas for many patients thirty or more seizures were described. In any case, all the available (and reliable) descriptions of all spontaneous minor and major seizures for each patient were taken into consideration. Eventually, individual patterns and

TABLE 1

LATERALIZATION OF PRESUMED EPILEPTOGENIC PROCESS ON THE BASIS OF ELECTROGRAPHIC (EEG), CLINICAL (AND/OR RADIOLOGICAL) AND ANATOMOPATHOLOGICAL CRITERIA

	Unilateral	Bilateral or non-lateralized	Negative	+ Anatomical + Clinical	+ EEG + Clinical	+ EEG + Anatomical	+ Anatomical	+ Clinical	+ EEG	Only	Conflicting with clinical	Conflicting with EEG
EEG	173 (134 + 39)[a]	14	—	46 (42 + 4)	—	—	10 (8 + 2)	53 (40 + 13)	—	45 (30 + 15)	19 (14 + 5)	—
Clinical	121 (110 + 11)[b]	12	54	—	—	46 (45 + 1)	N.D.[c]	—	53 (47 + 6)	4 (3 + 1)	—	19 (16 + 3)
Anatomical	57	—	130	—	46	—	—	N.D.[c]	10	N.D.[c]	1	0

[a] Electroencephalogram showed some bilateral features but with definite one-sided predominance of epileptiform discharges in 39 patients.
[b] In 11 patients the lateralization was based exclusively on radiological criteria.
[c] No data.

association thereof in any given ictal episode were tabulated and analyzed in relation to localization and lateralization of the epileptogenic focus. As previously mentioned, these were mainly decided upon on the basis of the interictal EEG findings, integrated with neurological data (exclusive of the seizure patterns themselves), X-ray studies and, when available, pathological findings.

Clinical neurological findings were totally negative in 54 (or 29%), and the radiological examination (including air and contrast studies in a considerable number of cases) was uninformative in 164 (or 87.5%) of the patient population. Type and incidence of the objective findings in the other patients are shown in Table 2. Clinical (exclusive of seizure patterns) and/or X-ray evidence that one or the other hemisphere might be involved in the epileptogenic process was present in 121 patients (or about 65%) (see Table 1).

AGE

The median age of the patient population at the time each subject was first referred to the EEG Laboratory was within 21 to 25 years. The age distribution is shown in Figure 1.

The median age at which 181 of these patients had their first seizure (such information was not available in the other 6 patients) was in the 11–15 years group (minimum less than 1 year, maximum over 60 years). The median time for duration of the seizure disorder in these patients was 6–8 years (minimum less than 1 year, maximum over 30 years).

Clearly lateralized epileptiform discharges could be observed in the EEG of patients regardless of their age. However, a record with features suggestive of a centrencephalic involvement (with or without asymmetries—typical petit mal was excluded from this study) was found in 20 patients, but only 3 of these were older than 25 years (see Figure 1) [see also Gabor and Ajmone Marsan (5)]. In none of these 20 patients were the seizures secondary to an expanding lesion [see, however, Ajmone Marsan and Lewis (2)].

ETIOPATHOLOGY

The pathogenesis was unknown in 87 (or 46.5%) of the cases. In the remaining 100 patients the probable etiopathological factors were distributed as follows (number of patients in parenthesis): intracranial expanding lesions (glioma, astrocytoma, meningioma, brain metastasis), definite (30) probable (9); encephalopathies (including birth trauma, head injury, postsurgery condition) (15); encephalitis and meningitis (15); vascular malformations and lesions (9); atrophy, cyst, porencephaly (15); and miscellanea (7).

In those patients in whom lateralization of the epileptogenic process was indicated by both EEG and clinical (and/or X-ray) findings, the underly-

TABLE 2

TYPE AND INCIDENCE OF CLINICAL (AND RADIOLOGICAL) FINDINGS IN TOTAL PATIENT POPULATION AND IN THE VARIOUS ELECTROENCEPHALOGRAM LOCALIZATION GROUPS[a]

Clinical findings[b]	Total population (N = 187)	Frontal (N = 46)	Fronto-central (N = 64)	Central (N = 33)	Centro-parietal (N = 40)	Para-sagittal (N = 71)	Temporal (secondary) (N = 37)	Diffuse or multifocal (N = 27)	Frontopolar (N = 25)
Hemiplegia	86 (46)	19 (41)	29 (45)	16 (48)	22 (55)	27 (38)	16 (43)	7 (26)	10 (40)
Hemihypoesthesia	33 (17)	6 (13)	10 (16)	4 (12)	13 (32)	11 (15)	6 (16)	2 (7)	4 (16)
Hemiatrophy	23 (12)	8 (17)	8 (12)	2 (6)	5 (12)	10 (14)	5 (13)	2 (7)	1 (4)
Visual field defect	10 (5)	— (—)	3 (5)	1 (3)	6 (15)	3 (4)	4 (11)	1 (4)	1 (4)
Miscellanea[c]	46 (25)	13 (28)	19 (30)	6 (18)	7 (17)	18 (25)	9 (24)	5 (18)	5 (20)
Behavior disorders or mental retardation	19 (10)	7 (15)	4 (6)	2 (6)	4 (10)	7 (10)	5 (13)	6 (22)	3 (12)
X-Ray and/or scan pos.	23 (12)	5 (11)	9 (14)	3 (9)	4 (10)	8 (11)	2 (5)	3 (11)	1 (4)
Clinical: negative	54 (29)	11 (24)	20 (31)	11 (33)	10 (25)	23 (32)	8 (21)	11 (40)	5 (20)

[a] The first four groups all include different patients; these same patients (plus 4) are redistributed in the remaining groups (see text). N = number of patients. Figures in parenthesis are percentages.

[b] More than one symptom can be present in the same patient.

[c] Including aphasia, paraplegia, nystagmus, ataxia, dysmetria, hyper-reflexia, Babinski, extrapyramidal signs, microcephaly.

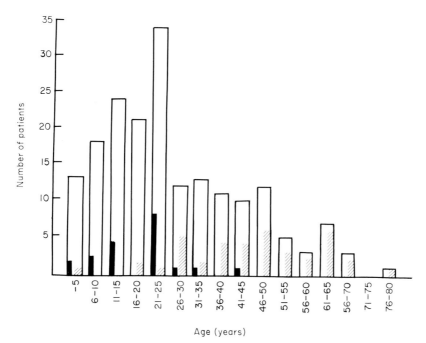

Figure 1. Age distribution in the patient population. [Age is that of the patient at his first electroencephalographic (EEG) examination.] Black columns: number of patients with EEG showing also, or mainly, paroxysmal discharges with centrencephalic features (exclusive of typical petit mal patterns). Columns with diagonal stripes: number of patients with expanding intracranial lesions.

ing etiopathological factor was known or could be reasonably suspected in 70% of the cases. In those patients in whom the lateralizing evidence was exclusively electrographic (neurological and X-ray findings being totally negative), an etiopathological factor was known or suspected in only about 40% of the cases. Of the 14 patients with EEG bilateral paroxysmal abnormalities, etiopathology was known in 7 (in 3 of which neurological lateralizing signs were also present). Among the 39 patients in which the epileptogenic factor was an expanding intracranial lesion, 36 had clearly lateralized electrographic paroxysmal discharges. The remaining 3 patients had bilateral EEG features (but with unilateral predominance in 2). Confirming a well-known fact was the finding that the presence of an expanding lesion as the probable etiological factor in focal seizures was exceptional below 26 years of age (4 out of 110 cases or 3.6%) (see Figure 1).

RESULTS

Seizure Patterns: Generalities

AURA

In 53 patients (28%), no aura was ever reported. In each of the remaining 134 patients, some (or all) seizures were preceded by subjective sensations of various types. These have been subdivided into the following seven categories (J through P in Tables 3 and 5), each patient presenting one or several types of aura in his seizures.

J. Somatosensory Aura. Sensation involving limbs, face, or other parts of the body, on one or the other side only, was reported by 66 patients (or 35%) in the form of (number of patients in parenthesis): paresthesias ("tingling," "pins and needles," "bug crawling," "prickling, "tickling") (33); numbness-dullness (31); pain (9); burning (5); electricity (5); feeling of weakness (5); tightening (3); drawing-pulling (3); vibration (2); others (shaky, throbbing, swelling, heaviness, lightness, undefined) (9). Different forms of sensations were not uncommonly reported by the same patient in different seizures.

K. Cephalic Aura. Such a sensation was reported by 32 patients (or 17%) in the form of pain (8 times), lightheadedness (7), warmth (4), numbness (2), and various sensations (pounding, whirling, largeness, tightness, shakiness, electricity) (1 each) or as an undefined or funny feeling (8).

L. General Body Sensation. Such an aura was reported by 26 patients (or 14%). It consisted of nonlocalized, different sensations, either undefinable (5) or variously described as drawing or pulling (5), warm or cold (5), electric shock (5), tightness (3), or various sensations (numbness, body separation, "immobility," "swirling," general muscle cramp) (1 each).

M. Specific Sensory Aura. Twenty-nine patients (or 15.5%) reported a total of thirty-seven types of such sensations: vertiginous (14), visual (9), auditory (6), gustatory (6), olfactory (2).

N. Visceral Sensations. These were noted in a total of 38 patients (or 20%). An epigastric aura was reported by 28 patients (or 15%). Various types of other sensations (throat, abdominal, hunger) and/or profuse sweating, salivation, urge to urinate, marked blushing or pallor were present in 20 patients (or 10.5%).

O. Psychic aura. Illusions (including "déjà-vu" phenomena), hallucinations, and forced thinking occurred in 24 patients (or 13%).

P. Various Feelings. Forty patients (or 21%) reported a variety of feelings of a psychological-emotional nature, immediately preceding an ictal episode. These were generally difficult to define or categorize and included: strangeness, fright, tension, anxiety, discomfort, tiredness, nervousness, and so on.

AUTOMATISMS

Seizure patterns including automatic behavior were observed in 85 patients (or 45%). Prominent automatisms and/or seizures consisting of a pure automatism were present in 40 of such patients. In cases in whom the seizure also included motor tonic or clonic phenomena, automatic behavior would appear as the earliest manifestation (or immediately after

TABLE 3

SEIZURE PATTERNS: INCIDENCE IN TOTAL PATIENT POPULATION AND IN RELATION TO VARIOUS CLINICAL FINDINGS[a]

Seizure patterns[b]	Total population (N = 187)	Clinical negative (N = 54)	Hemiplegia (N = 86)	Hemihypoesthesia (N = 33)	Hemiatrophy (N = 23)	Visual field defect (N = 10)	Behavior disorder–mental retardation (N = 19)
A. Clonic	100 (53)	22 (41)	54 (63)	21 (63)	12 (52)	7 (70)	5 (26)
B. Clonic + H.E. adver.	39 (21)	10 (18)	19 (22)	8 (24)	6 (26)	— (—)	3 (16)
C. Clonic + tonic	35 (19)	12 (22)	19 (22)	9 (27)	5 (21)	4 (40)	1 (5)
D. Clonic + tonic + H.E. adver.	31 (16)	5 (9)	19 (22)	7 (21)	6 (26)	3 (30)	1 (5)
Clonic: total	124 (66)	32 (59)	63 (73)	24 (73)	15 (65)	8 (80)	6 (31)
E. Tonic unilateral	43 (23)	12 (22)	20 (23)	11 (33)	9 (39)	3 (30)	2 (10)
F. Tonic unilateral + bilateral	26 (14)	10 (18)	10 (11)	8 (24)	5 (21)	2 (20)	2 (10)
G. Tonic unilateral + bilateral + H.E. adver.	46 (24)	12 (22)	22 (25)	5 (15)	9 (39)	3 (30)	5 (26)
H. Tonic bilateral + H.E. adver.	25 (13)	9 (16)	8 (9)	4 (12)	3 (13)	2 (20)	6 (31)
I. H.E. adver.	57 (30)	18 (33)	25 (29)	9 (27)	9 (39)	2 (20)	6 (31)
Tonic: total	117 (62)	33 (61)	52 (60)	20 (60)	19 (83)	5 (50)	14 (74)
H.E. adver.: total	109 (58)	26 (48)	51 (59)	19 (57)	18 (78)	5 (50)	13 (68)
J. Aura: somatosensory	66 (35)	15 (28)	40 (47)	18 (54)	12 (52)	6 (60)	4 (21)
K. Aura: cephalic	32 (17)	12 (22)	13 (15)	9 (6)	4 (17)	3 (30)	— (—)
L. Aura: general body	26 (14)	8 (15)	12 (14)	8 (24)	6 (26)	1 (10)	1 (5)
M. Aura: sensory	29 (15)	6 (11)	14 (16)	6 (18)	6 (26)	4 (40)	2 (10)
N. Aura: visceral	38 (20)	8 (15)	19 (22)	10 (30)	9 (39)	3 (30)	4 (21)
O. Aura: various feelings	40 (21)	4 (7)	16 (18)	10 (30)	7 (30)	1 (10)	2 (10)
P. Aura: psychic	24 (13)	9 (16)	6 (7)	5 (15)	2 (9)	1 (10)	3 (16)
Q. Automatic phenomena	85 (45)	26 (48)	33 (38)	13 (39)	11 (48)	4 (40)	11 (58)
R. Pure automatism	40 (21)	14 (26)	13 (15)	5 (15)	4 (17)	— (—)	6 (31)

[a] Figures in parenthesis are percentages. N = number of patients.

[b] H.E. adver. = head and eyes tonic adversion.

an aura, if the latter was present) in 25 patients, whereas it was preceded by motor patterns in 24 patients. Various forms of automatisms were observed, and the same patient might exhibit either one single or several forms in the course of any given ictal episode. The following types of automatic behavior were observed in order of incidence (number of patients): gestural (60); ambulatory (38); alimentary (33); mimetic (22); verbal (18); laughing (11); complex movements and/or violence (9); and complex and organized activities (7).

SPEECH DISTURBANCES

In the case of 85 patients, on the basis of direct observation and testing during their ictal episode(s), or of specific statements in the available description, there were definitely no alterations of speech during or following the seizure. In 19 patients (or about 10%), aphasia was present, either ictal or postictal. Loss of articulation or speech arrest occurred in 51 patients (or 27%). In total, 67 different patients showed either aphasia or speech arrest or both. Twenty-eight additional patients had slurred speech (19 ictal, 9 postictal). The remaining patients only presented "moaning" or a cry in the course of their attack(s).

MOTOR PATTERNS

Of 187 patients, 19 (or about 10%) had no partial motor phenomena (exclusive of automatic movements) and/or only had generalized grand mal convulsions or generalized tonic seizures. Of the 168 patients with seizures consisting of motor manifestations (other than grand mal), 106 (or 63%) showed at least two and, often, three or more different patterns. All these various partial motor phenomena have been subdivided, for purposes of description and analysis, into nine categories including three main types (clonic, tonic, and head and eyes adversive movements) and several combinations thereof (see A through I in Tables 3 and 5):

   A. Pure clonic unilateral
   B. Clonic unilateral + head and eyes adversive
   C. Clonic unilateral + tonic unilateral and/or bilateral
   D. Clonic unilateral + tonic (unilateral or bilateral) + head and eyes adversive
   E. Tonic unilateral
   F. Tonic unilateral + bilateral
   G. Tonic unilateral + head and eyes adversive
   H. Tonic bilateral + head and eyes adversive
   I. Head and eyes adversive (only)
The incidence of these categories of motor patterns in the general patient population is shown in Tables 3 and 5. Clonic patterns were present in some or all seizures of 124 patients and seizures consisting of either tonic

postures or head and eyes adversions or both (without motor clonic components) occurred in 117 cases. (The same patients might show either type of motor pattern in different ictal episodes.) Patients with seizure motor patterns consisting always of clonic phenomena ($\pm$ tonic and $\pm$ head and eyes adversion) were 51 (or 27%). Patients with motor patterns consisting only of tonic phenomena ($\pm$ head and eyes adversion), without clonic movements in any of their seizures were 44 (or 23.5%). In 73 patients (or 39%) both types of seizures (i.e., with tonic and clonic phenomena) were observed.

Seizure Motor Patterns: Lateralizing Features

Motor patterns were characterized by lateralizing features in 160 patients. Of these, 82 cases had features that were exclusively unilateral and consistent as to the involved side in all their seizures. These included different patterns of motor phenomena in 39 patients, whereas the same, single seizure type repeatedly occurred (or only one ictal episode was observed) in 43 patients. In these two subgroups, however, all motor features were consistent in their lateralization, regardless of whether the seizures consisted of multiple different or of a single pattern.

In 78 patients, the involved side might shift in different seizures or different types of motor patterns might involve both sides asymmetrically (for example, tonic extension of the right arm with head and eyes turning to the left) in the course of the same ictal episode. Several different seizure types were observed in 66 patients, and the same complex seizure pattern would include lateralizing motor features pointing to both sides in 12 patients.

In the remaining 27 of the total 187 patients, lateralizing features were never observed, motor phenomena being absent or bilateral and symmetrical in all of their seizures. Of these, a single (or the same) seizure pattern was reported in 7 patients.

An attempt was made to evaluate the lateralizing reliability (especially in relation to the lateralization based on EEG interictal findings) of thirteen types of individual motor phenomena which have been observed (isolated or in the different combinations of patterns mentioned in the preceding section) in the course of various ictal episodes. In order to make such an evaluation, the lateralization of the epileptogenic lesion was first established independently on the basis of EEG, anatomopathological and clinical-radiological criteria (exclusive of the seizure patterns themselves). Such lateralization was obtained by at least one, but often two or all these three criteria, as indicated in Table 1. Thus, after exclusion of the 14 cases in whom the EEG findings had failed to disclose any lateralizing feature (bilateral abnormalities or patterns strongly suggestive of a centrencephalic involvement) and of 19 cases in whom the lateralization derived from EEG criteria was in conflict with that suggested by the clinical findings, a total of 154 patients could be utilized to assess the lateralizing value of the various ictal motor phenomena. Of these patients, 71 had seizures in which the motor patterns—no matter whether similar or different in type and association—consistently indicated a lateralization which was compatible with that indicated by the above criteria. On the basis of these same criteria, the lateralizing features of the various ictal motor phenomena were all inconsistent (that is, ipsilateral) in 7 patients, whereas in 59 patients the motor patterns were characterized by features suggestive of both right- and left-sided involvement in the same or in different seizures. Motor patterns were either absent or bilateral and symmetrical in the remaining 17 patients.

The lateralizing reliability of each of the thirteen individual motor phenomena is indicated in Table 4. This table shows the number of patients with seizures including each motor phenomenon, and the incidence of its lateralization (i.e., always contralateral, always ipsilateral, or both ipsi- and contralateral) as indicated by the analysis of all ictal episodes in each patient. The contralateral-ipsilateral ratios and the levels of statistical significance, if any, of the lateralizing validity of each phenomenon are also shown in this table. Note how certain of these motor patterns have an unquestionable contralateral predominance (to the preestablished location of the epi-

TABLE 4
LATERALIZING RELIABILITY OF VARIOUS ICTAL MOTOR PATTERNS[a]

Motor pattern	Contra-lateral	Ipsilateral or contra-lateral + ipsilateral	Ratio contralateral/ ipsilateral	Significance probability[b]	Chi square
Head tonic adversion	45	40	1.12	—	0.19
Eyes tonic adversion	35	31	1.13	—	0.14
Tonic					
Arm extension	24	12	2.00	—	3.36
Arm flection	35	13	2.69	<0.01	9.19
Hand extension	7	2	3.50	—	1.78
Hand flection	17	7	2.43	—	3.38
Leg extension	22	6	3.67	<0.01	8.04
Leg flection	6	9	0.67	—	0.07
Face	9	6	1.50	—	0.12
Clonic					
Face	53	8	6.62	<0.01	31.7
Arm	61	10	6.10	<0.01	35.4
Hand	34	5	6.80	<0.01	20.1
Leg	57	10	5.70	<0.01	31.6

[a] Contralateral and ipsilateral refer to the side of the electrographic focus of interictal epileptiform activity. These data are based on all seizures observed in 154 patients (see text). Any one of these thirteen motor patterns might have occurred either once or several times in the seizure(s) of any given patient; in the latter case the pattern could be consistently contralateral, consistently ipsilateral, or shift side in different ictal episodes.

[b] Obtained from testing the hypothesis of no lateralizing value.

leptogenic focus) and a statistically significant lateralizing value (that is, all types of clonic movements, tonic extention of one leg, tonic flection of one arm), whereas others have an almost equal ratio of contralateral versus ipsilateral location, and no lateralizing value can be demonstrated by statistical tests.

One-hundred and six patients out of 154 (or 69%) had unilateral clonic motor patterns in the course of at least one ictal episode. In 37 of such patients the clonic movements also occurred in association with tonic adversion of head and eyes, and in 10 they were always preceded by this tonic pattern. The clonic convulsions were in most instances (86.5%) consistently and exclusively contralateral to the electrographic focus in the 59 patients in whom this pattern was not accompanied by tonic adversion: in some seizures of 7 patients the clonic movements occurred also and in 1 only ipsilaterally. Of the 47 patients in whom such movements were always or often associated with a tonic adversion of head and eyes, consistent contralateral features were observed only in 23 (or 49%): ipsilateral clonic movements occurred in some seizures of 8 patients, ipsilateral adversion in some seizures of 10 patients, and both clonic and tonic adversion movements were ipsilateral in those of 10 patients. In summary, and considering only the motor clonic patterns, the ratio of their contralateral versus ipsilateral side of appearance was 51/8 (6.4) in those patients in whom the seizure consisted exclusively of such pattern, whereas it was 31/16 (1.95) in cases in whom the same motor pattern was associated with tonic head and eyes adversion. In the latter situation, the ratio of contra- versus ipsilateral head and eyes adversion was 27/20 (1.35).

ADDITIONAL LATERALIZING INFORMATION

Of the 154 patients who could be utilized (see preceding section), 57 had somatosensory auras preceding their seizures. Of these auras, only 2 were ipsilateral to the side of the epileptogenic focus. In 32 of the 55 patients with contralateral auras, the motor seizure patterns were also consistently in the contralateral side, and in 21 the motor patterns would be shifting from one to the other side in different ictal episodes or show bilateral, asymmetrical features in the same episode. Thus, of the 71 patients with seizure motor patterns consistently contralateral to the side of the epileptogenic focus, 32 had an additional confirmation of such lateralization by the occurrence of a somatosensory aura, whereas only 1 had his lateralization "weakened" by the presence of an ipsilateral aura. Of the 59 patients with seizure motor patterns shifting from one to the opposite side, a somatosensory aura "helped" in reinforcing the contralateral location of the focus in 21.

Of the 17 patients in whom motor phenomena were absent or without lateralizing features, a somatosensory aura contralateral to the focus was reported by 2.

Ictal or postictal speech disturbances (see above) could not be utilized for purposes of lateralization in this study due to the incomplete or questionable information concerning the side of cerebral dominance in a too large number of patients.

Seizure Patterns: Localization of Epileptogenic Foci

On the basis of their EEG interictal findings, all (except 4) patients were subdivided into four groups according to the main and most consistent brain localization of the paroxysmal abnormalities: (I) frontal (46 patients), (II) frontocentral (64), (III) central (33), (IV) centroparietal (40). The same patients (plus 4) were also distributed, according to different localization criteria, in four additional groups: (V) with parasagittal involvement (71 patients), (VI) with probable secondary involvement of temporal regions (37), (VII) with prominent diffuse or multifocal abnormalities in addition to the main focus (27), and (VIII) with (only or also) frontopolar involvement (25).

The distribution of clinical findings (exclusive of the seizure episodes) in these eight groups is shown in Table 2. Worth noting are the following points. (*a*) A relatively high percentage of patients with a normal neurological examination were found in the group of diffuse EEG abnormalities. This group would also tend to show a relatively greater number of patients with mental retardation and/or behavior disorders, and the smallest percentage of cases with hemiplegia and/or hemihypoesthesia. (*b*) The largest incidence of patients with sensory deficits was, as expected, in the group of centroparietal foci; a relatively larger number of patients in this same group as compared to all the other groups combined, also showed visual field defects. (This sign, however, only occurred in about 5% of the entire patient population.) (*c*) The incidence of hemiatrophy, on the other hand, did not seem to be significantly higher in patients of the centroparietal group. Such sign was present in only 1 patient (or 4%) of the group with electrographic evidence of frontopolar involvement.

The incidence of the various auras, automatisms, and different combinations of motor seizure patterns in the patients of each of these same eight groups is shown in Table 5. Table 6 compares such incidence between each individual group and the entire patient population, indicating those items for which the difference in incidence (either higher or lower) is statistically significant. Worth noting are the following findings. (*a*) Somatosensory auras occurred rarely in patients with epileptogenic foci in the frontal and frontopolar regions. An aura consisting of various general body sensations seems to be particularly common with foci in the frontopolar area. (*b*) There was a low incidence of clonic motor patterns in seizures originating from these same frontal regions. (*c*) Frontal foci would show a significantly high incidence of psychic auras. (*d*) Seizures originating from frontal foci tend to be characterized by adversive turning of head and eyes, with or without bilateral tonic motor patterns, as well as by frequent automatic behavior. The latter is particularly prominent when the epileptiform activity involves the frontopolar regions: in such cases not only are automatic phenomena common, but there is also a significantly higher incidence of seizures consisting exclusively of automatisms than in the overall patient population. (e) Seizures originating from epileptogenic foci localized in the central region show a high incidence of unilateral clonic and tonic motor patterns. (f) The same is true when the foci are in the parasagittal region in which case, however, clonic movements tend to be preferentially preceded by, or associated with, tonic adversion of head and eyes; in parasagittal foci, this last pattern would also occur as the only partial motor phenomenon of a seizure (with or without a final grand mal episode) in a high percentage of cases. (g) When the centroparietal regions are involved, there is a significantly high incidence of somatosensory auras and an equally significant low incidence of automatisms. (h) When the epileptiform activity is not limited to the supra-Sylvian regions but also appears over temporal structures, the incidence of visceral and especially epigastric auras is significantly higher and also higher is the incidence of auras involving specific sensory modalities (visual, auditory, olfactory, gustatory).

Table 6 also shows the significantly different incidence of several of these signs and patterns between any given group of patients and each one of the other groups. Thus, for instance, in one case in which the differential localization diagnosis of the epileptogenic focus is between frontal and central or centroparietal, the occurrence of automatisms would strongly suggest a frontal location. On the other hand, in the same hypothetical case, the occurrence of clonic motor patterns (with or without head and eyes tonic adversion) would support the central or centroparietal location. Such a diagnostic conclusion would be further reinforced by the presence of a somatosensory aura. Worth mentioning is the predominance of seizures with automatic components or consisting exclusively of automatisms in the group of patients with electrographic evidence of frontopolar involvement. This finding had already been stressed in comparing this group with the entire patient population, but it is interesting to note that the incidence of automatisms is also significantly higher in this group when it is compared to each of the other individual groups, including that of patients with EEG evidence of both supra-Sylvian and temporal lobe involvement.

Additional Findings Related to Seizure Patterns

SEIZURES WITHOUT PARTIAL MOTOR MANIFESTATIONS

The 27 patients in whom the motor seizure pattern(s) failed to provide any lateralizing clue or in whom no motor phenomena were present, appeared to be fairly evenly distributed among the various EEG diagnostic

TABLE 5

SEIZURE PATTERNS: INCIDENCE IN TOTAL POPULATION AND IN THE VARIOUS ELECTROENCEPHALOGRAM LOCALIZATION GROUPS[a]

Seizure patterns	Total population (N = 187)	Frontal (N = 46)	Fronto-central (N = 64)	Central (N = 33)	Centro-parietal (N = 40)	Para-sagittal (N = 71)	Temporal (secondary) (N = 37)	Diffuse or multifocal (N = 27)	Fronto-polar (N = 25)
A. Clonic	100 (53)	17 (37)	38 (59)	18 (54)	25 (62)	37 (52)	19 (51)	13 (48)	8 (32)
B. Clonic + H.E. adver.	39 (21)	2 (4)	18 (28)	8 (24)	10 (25)	21 (30)	8 (22)	8 (30)	3 (12)
C. Clonic + tonic	35 (19)	2 (4)	11 (17)	11 (33)	10 (25)	20 (28)	5 (13)	5 (18)	2 (8)
D. Clonic + tonic + H.E. adver.	31 (16)	2 (4)	14 (22)	6 (18)	8 (20)	14 (20)	7 (19)	7 (26)	4 (16)
Clonic: total	124 (66)	20 (43)	50 (78)	25 (76)	27 (67)	50 (70)	22 (59)	16 (59)	12 (48)
E. Tonic unilateral	43 (23)	10 (22)	19 (30)	8 (24)	6 (15)	20 (28)	7 (19)	5 (18)	5 (20)
F. Tonic unilateral + bilateral	26 (14)	10 (22)	7 (11)	3 (9)	6 (15)	12 (17)	7 (19)	3 (11)	5 (20)
G. Tonic unilateral + bilateral + H.E. adver.	46 (24)	14 (30)	17 (27)	8 (24)	6 (15)	22 (31)	11 (30)	9 (33)	10 (40)
H. Tonic bilateral + H.E. adver.	25 (13)	11 (24)	5 (8)	5 (15)	4 (10)	12 (17)	5 (13)	6 (22)	4 (16)
I. H.E. adver.	57 (30)	22 (48)	20 (31)	8 (24)	8 (20)	27 (38)	14 (38)	11 (41)	10 (40)
Tonic: total	117 (62)	38 (82)	45 (70)	17 (51)	16 (40)	53 (74)	29 (78)	18 (66)	21 (84)
H.E. adver.: total	109 (58)	32 (69)	40 (62)	18 (54)	18 (45)	49 (69)	27 (73)	21 (78)	18 (72)
J. Aura: somatosensory	66 (35)	8 (17)	20 (31)	15 (45)	21 (52)	24 (34)	8 (22)	6 (22)	4 (16)
K. Aura: cephalic	32 (17)	8 (17)	11 (17)	9 (27)	3 (7)	14 (20)	8 (22)	6 (22)	5 (20)
L. Aura: general body	26 (14)	9 (20)	12 (19)	2 (6)	3 (7)	10 (14)	8 (22)	5 (18)	8 (32)
M. Aura: sensory	29 (15)	5 (11)	10 (16)	3 (9)	10 (25)	9 (13)	10 (27)	6 (22)	4 (16)
N. Aura: visceral	38 (20)	10 (22)	13 (20)	6 (18)	9 (22)	16 (22)	13 (35)	6 (22)	3 (12)
O. Aura: various feelings	40 (21)	12 (26)	13 (20)	7 (21)	7 (17)	11 (15)	11 (30)	9 (33)	9 (36)
P. Aura: psychic	24 (13)	10 (22)	7 (11)	3 (9)	4 (10)	7 (10)	4 (11)	7 (26)	4 (16)
Aura: absent	53 (28)	14 (30)	19 (30)	9 (27)	9 (22)	18 (25)	9 (24)	10 (37)	7 (28)
Q. Automatic phenomena	85 (45)	28 (61)	34 (53)	10 (30)	10 (25)	33 (46)	23 (62)	17 (63)	21 (84)
R. Pure automatism	40 (21)	14 (30)	17 (27)	3 (9)	4 (10)	15 (21)	6 (16)	9 (33)	11 (44)

[a] Figures in parenthesis are percentages. N = number of patients. (See Table 6 for statistically significant figures.)

[b] H.E. adver. = head and eyes tonic adversion.

TABLE 6

SEIZURE PATTERNS: COMPARISON OF THEIR INCIDENCE BETWEEN ELECTROENCEPHALOGRAM LOCALIZATION GROUPS[a] AND BETWEEN EACH GROUP AND THE TOTAL PATIENT POPULATION[b]

	I Frontal	II Fronto-central	III Central	IV Centro-parietal	V Para-sagittal	VI Temporal (secondary)	VII Diffuse or multifocal	VIII Fronto-polar
vs All groups	(A)*, (B)*(C)* (D), H, I, (J)*, P, Q	(H)	C	J*, (Q)*(R)	B, C, I	M, N, Q	P, Q	(A), (J), L*, Q* R*
vs Group I		B*	B*, B*, J*	B*, C*, J*	B*, C*	B*	B*, D*	Q*
vs Group II	H*	—						Q*
vs Group III	Q*		—	—				L*, Q*, R*
vs Group IV	Q*	Q*					Q*	Q*, R*
vs Group V				J*	—		Q*	O*, Q*, R*
vs Group VI				J*		—		R*
vs Group VII				J*	—		—	
vs Group VIII	A*							—

[a] The first four groups all include different patients (plus 4) are redistributed in the remaining groups.

[b] The individual seizure patterns of Table 5 are referred here by capital letters. Only significant results are included in this table and should be interpreted as "is significantly greater than." In the comparison between each group and the entire patient population, the letters in parenthesis should be interpreted as "is significantly smaller than." Letters with asterisk indicate comparison between groups with corresponding seizure pattern is significant at 0.05 level by the same test. Absence of asterisk indicates significance at 0.01 level by a normal deviate test.

groups. The percentages varied between 8 and 20%, with the largest in the group of centroparietal foci and the smallest in that of frontocentral foci. These differences were not tested for statistical significance.

In 13 of these patients, the electrographic localization was clear-cut and consistent, and in additional 7 patients the EEG discharges were bilateral but with unilateral predominance. In 12 patients there were also neurological or X-ray signs of unilateral involvement.

TONIC ADVERSION OF HEAD AND EYES

Seizures consisting of this pattern only, with no other motor component, were observed at least once in 44 patients (or 23.5%). In about 75% of these, the electrographic focus was either frontal or frontocentral. Other ictal episodes in 10 of these 44 patients and in 13 other subjects, would consist of head and eyes adversive movements followed by a generalized tonic (and clonic) convulsion. A frontal or frontocentral EEG focus was also present in over 90% of these 23 patients. On the other hand, only 6 of the 73 patients with foci located in the central or centroparietal region, had seizure patterns consisting exclusively of grand mal preceded by tonic adversion of head and eyes (and in 3 of these there was EEG evidence of parasagittal or diffuse involvement).

Seventy-eight patients (or about 42%) never showed tonic head and eyes adversive movements in the course of their seizure(s). The lowest incidence of seizures without such motor pattern was found in the group of 71 patients with EEG evidence of parasagittal involvement (15, or 21%), whereas the highest incidence was noted in the group of 40 patients with centroparietal foci (22, or 55%). However, the location of the epileptogenic focus, as suggested by EEG data, did not appear to be significantly related to these negative findings.

MOTOR SEIZURE PATTERNS WITH BILATERAL DISTRIBUTION

Ictal episodes consisting of adversive head and eyes movements, accompanied by a variety of complex tonic postures and/or clonic convulsions of more-or-less limited sectors of both sides of the body occurred rather commonly. Thirty-nine patients showed, at least once, bilateral but asymmetrical motor components in the course of the same ictal episode; that is, features suggesting a possible participation of the two hemispheres or the activation of both ipsi- and contralateral mechanisms in the involved hemisphere. This finding was observed in about one-fifth of the entire patient population, and this incidence was similar in the eight groups of patients characterized by a common EEG localization of the epileptogenic process. Nevertheless, in 18 of these 39 patients (or 46%), the electrographic features were suggestive of a primary midline- parasagittal involvement.

In 48 patients, including 18 of the preceding series of 39, some seizures were characterized by motor phenomena which—regardless of the complexity of their patterns—were clearly unilateral, but the involved side would shift in different ictal episodes; that is, suggesting a left hemispheral origin in one and a right hemispheral origin in another seizure or vice versa. The EEG findings in this group of patients showed a relatively high percentage (36%) of bilateral patterns (with or without a clear hemispheral predominance) and, in 5 other patients, the electrographic evidence of lateralization was in conflict with that suggested by clinical neurological signs. In relation to the cortical localization of epileptiform discharges, the occurrence of seizures with motor patterns indicative of both right and left hemispheral origin, was found in a similar proportion of patients (20–25%) in all but one of the eight groups. The only group with a slightly higher incidence was the group of patients with EEG evidence of diffuse-multifocal involvement: such seizures would occur in over half of the members of this group. Worth mentioning is also the fact that 23 out of the 48 patients (or 48%) had EEG evidence suggestive of a midline-parasagittal involvement.

SEIZURE PATTERNS AND CLINICAL FINDINGS

Table 2 shows the incidence of the various auras, automatisms, and motor patterns in the seizures of patients in relation to their clinical findings. The following trends, not tested for statistical significance, are suggested. (a) The occurrence of a somatosensory aura seems to be relatively higher when patients have a hemihypoesthesia or a visual field defect, whereas it is less likely in patients with negative neurological findings or with mental retardation and/or behavior disorders. (b) Patients with the latter finding have the highest incidence of automatic phenomena and of seizures consisting exclusively of automatisms. On the other hand, a pure automatism was never observed in the 10 patients with visual field defect. (c) Patients with mental retardation and/or behavior disorder also tend to have the smallest incidence of motor unilateral clonic and/or tonic patterns, the motor phenomena in their ictal episodes consisting most frequently of bilateral tonic movements with adversion of head and eyes. (d) The highest incidence of clonic patterns is found in patients with hemiplegia, hemihypoesthesia, and visual field defects, whereas simple unilateral tonic postures of the limb(s) and simple adversion of head and eyes tend to predominate in patients with hemiatrophy.

DISCUSSION

The present study has confirmed the clinical impression of a much greater complexity and variability than one might expect, on the basis of textbook descriptions, in the pattern of so-called "partial (or focal) seizures with elementary expression," resulting from epileptogenic processes in the frontal and peri-Rolandic regions. Furthermore, repeated observations in a number of cases have shown that similar or practically indistinguishable seizure patterns can result, regardless of the specific electrographic location of the primary epileptogenic process within this relatively extensive supra-Sylvian area of the cerebral hemisphere. The study has also confirmed the fact that the numerous ictal episodes which one observes in certain patients may be characterized either by a single, stereotyped pattern or, more often, by multiple and rather different patterns. In addition, in the same or in different ictal episodes of a considerable number of patients, such patterns may include features that could suggest a possible primary involvement of either hemisphere, in spite of the often clear and consistent electrographic and clinical evidence of a unilateral location of the epileptogenic process.

These findings are unquestionably puzzling and, in most cases, do not lend themselves to a logical interpretation. Some of these could be the consequence of possible misinterpretations of the electrographic data or, more probably, simply reflect the inadequacy of scalp EEG to provide with precision location and extent of the epileptogenic process; for instance, in differentiating a purely cortical from a corticosubcortical or even primarily subcortical involvement. It should also be kept in mind that only the electrographic interictal manifestations have been utilized for the localization of an epileptogenic process, since recordings during the occurrence of spontaneous ictal episodes could be obtained only sporadically. On the other hand, the information provided by the simultaneous EEG monitoring of induced seizures had proved similarly inadequate for a satisfactory interpretation of most findings, in a previous study (1). Whatever limitations might be implicit in the methods and criteria which have been employed here to localize and lateralize an epileptogenic focus, these would only account for some of the present findings; a convincing interpretation would still be wanted for the large majority of the findings.

Although our knowledge of the pathophysiology of the epileptogenic process remains fragmentary, its diagnostic localization and lateralization continues to depend almost exclusively on the correct interpretation of the functional manifestations of the process, both central (i.e., electrographic) and peripheral (i.e., subjective and objective) phenomena that constitute the seizure patterns. One of the purposes of this study was to improve our understanding of—and thus better utilize—all the possible information provided by the clinical seizure patterns, for the solution of practical diagnostic problems. This goal was only partially fulfilled, and the localization of an epileptogenic process will keep presenting a challenge in many individual situations. On the basis of our findings, however, it should be possible in the future to utilize a larger number of data, in a more reliable way, or, alternatively, to minimize the significance of other data and thus substantially increase the probability of a correct diagnosis.

In the matter of some thirteen seizure motor patterns with unilateral distribution, for instance, it has been possible to establish the relative significance of each of them for the lateralization of the epileptogenic process presumably responsible for their occurrence. This set of data clearly shows the highly reliable lateralization value of certain patterns (such as unilateral clonic convulsions of limbs and face), the total unreliability of others (such as tonic flection of one leg) and the very questionable value of still other patterns (such as tonic adversive turning of head and eyes, tonic contraction of one side of the face, or tonic extension of one arm). Thus, if a patient shows in one of his ictal episodes a tonic turning of head and eyes to the right, and in the course of another seizure, clonic movements of the left arm, the lateralizing significance of the former pattern should be questioned or deemphasized, the probability being fairly high that the epileptogenic focus is on his right hemisphere. In contrast, cases in whom clonic movements of one limb or hemiface are preceded by, or associated with, a tonic adversion of head and eyes in the course of the same ictal episode, are more difficult to interpret. Such patients tend to show a high incidence of conflicting lateralizing features, not only in the tonic adversive pattern but also in the clonic pattern. The possibility of bilateral epileptogenic processes should be considered in such cases, even when the electrographic evidence seems clearly to indicate a unilateral involvement.

The lateralizing value of a somatosensory aura was consistently very high. Such an aura was reported by more than one-third of patients showing a definite unilateral focus in their EEG, and the incidence of its occurrence in one sector of the hemibody ipsilateral to the side of the electrographic focus was less than 4%.

The high lateralizing value of the aura which, by definition, is the earliest sign of a seizure, might suggest that some of the various motor patterns carried with them no lateralizing validity purely because these were the peripheral expression of spread of epileptic activation to other cortical regions situated within the opposite hemisphere. Being aware of this possibility, we have avoided including in our analysis any motor pattern that might appear later in the course of an ictal episode. Most of the thirteen motor phenomena listed in Table 4 occurred either as a single isolated phenomenon or, when associated with others, simultaneously. In those cases in which, for instance, a contralateral tonic adversion of the head was followed, after a few seconds, by an ipsilateral tonic adversion, the latter was not included in the data and the pattern was tabulated only as "contralateral."

The localizing value of the various seizure patterns, either taken in isolation or in their complex combination was, in general, less easy to assess than their lateralizing value. The reason for this should probably be looked for, at least in part, in the fact that the EEG evidence, itself, was clearly indicative of an epileptogenic process localized to a specific, circumscribed region in only a relatively small number of cases. The electrographic findings in the large majority of patients would suggest that the process involved more than one cortical region. Thus, in most cases, one had to rely on subjective interpretations of the tracings to determine the site of the most important or primary focus. On the basis of such interpretation, patients were then assigned to a given group of regional localization, without it being possible, however, to avoid a certain degree of overlap between the different groups. In view of this situation, the various correlative analyses of seizure patterns, which were eventually carried out in the individual members of each group for comparison with those of the other groups, could hardly be expected to yield results sufficiently clear-cut and of an absolute pathognomonic significance, to be subsequently utilized as crucial criteria in cases where the differential topographical diagnosis of the epileptogenic focus presents a problem.

In spite of these limitations, it has been possible to establish, at least on a statistical basis, the preferential frequency of occurrence (or, alternatively, the scarcity) of certain patterns in the seizures resulting from epileptogenic processes of specific cortical locations. Thus, for instance, the presence of a somatosensory aura would make a frontopolar or purely frontal origin rather unlikely, whereas the presence of a psychic aura would strongly suggest such an origin. Similarly, an epileptogenic lesion involving exclusively these same regions would seldom manifest itself with clonic (Jacksonian) movements but, quite frequently, with seizures characterized by a tonic adversion of head and eyes with or without complex tonic postures of the limbs of both sides [see, also, Fegersten and Roger (4).] The findings related to the preceding example, although proving the localizing value (or lack thereof; see Table 6) of a number of seizure patterns, could hardly be defined as strikingly original. Indeed, most of such findings have been well known even before the detailed analysis carried out by Penfield [see Penfield and Jasper (8)].

However, some similar findings were less well established, at least in our experience. Thus, the significantly high incidence of automatic phenomena (and also of ictal episodes consisting exclusively of automatisms), in the case of frontal and especially frontopolar epileptogenic lesions, was rather surprising. In fact, the statistical significance of such incidence held true not only in comparisons between these groups and the total patient population, but also when these groups were compared with that of patients with evidence of temporal lobe involvement. In spite of the fact that cases with pure temporal lobe foci have not been included in the present study, such findings appear rather interesting.

The high incidence of somatosensory auras in the group of patients with centroparietal foci is not surprising. Although such an aura occurred also in a considerable number of patients with pure central and with centroparasagittal foci, its higher incidence was statistically significant only for the group of centroparietal lesions, both in relation to the entire patient population and in relation to various individual groups (especially those of patients with frontal involvement). Thus, in a case in whom the differential diagnosis of the location of an epileptogenic process is between centroparietal and frontal, the occurrence of a somatosensory aura would strongly favor the former, and this diagnosis would be reinforced by the presence of unilateral clonic movements and by the total absence of automatic phenomena.

These and other analogous findings should simply be interpreted as indicating that some seizure patterns or signs tend to occur preferentially, whereas others are rather uncommon, in any given group of patients in whom the epileptogenic process involves primarily certain cortical regions. The relation between site of the cortical focus and seizure symptomatology tends to be in the direction of that suggested by cortical physiology and is in general agreement with the commonly accepted notions of clinical neurology. On the other hand, and in spite of the statistical significance of some of the figures, this study has clearly demonstrated that each and every sign or pattern can indeed occur in the course of seizures of some members of each different group of patients. Therefore, the localizing value of individual auras, motor patterns, or automatisms should never be considered as crucial but, simply, suggestive. Only the coexistence (and absence) of a number of these specific signs and patterns in the seizure(s) of any given patient would permit reaching a reliable diagnostic localization conclusion which might confirm (or, occasionally, contradict) that derived from the interpretation of the electrographic findings.

SUMMARY

1. The patterns of a large number of ictal episodes in 187 patients with electrographic evidence of a focal epileptogenic process in the frontocentroparietal regions have been analyzed and correlated with the presumed site and side of such processes. Age, etiopathology, clinical findings (exclusive of the seizure patterns), and other data have also been taken into consideration.

2. For this analysis, the following seizure patterns (and association thereof) have been considered: auras (seven types), motor phenomena (nine main types), and automatic phenomena. On the basis of the localization of interictal paroxysmal discharges in their EEG, the patients have been subdivided in four main groups (frontal, frontocentral, central, and centroparietal) and also into four other overlapping groups emphasizing particular or addition localizations (parasagittal, secondary temporal, diffuse or multifocal, and frontopolar).

3. The lateralizing reliability of thirteen types of individual motor phenomena, occurring in various ictal episodes, was evaluated in 154 patients in whom it had been possible to establish with reasonable certainty the hemispheral side involved by the epileptogenic process, on the basis of

EEG, anatomopathological, and clinical–radiological criteria. A somatosensory aura was found to have the highest localizing value (being contralateral to the side of the presumed epileptogenic lesion in over 96% of the 57 patients reporting it).

4. Epileptogenic processes localized to certain cortical regions tend to manifest themselves with (or without) certain seizure patterns. The higher (or lower) incidence of many of such seizure patterns in the different groups of patients with a common regional (electrographic) localization of their epileptogenic process, was statistically significant. On the other hand, the incidence of other patterns did not seem to bear any significant relationship with the site of the interictal EEG focus.

5. These and other findings have been discussed in relation to their practical diagnostic implications.

REFERENCES

1. Ajmone Marsan, C., and Abraham, K., A seizure atlas. *Electroenceph. clin. Neurophysiol.*, 1960, Suppl., **15**: 1–215.
2. Ajmone Marsan, C., and Lewis, W. R., Pathological findings in patients with EEG "centrencephalic" patterns. *Neurology (Minneap.)*, 1960; **10**: 922–930.
3. Ajmone Marsan, C., and Zivin, L. S., Factors related to the occurrence of typical paroxysmal abnormalities in the EEG records of epileptic patients. *Epilepsia*, 1970, **11**: 361–381.
4. Fegersten, L., and Roger, A., Frontal epileptogenic foci and their clinical correlations. *Electroenceph. clin. Neurophysiol.*, 1961, **13**: 905–913.
5. Gabor, A. J., and Ajmone Marsan, C., Co-existence of focal and bilateral diffuse paroxysmal discharges in epileptics. *Epilepsia*, 1969, **10**: 453–472.
6. Gastaut, H., Epilepsies. In: *Encyclopédie Médico-Chirurgicale*, Paris, 1963: 1–44.
7. Kennedy, W. A., Clinical and electroencephalographic aspects of epileptogenic lesions of the medial surface and superior border of the cerebral hemisphere. *Brain*, 1959, **82**: 147–161.
8. Penfield, W., and Jasper, H. H., *Epilepsy and the Functional Anatomy of the Human Brain*. Little, Brown, Boston, 1954.
9. Penfield, W., and Kristiansen, K., *Epileptic Seizure Patterns*. Thomas, Springfield, Illinois, 1951.
10. Rasmussen, T., Surgical therapy of frontal lobe epilepsy. *Epilepsia*, 1963, **4**: 181–198.
11. Zivin, L., and Ajmone, Marsan, C., Incidence and prognostic significance of "epileptiform" activity in the EEG of non-epileptic subjects. *Brain*, 1968, **91**: 751–778.

PROBLEMS OF ANALYSIS AND INTERPRETATION OF ELECTROCEREBRAL SIGNALS IN HUMAN EPILEPSY. A NEUROSURGEON'S VIEW

GIAN FRANCO ROSSI*

Istituto di Neurochirurgia, Università Cattolica del Sacro Cuore, Rome, Italy

The prime object of surgical treatment of epilepsy is the removal of the causal brain pathology and of the brain tissue giving origin to the paroxysmal discharge responsible for the seizure, namely, the epileptogenic zone. If only one epileptogenic zone is found responsible for the epileptic syndrome, surgery can lead to the definitive disappearance of the seizures. Surgery may be taken into consideration also in order to interrupt the pathway or pathways of propagation of the paroxysmal discharge from the epileptogenic area to other cerebral regions. In this latter case, surgical treatment aims at preventing diffusion and generalization of the epileptic discharge but does not suppress it. In any case, it is apparent that the first necessary prerequisite for surgical treatment of epilepsy is the identification and accurate spatial location of the epileptogenic zone.

There are patients in whom the clinical characteristics of the seizure itself bring sufficient or strong evidence. This is the case, for instance, of typical Jacksonian motor seizures or, more generally, of the partial seizures characterized by what has been called "simple symptomatology" [see the recent classification proposed by an international committee (34)]. In many epileptic patients, however, the clinical seizure pattern is of such complexity as to make recognition of its precise site of origin within the brain and, in many cases, even of the hemisphere in which it originates, very hard or unreliable. If we take into consideration here only the cases which do not show clinically and neuroradiologically any obvious gross brain lesion, the main possibilities of finding where the epileptogenic zone is located depend on electrophysiological exploration of the brain.

The great help provided by electroencephalography in the diagnosis of

* The personal research reported in the present article was supported by the Consiglio Nazionale delle Ricerche, Contract No. 70.1817.04, and by the Programma Speciale Tecnologie Biomediche, Consiglio Nazionale delle Ricerche. I wish to thank Drs. A. Gentilomo and G. Colicchio for their help in selection and analysis of the stereoelectroencephalographic material, and Drs. G. Rosadini, B. Cavazza, and F. Ferrillo of the Centro di Neurofisiologia Cerebrale of the Consiglio Nazionale delle Ricerche, Genoa, for the computer analysis of part of the records.

epilepsy is well known. Very good results can be reached, particularly when the standard electroencephalogram (EEG) is integrated with electroencephalographic examinations performed under particular conditions already discussed by us at length elsewhere (5, 60): during nocturnal sleep, during intravenous injection of convulsant drugs, and during intracarotid and intravertebral injections of barbiturates or convulsants.

It is also well known that conventional electroencephalography based on recording of brain electrical activity through electrodes applied on the scalp has great limitations. Epileptic discharges occurring in deeply located brain structures—and even in the cortex (1, 21)—may not be revealed by scalp electrodes. Furthermore, scalp-recorded ictal discharges can result from the propagation to the brain surface of ictal activity arising deeply and not detectable. Misleading interpretations may follow. Direct recording from the exposed cerebral cortex or electrocorticography only partially obviates these difficulties. For these reasons, during the fifties, methods for exploration of electrocerebral activity of man through electrodes directly inserted into the brain, stereoelectroencephalography (10), were developed (4, 8, 11, 13, 19, 20, 24, 25, 27, 32, 36, 38, 40, 41, 43, 44, 46, 48, 50, 58, 64, 68, 72, 73, 75). Indeed the experience obtained so far has proved that stereoelectroencephalography can substantially help the neurosurgeon in getting a more precise picture of the epileptic phenomena and in planning the strategy for surgical treatment.

Considered as a whole, the electrophysiological technologies are today sufficiently developed to allow the collection of a number of data; however, anyone who is familiar with electroencephalography, and even more with stereoelectroencephalography, knows very well how many and multiform can be the abnormal electrocerebral events recorded from the brain of the epileptic patient. Potentially, each one of these events should provide information about the epileptogenic state of the cerebral structure from which it is recorded. The mode of occurrence of the epileptic potentials, their changing behavior during prolonged recording, their spatial distribution, their reciprocal interrelations should reflect the dynamic features of the epileptic process and the relative role that the different cerebral structures play in the epileptic syndrome of the patient under examination.

We are faced here with the problem of the analysis and interpretation of the epileptic electrocerebral signals. For as stated at the beginning, from a neurosurgical point of view, the problem is that of extracting from these signals the information necessary to reach identification of the epileptogenic zone. The problem is certainly not an easy one. Obviously, the present report does not presume to offer or suggest its solution. Its aim is simply that of making an attempt, based on personal experience, to focus on some of the aspects of the problem for discussion.

The material presented is taken from stereoelectroencephalographic recordings in epileptic patients hospitalized in our Institute. All of them were considered as possible candidates for surgical treatment because of the failure of pharmacological therapy to control their frequently occurring seizures. In most of the cases, the latter were of temporal lobe origin.

Procedure

Multipolar electrodes (several Teflon-insulated stainless-steel wires, 0.10 mm in diameter, bound together to form a shaft) were implanted, with the help of the Talairach's stereotaxic instrument, into cerebral structures preselected on the basis of the clinical characteristics of the seizures and of several electroencephalographic examinations, according to criteria previously reported (22, 52, 53, 54, 59, 60, 61).

A comment on the relative importance of "acute" versus "chronic" stereoelectroencephalographic exploration will introduce our discussion. An analysis of some of the aspects of the electrocerebral epileptic signals will follow. For this purpose, the electrical abnormalities recorded in epileptics will be subdivided into two main groups: the ictal and the interictal ones. The two groups will be considered separately.

Duration of the Stereoelectroencephalographic Recording

In standard electroencephalography a well-known criterion for judging the physiopathological origin and diagnostic significance of a given epileptic abnormality is the consistency of the phenomenon in time. Repeated occurrence with the same or similar electrophysiological and topographical characteristics gives value to the finding; sporadic or occasionally occurring abnormalities are, on the contrary, of little help. On this account, long-lasting and often repeated EEGs are required. In our opinion, as well as in that of many others (56, 58, 63; and, in addition, 3, 7, 14–18, 21, 23, 26, 29, 33, 39, 45, 47, 57, 62, 66, 71, 74) the same criterion has to be applied when performing stereoelectroencephalographic examinations and when attempting an interpretation of the meaning of the electrocerebral epileptic signals recorded from depth.

An example (Case 1) of the importance of repeated recording is given in Figure 1 in which two samples of the stereoelectroencephalographic recording taken from a young man suffering from partial seizures with complex symptomatology are reproduced. It was found necessary to explore both temporal lobes and both supplementary motor areas because of some clinical aspects of the seizures. Electrodes were, therefore, chronically implanted in these structures. On the first day after implantation, electrical ictal activity was recorded only from the left supplementary motor area (left part of Figure 1): short-lasting discharges of the type illustrated were repeatedly observed during the day. The next day, the ictal activity from the left supplementary motor area was no longer present. Finally, on the third day, ictal discharges occurred in the left amygdala (right part of

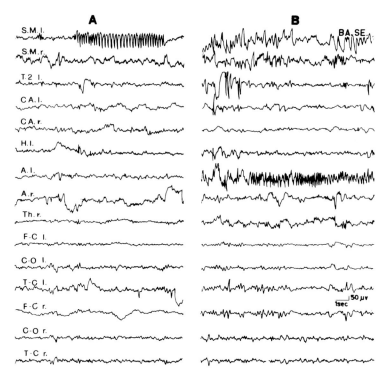

Figure 1. Depth (channels 1 to 9) and scalp (channels 10 to 15) recording from a patient suffering from partial seizures with complex symptomatology (Case 1). (A) First day after electrode implantation; ictal electrical discharge from left supplementary motor area. (B) Two days after A; ictal discharge from the left amygdala. S.M., supplementary motor area; T.2., second temporal convolution; C.A., Ammon's horn; H., hippocampal gyrus; A., amygdala; Th., centromedian thalamic nucleus; F-C, frontocentral; C-O, centro-occipital; T-C, temporocentral; l, left; r, right.

Figure 1), in one instance heralding a clinical seizure. In the case just illustrated, the existence of an unique epileptogenic zone involving the left supplementary motor area only, might have been suspected on the basis of an acute or 1-day examination. It was only by continuing the examination for some days that ictal discharges originating from other structures could be noticed. Other examples of the utility of protracting the stereoelectroencephalographic analysis for several days will be given later.

Anatamomicroscopical controls of surgical specimens have shown that the damage to nervous tissue caused by chronically implanted electrodes is minimal (7, 28, 33, 57), and this was confirmed by our own experience.

Nevertheless, some disadvantages of the use of chronically implanted electrodes have to be mentioned. First of all, chronic implantation potentially increases the risk of infection. This can be avoided by appropriate care. Actually, in our experience, infection in the epileptic patients with implanted electrodes is lower than in other neurosurgical operations. A second and more relevant disadvantage of chronic stereoelectroencephalographic examination is the lessened flexibility of spatial brain exploration. This is due to the usually lower number of exploring electrodes in chronic than in acute stereoelectroencephalography and the possibly frequent changes in position of each electrode in acute but not in chronic exploration. This is perhaps the main reason why acute stereotaxic exploration is considered preferable to the chronic one for several scientists (10). These limitations of chronic stereoelectroencephalography are partially overcome by the use of multipolar electrodes and, above all, by accurate study of the patient prior to implant, which would provide the necessary information for the careful planning of exploration strategy.

Summing up, in our opinion, the balance between acute and chronic exploration is in favor of the latter. According to our experience, in many patients there is a great variability of the epileptic picture. Different epileptic phenomena may be recorded either on different days, the conditions of the patient being apparently similar (as in the example illustrated above), or on the same day in relation to changes of the patient's conditions: physiological sleep or particular emotional situations or drug administration, all of which obviously influence the epileptic pattern (some examples will be given later). The chances of getting a more complete and precise picture of the epileptic process are, therefore, increased by prolonged recording. Radiotelemetry of the recorded electrocerebral activity further extends the possibilities of examining the patient in several conditions, as stressed by Dr. Crandall in this volume (see also 42, 45, 65).

RECORDING OF ICTAL ELECTRICAL ACTIVITY

In agreement with many other neurosurgeons and electroencephalographers, we believe that the recording of epileptic ictal discharges is of very great value (10). Indeed, the ictal discharge can be regarded as the electrocerebral signal most directly indicative of the epileptogenic state of a neuronal population. Two examples of two different situations leading to two completely different interpretations of the epileptic process will be given.

Figure 2 illustrates the EEG and stereoelectroencephalographic records from a young man suffering from partial seizures with complex symptomatology (Case 2). The clinical characters of the seizures pointed to their origin from the temporal lobe but did not indicate the side. Likewise, the scalp EEG did not help. Several electrodes were implanted in the temporal structures of both sides; one electrode in the centromedian thalamic nucleus. A well-organized ictal discharge is seen to arise from the anterior part of the left hippocampal gyrus and then propagate to the posterior part of the same structure. Nothing appears on the scalp EEG. During the discharge the patient felt what could be considered the "aura" usually preceding his seizures. This pattern was recorded several times during 10 days. Figure 3 reproduces another sample of the stereoelectroencephalo-

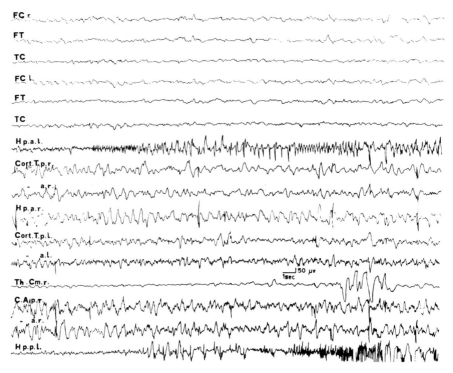

Figure 2. Scalp electroencephalogram (EEG) (channels 1 to 6) and stereoelectroencephalographic recording (channels 7 to 16) from a patient suffering from partial seizures with complex symptomatology (Case 2). An ictal discharge arises from the anterior part of the left hippocampal gyrus and later involves the posterior part of the same structure. The patient experiences an "aura." No ictal activity appears in the recordings from the other deep structures nor in the scalp EEG. FC, frontocentral; FT, frontotemporal; TC, temporocentral; Hp., hippocampal gyrus; Cort. T., temporal neocortex; Th.Cm., centromedian thalamic nucleus; C.A., Ammon's horn; a., anterior; p., posterior; r., right; l., left.

graphic record taken from the same patient during Megimide activation. Here again, an ictal discharge appears at the level of the anterior part of the left hippocampal gyrus and quickly propagates to other temporal structures, at first in the left and then in the right hemisphere. A typical clinical seizure accompanied the electrical discharge. Finally, the electrical stimulation of the same anterior part of the left hippocampal gyrus proved to be the one which could elicit epileptic discharges with the lowest threshold.

Summing up, the most relevant findings in the case just illustrated were that (a) the spontaneous ictal discharges occurred always and only from the same cerebral structure; (b) the ictal discharges induced by the intravenous injection of a convulsant drug also came from the same structure; and (c) the same structure was the most sensitive to direct electrical stimulation. The evidence that this structure belonged to the epileptogenic zone

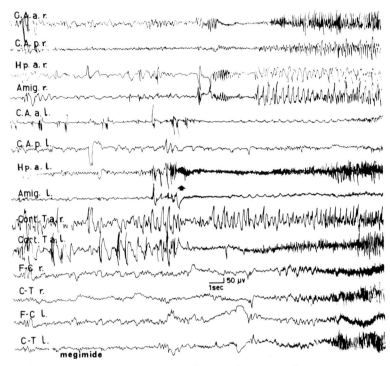

Figure 3. Same patient as in Figure 2 (Case 2). Megimide activation (10 cc). An ictal discharge arises from the anterior part of the left hippocampal gyrus then quickly generalizes. The arrows mark the beginning of the clinical seizure. C.A., Ammon's horn; Hp., hippocampal gyrus; Amig., amygdala; Cort. T., temporal neocortex; F-C, frontocentral; C-T, centro-temporal; a., anterior; p., posterior; r., right; l., left.

responsible for the epileptic syndrome of the patient was thus considered sufficient. This young man was operated upon for a left anterior temporal lobectomy and the seizures completely disappeared. In other words, this can be considered an "easy" case.

Let us now take into consideration a completely different picture. The case has been briefly mentioned before (Case 1) when discussing the utility of prolonged stereoelectroencephalographic examination. As we have seen (see Figure 1), ictal discharges were recorded on different days from the left supplementary motor area and from the left amygdala. The latter was found to give rise to a clinical seizure. Figure 4 illustrates the effect of Megimide intravenous injection in the same patient: an ictal electrical discharge, accompanied by a clinical seizure, arises from the right amygdala. The clinical characteristics of the seizure were quite similar to those of the previously observed seizure originating from the left amygdala.

To sum up, the analysis of the ictal activity in this patient did not appear to indicate the existence of an unique epileptogenic zone responsible for the whole epileptic syndrome. The possibility of a "multifocal" origin of such a syndrome had to be considered. The results of direct electrical stimu-

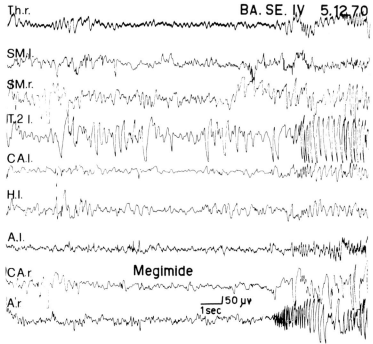

Figure 4. Same patient as in Figure 1 (Case 1). Megimide activation (15 cc). Ictal discharge accompanied by clinical seizure arising from the right amygdala and then involving other temporal structures of the ipsi- and contralateral side. Th., centromedian thalamic nucleus; SM., supplementary motor area; T.2, second temporal convolution; CA., Ammon's horn; H., hippocampus; A., amygdala; r., right; l., left.

lation appeared to support such a view. The case was judged unsuitable for surgical treatment.

RECORDING OF INTERICTAL ABNORMALITIES

The case just illustrated, in which it appeared that ictal epileptic discharges could take origin from different cerebral structures, is relevant to the third part of our discussion. This will deal with the interpretation and possible utilization of the stereotactically recorded interictal epileptic activity.

As is well known, opinions differ considerably in this regard. On the one hand (9, 10, 49, 67), it has been stated that the interictal epileptic potentials cannot be of substantial help in elucidating the mechanism of origin of the epileptic syndrome. This view is based on the fact that they are often too multifarious and too dispersed anatomically; they can have been propagated from other structures rather than originating from the recorded site; their morphology can hardly help in differentiating between primary or secondary origin; and so on. On the other hand [see, for instance,

Penfield and Jasper (51)], it has been suggested that information of diagnostic utility can be gained by careful analysis of morphology and amplitude; possible association with abnormal background electrical activity; time relations between potentials recorded from different cerebral structures, and rate of discharge.

An attempt was made to analyze whether or not, and in what way one might find electrophysiological criteria helpful in identifying the relative importance of the many and multiform interictal signals. An analysis of our material brought into evidence some data which I consider useful to report here. In particular, the following four points will be taken into consideration: (a) rate of discharge or amount of interictal epileptic potentials; (b) regularity or stability of interictal epileptic discharges; (c) characteristics of background nonepileptic electrical activity; (d) time relationships among interictal epileptic potentials recorded from different brain structures.

Amount of Interictal Epileptic Potentials

A relatively simple example appears apt for beginning our discussion. It is taken from a patient (Case 3) presenting epileptic seizures of psychomotor type, with typical automatisms, which were considered to be of temporal origin. The clinical aspects of the seizures as well as in the scalp-recorded EEG, which showed bilateral temporal spiking, did not lateralize the temporal lobe involved. Figure 5 illustrates recordings made by depth electrodes between seizures: isolated epileptic potentials occur in several of the temporal structures explored; most of them appear to lack any obvious time relation. However, the rate of discharge or, in other words, the amount of interictal epileptic activity is definitely more abundant in the left Ammon's horn. Figure 6 reproduces one of the typical ictal discharges found in the same patient, in this case provoked by a small amount of Megimide. There is no doubt that the discharge arises from the same structure, namely, the left Ammon's horn, which is the site of the most intense interictal epileptic activity. Two years ago, left temporal lobectomy was performed, and the patient has been free from seizures since.

In this case, therefore, we find an indication that the rate of discharge or the amount of interictal epileptic potentials can throw some light on the epileptogenicity of the explored cerebral structures.

In the following case (Case 4) the interpretation of the stereoelectro-encephalographic findings is more difficult. Electrodes were chronically implanted in temporal and frontal structures of both hemispheres in a young lady suffering from partial seizures with complex symptomatology, as well as from generalized convulsive seizures. Figure 7 shows an ictal discharge arising on a background of intense diffuse spiking in the right Ammon's horn following intravenous injection of Cardiazol (Metrazol). In contrast, Figure 8 shows that, during the same recording session, another seizure

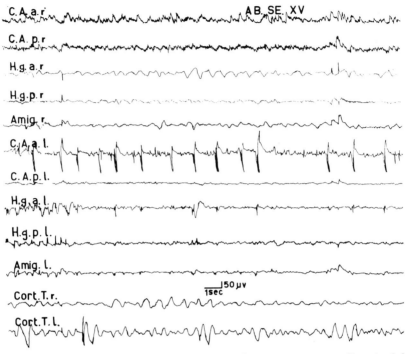

Figure 5. Stereoelectroencephalographic record of a patient eventually cured by left temporal lobectomy (Case 3). Interictal epileptic potentials are recorded from several temporal structures, mainly on the left side, and particularly from the anterior part of the left Ammon's horn. C.A., Ammon's horn; H.g., hippocampal gyrus; Amig., amygdala; Cort. T., temporal neocortex; a., anterior; p., posterior; l., left; r., right.

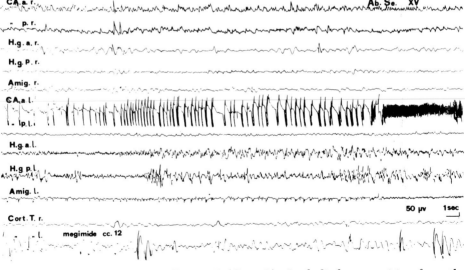

Figure 6. Same patient as in Figure 5 (Case 3). Ictal discharges arising from the anterior part of the left Ammon's horn following Megimide intravenous injection (12 cc). C.A., Ammon's horn; H.g. hippocampal gyrus; Amig., amygdala; Cort. T., temporal neocortex; a., anterior; p., posterior; r., right; l., left.

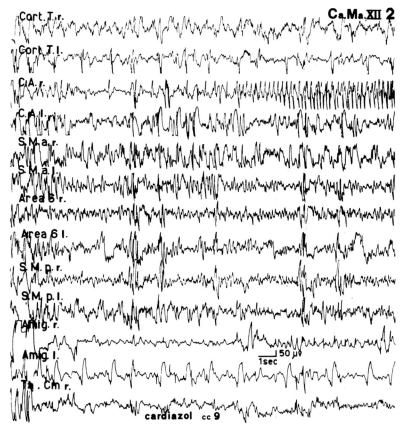

Figure 7. Stereoelectroencephalographic recording from a patient suffering from partial seizures with complex symptomatology and also from generalized seizures (Case 4). Cardiazol activation. On a background of abundant and diffuse epileptic potentials an ictal discharge appears in the right Ammon's horn. Cort. T., temporal neocortex; C.A., Ammon's horn; S.M., supplementary motor area; Area 6, frontal area 6; Amig., amygdala; Th.Cm., centromedian thalamic nucleus; l., left; r., right; a., anterior; p., posterior.

discharge occurs in left temporal neocortex, perhaps accompanied by a less evident discharge from the left amygdala. Finally, Figure 9 reproduces the stereoelectroencephalogram recorded shortly after the previous ones and shows another and more important seizure discharge involving at first the frontal structures and later the temporal neocortex. Repeated examinations, performed during several days, confirmed that ictal discharges, followed by clinical seizures, could arise from different brain sites (see also Figures 11 and 12). An interesting behavior of the interictal activity was noticed. Figure 10 reproduces a typical sample of the interictal pattern, showing that, although epileptic potentials occur in several structures of both temporal lobes and also in the frontal lobes, there is an obvious numerical prevalence in the Ammon's horn of the right side. As shown in Figure 11, the record obtained on a different day confirms this finding

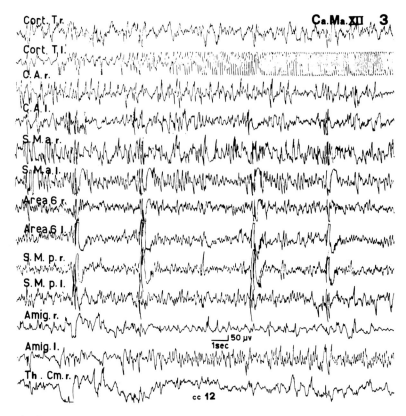

Figure 8. Same patient as in Figure 7 during the same recording session. Another ictal discharge now arises from the left temporal neocortex, perhaps accompanied by ictal activity in the ipsilateral amygdala. Cort. T., temporal neocortex; C.A., Ammon's horn; S.M., supplementary motor area; Area 6, frontal area 6; Amig., amygdala; Th.Cm., centromedian thalamic nucleus; r., right; l., left; a., anterior; p., posterior.

and in addition shows that ictal electrical activity can originate from the same structure.

To sum up, stereoelectroencephalography, in this patient, shows that (*a*) ictal epileptic discharges can arise from both right and left temporal lobes and from the frontal lobe and (*b*) the interictal epileptic activity is definitely more conspicuous in the right temporal lobe and precisely in the Ammon's horn.

When we examined the patient, we decided that the indications given by the ictal activity deserved more consideration. Therefore, the patient was not operated upon. A few months later, she was brought into the hospital in a comatose state, which was due to protracted epileptic status. She died a few hours after hospitalization. Autopsy was performed. A large and old lesion was found within the tip of the right temporal lobe, that is, on the cerebral region from which sustained interictal epileptic activity had been recorded.

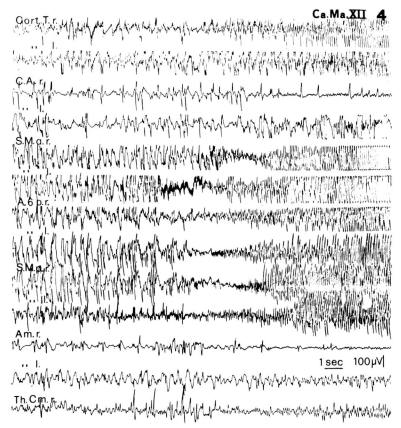

Figure 9. Same patient as in Figures 7 and 8 during the same recording session. A new ictal discharge appears to arise from the frontal structures (beginning from the left supplementary motor area, then involving the right one and area 6 of both sides) and, later, the temporal neocortex bilaterally, with final generalization. Cort. T., temporal neocortex; C.A., Ammon's horn; S.M., supplementary motor area; Area 6, frontal area 6; Am., amygdala; Th.Cm., centromedian thalamic nucleus; r., right; l., left; a., anterior; p., posterior.

Regularity or Stability of Interictal Epileptic Potentials

Interesting information can be obtained from the behavior of the interictal discharges recorded in different physiological or pharmacological conditions. In our experience, the brain structures constituting the epileptogenic zone have a tendency to generate epileptic potentials interictally with a certain regularity or stability independently of the condition of the patient. Two types of examples can be given.

1. As is well known, the variations of cerebral functional organization occurring during sleep influence epileptic activity (5, 6, 55). The interictal epileptic potentials recorded from the epileptogenic zone appear to be less affected than those recorded from other brain sites. Let us take into consideration again the stereoelectroencephalogram recorded from the patient

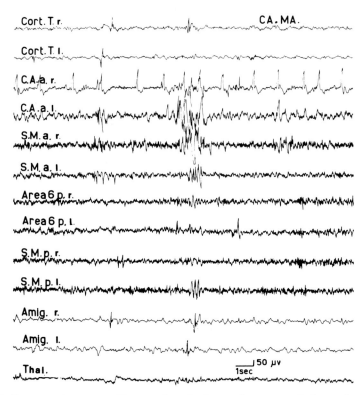

Figure 10. Same patient as in Figures 7 to 9. Stereoelectroencephalographic recording obtained a few hours before the Cardiazol activation illustrated in the previous figures. Interictal epileptic potentials are recorded from several structures but are particularly abundant from the anterior part of the right Ammon's horn. Cort. T., temporal neocortex; C.A., Ammon's horn; S.M., supplementary motor area; Area 6, frontal area 6; Amig., amygdala; Thal., thalamus; r., right; l., left; a., anterior; p., posterior.

previously discussed (Case 4), in whom a left temporal lesion was found at autopsy. The recordings from the right and left Ammon's horns are illustrated in Figure 12 and confirm what was reported above. Ictal discharges can be seen in both structures during wakefulness (A and B). Particularly interesting is the behavior of the interictal activity. That recorded from the right Ammon's horn is always present, independently of the state of the patient, that is, during wakefulness (C), during slow wave sleep (D), and during rapid eye movement (REM) sleep (E). The activity recorded from the left Ammon's horn, on the contrary, appears to undergo marked variations: rare during wakefulness, greatly increased during sleep stage II, and almost absent during REM sleep.

2. Anticonvulsive medication obviously reduces epileptic activity. We have examples that the interictal epileptic discharges recorded from the epileptogenic zone are less affected than those recorded from other brain sites. Figure 13, taken from a patient suffering from right temporal epilepsy (Case 5), reproduces (on the left) a specimen of the stereoelectroencepha-

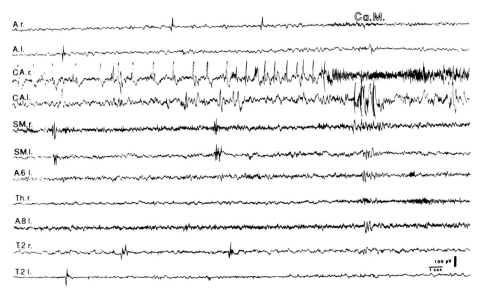

Figure 11. Same patient as in Figures 7 to 10. Stereoelectroencephalogram recorded 2 days later. Abundant interictal epileptic activity is still recorded from the right Ammon's horn. An ictal discharge arises from the same structure. A., amygdala; C.A., Ammon's horn; S.M., supplementary motor area; A.6, frontal area 6; T.2, second temporal convolution; r., right; l., left.

logram recorded 6 days after withdrawal of antiepileptic medication: epileptic potentials occur in the right and left hippocampal gyrus, with involvement of the Ammon's horn on the left side. On resumption of the pharmacological anticonvulsive treatment, the interictal epileptic activity appears, some days later, to be confined to the right hippocampal gyrus (right part of the figure).

What has been reported above draws attention to a particular phenomenon: the stability of epileptic potentials recorded between seizures from a certain brain structure.

Background Nonepileptic Electrical Activity

The finding of a circumscribed disorganization of the background rhythm and of slow waves is commonly regarded as indicative of a brain lesion. The phenomenon is so well known that it does not require any particular comment (10, 51, 58). Our experience confirms the great help provided by the recording of these electrical signs, as well as by the analysis of their relations with irritative potentials, in order to define correctly the physiopathological basis of the epileptic syndrome. Brain pathology, such as small tumors that had escaped recognition on the neuroradiological examinations, could be located by stereoelectroencephalographic recording (10).

Power spectral analysis might help in bringing into evidence lesional aspects of the background electrical activity. An example is given in Figure 14, reproducing the power spectrum of the electrical activity recorded from

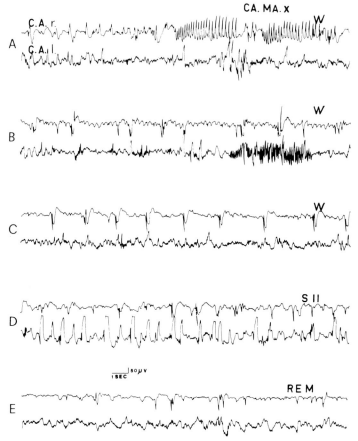

Figure 12. Same patient as in Figures 7 to 11. The recordings from right and left Ammon's horn are reproduced. Ictal discharges arise from both structures during wakefulness (A and B). Interictal activity as well is recorded from both structures; however, whereas that recorded from the right Ammon's horn is relatively unaffected by the sleep–wakefulness cycle (C, wakefulness; D, stage II of sleep; E, rapid eye movement (REM) sleep), the contralateral one undergoes marked variations. C.A., Ammon's horn; r., right; l., left.

the left Ammon's horn, right anterior hippocampal gyrus, and right uncus in a patient (Case 6) presenting psychomotor seizures and who was later completely cured by right anterior temporal lobectomy. At operation a small glioma was found within the anteromedial part of the temporal lobe. The power spectrum analysis shows the presence of slow electrical activity in the depth of the right temporal lobe (the spectrum peaks at about 2 cps.), this being particularly abundant in the uncus.

Time Relations among Interictal Epileptic Potentials of Different Cerebral Structures

A fourth possible way to get information about the dynamic properties of the epileptic process is by the analysis of the time relations among inter-

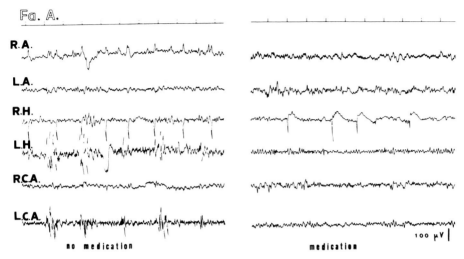

Figure 13. Interictal epileptic activity from the right and left (R and L) amygdala (A), hippocampal gyrus (H), and Ammon's horn (C.A.) in a patient suffering from partial seizures with complex symptomatology (Case 5). When no antiepileptic drugs are given (left part of the figure), epileptic potentials are recorded from both right and left temporal structures; following antiepileptic medical treatment, the epileptic potentials remain confined to right hippocampal gyrus.

ictal epileptic potentials recorded from different brain structures. For this purpose, we found the method developed by Rosadini and co-workers (30, 31) convenient and reliable. This technique is appropriate for defining the average morphology of the epileptic potentials and their average temporal relationship in multiple leads.

The electrocerebral activity is recorded on a multichannel magnetic tape. A PDP 12 computer with time clock and video monitor system is used

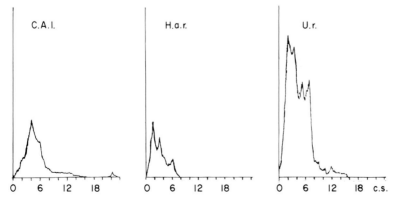

Figure 14. Power spectral analysis of the electrical activity of the left Ammon's horn (C.A.l.), right anterior hippocampal gyrus (H.a.r.), and right uncus (U.r.) recorded from an epileptic patient in whom right temporal lobectomy revealed a small glioma within the anteromedial part of the temporal lobe (Case 6). Slow electrical activity is definitely more abundant on the right deep temporal structures, and particularly in the uncus.

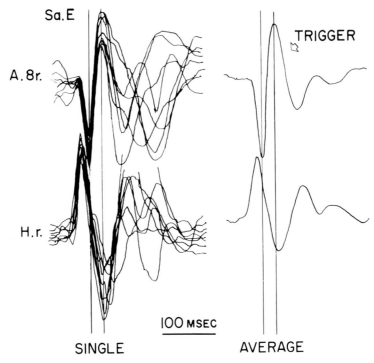

Figure 15. Time relations of interictal epileptic potentials from frontal area 8 (A. 8) and hippocampal gyrus (H) of the same side. On the left: superposition of eight potentials recorded oscilloscopically. On the right: average of the same potentials performed with the technique described by Ferrillo and co-workers (31, 30). The two vertical lines are used for the selection of the potentials to be averaged. (r., right)

for the elaboration. The technique is based on the following principles. First, a given type of epileptic potential recorded from one cerebral structure is selected as the "trigger" of the whole operation. Second, the digitized record runs on the video monitor of the computer; as the selected potential appears, the operator stops the tape and superposes two movable vertical reference lines on the epileptic potential in order to denote some of its neurophysiological characteristics, for instance the two peaks in the case of a diphasic potential (see Figure 15); the sample of the record is then stored in memory. Third, the tape is started again and then stopped when a potential with similar characteristics appears on the monitor; if the new potential fits with the reference lines previously fixed, it is put into memory and summated with the preceding one; if it is different it is discarded, and so on; simultaneously, a summation is performed of the electrical events occurring in the other channels.

An example of the results of such a technique is given in Figure 15. The recordings from frontal area 8 and from the hippocampal gyrus of the same side are reproduced. The epileptic potential from area 8 is selected

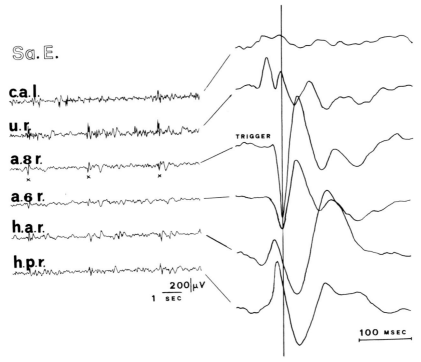

Figure 16. Average time relation of interictal epileptic potentials recorded from left Ammon's horn (c.a.l.), right uncus (u.r.), right area 8 (a.8 r.), right area 6 (a. 6 r.), anterior (h.a.r.) and posterior hippocampal gyrus (h.p.r.) of the right side in a patient suffering from psychomotor seizures who was later cured by right temporal lobectomy (Case 7). The epileptic potentials from right area 8 were used to trigger the averaging process. Note the particular temporal relations of the right-sided epileptic potentials brought out by the averaging process and the apparent lack of any relation between right and left potentials.

as the "trigger." The two vertical reference lines are superposed to the peaks of this diphasic spike to define it. On the left part of the figure the results of the single superposition of 8 of these selected spikes is reproduced together with the superposition of the simultaneously occurring epileptic potentials of the hippocampal gyrus. On the right, the results of averaging of the same potentials are given. In this case the average morphology as well as the average time relationship of the two potentials closely reflect the morphology and time relation of the single events.

Figure 16 illustrates what was obtained by applying this technique in one of our patients (Case 7). Epileptic potentials were recorded from deep temporal structures of both hemispheres as well as from frontal regions of the right hemisphere. On the stereoelectroencephalographic record, the left and right temporal spikes do not appear to be related in time. In contrast, the right temporal and frontal epileptic potentials seem to occur synchronously. On the right side of the figure the results are reproduced of

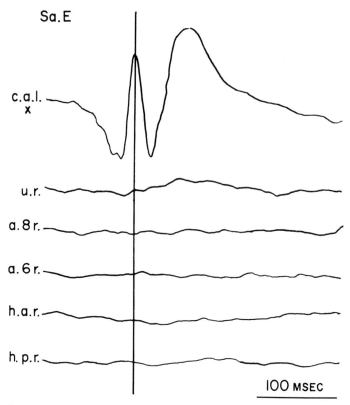

Figure 17. Same patient as in Figure 16. The epileptic potentials from left Ammon's horn (c.a.l.) were used to trigger the averaging process. The lack of any time relation with the right side epileptic potentials is confirmed. u.r., right uncus; a. 8 r., right area 8; a. 6 r., right area 6; h.a.r., anterior hippocampal gyrus; h.p.r., posterior hippocampal gyrus.

the averaging technique described above. The epileptic spike recorded from the right area 8 is used as a trigger. First of all, it is apparent that the epileptic potentials occurring in the left temporal lobe (left Ammon's horn) cannot be correlated with those on the right. Second, it appears that, although closely related in time, the potentials on the right side are not synchronous: (*a*) the temporal spikes precede the frontal ones, and (*b*) the spikes recorded from the uncus seem to precede all the others. This temporal sequence was confirmed by using as trigger of the averaging process spikes of other right structures. Finally, Figure 17 illustrates the results of averaging obtained from the same record by employing as a trigger the spikes recorded from the left Ammon's horn. The lack of time relations with the epileptic potentials of the contralateral hemisphere is obvious.

Summing up, this type of analysis appears suited to give an indication of the average time relationships among the interictal spikes occurring in different brain regions. Similar indications can be obtained by cross-correlation. We do not have enough material to judge whether the finding of a certain temporal sequence of interictal epileptic discharges from different brain structures actually reflects an epileptogenic hierarchy.

CONCLUSIONS

As stated at the beginning, the aim of the present report has been to present and discuss some of the problems of interpretation of the electro- cerebral signals recorded in epileptic patients, especially in view of eventual surgical treatment. Obviously, the final indication for surgery must depend on the integration of electrophysiological findings with many other data. The medical history of the patient, neurological and psychological status, neuroradiological examinations, clinical signs, frequency and severity of the seizures, sensitivity to antiepileptic pharmacological therapy, all have to be carefully analyzed and evaluated. However, in most of the patients who do not present gross brain pathology, electrophysiology remains the main source of information for the precise spatial location of the epilepto- genic zone. In these cases, the success of surgical treatment depends largely on the correct collection, analysis, and interpretation of the electrocerebral signals. In my opinion, it is likely that the still relatively high number of failures of surgery in curing epileptics might be reduced if our knowledge in this regard could be improved (10). The problem is not so much a technical one, but rather methodological and conceptual.

In fact, today the techniques for placing suitable electrodes in almost any brain site with satisfactory accuracy, for recording and storing electro- cerebral activity in such a way as to permit various types of analysis for relating the brain's electrical activity to the patient's behavior, are no longer a problem in specialized centers. However, we are still faced with many difficulties and uncertainties when trying to extract from the recorded sig- nals the information necessary for understanding the neural mechanisms responsible for the epileptic syndrome.

With the present report an attempt has been made to illustrate some of the aspects of this problem. The importance ascribed to prolonged record- ing, for instance, clearly reflects the view that the abnormal neural events leading to the seizure cannot be regarded as a simple or stereotyped mech- anism, but rather as a complex phenomenon varying in time under the influence of several factors, many of which certainly still escape our recog- nition. Likewise, the emphasis put on some aspects of the abnormal nonictal electrical abnormalities reflects the feeling we have that the study of ictal activity may not be sufficient. As stated before, we share the view of many other neurosurgeons on the importance of recording of ictal activity arising from a certain brain structure and of the tracing of the progressive involve- ment of other cerebral structures by the ictal discharge. At the present these phenomena appear to be the most useful for defining the epilepto- genic zone and the dynamic process of the epileptic seizures. Nevertheless, in some patients, the attempt to obtain a complete and convincing picture of the epileptic syndrome solely on the basis of the analysis of the ictal electrocerebral signals gives unsatisfactory results. The analysis of interictal potentials can, therefore, be helpful, in spite of the risks of sometimes getting from it misleading information. It is likely that an improvement in extracting correct information from interictal activity may be gained by computer analysis. Simple examples of the possible utilization of automatic elaboration of interictal electrocerebral signals have been given in the present report [see also Ferrillo *et al.* (30, 31)]. Previous and interesting contributions have been reported by others (2, 12, 14–18, 35, 37, 69). Obviously, one must have clearly in mind what to ask the computer; that is, one must define the details of the approach to the neurophysiological problem that the computer might help to solve.

The problems of analysis and interpretation of electrocerebral signals in epilepsy are many and can be faced in several ways. What has been reported above is only an example taken from the joint work of neurosurgeons and neurophysiologists on epileptic patients with implanted electrodes. The work in man, however, though very important, has to be kept within the limits of its exclusive clinical and therapeutic purposes. Many problems in epilepsy and many methodological approaches have to be left to animal experimentation.

SUMMARY

The problem of analysis of interpretation of electrocerebral signals in epileptic patients is approached from a neurosurgical point of view. The discussion centers on the electrophysiological criteria helpful in locating the epileptogenic zone through stereotaxically implanted electrodes, mainly in temporal lobe patients.

The utility of prolonged and repeated recording is emphasized.

Great importance is ascribed to the study of ictal discharges. Comparison of ictal activity occurring spontaneously and provoked by convulsive drugs or electrical stimulation appears useful.

The analysis of interictal electrical activity can integrate the information given by the study of ictal discharges. The importance of the study of background activity, of amount and stability in time of interictal epileptic potentials, of their behavior during physiological sleep or under the influence of drugs, as well as of time relations among potentials recorded from different brain sites, is pointed out. The use of the computer for particular analysis of the electrocerebral signals in epileptics can be helpful.

REFERENCES

1. Abraham, K., and Ajmone Marsan, C., Patterns of cortical discharges and their relation to routine scalp electroencephalography. *Electroenceph. clin. Neurophysiol.*, 1958, **10**: 447–461.

2. Adey, W. R., Elul, R. D., Walter, R. D., and Crandall, P. H., The cooperative behavior of neuronal population during sleep and mental tasks. Proc. Amer. EEG Soc. *Electroenceph. clin. Neurophysiol.*, 1967, **23**: 88.

3. Ajmone Marsan, C., and Abraham, K., Considerations on the use of chronically implanted electrodes in seizures disorders. *Confin. Neurol.*, 1966, **27**: 95–110.

4. Ajmone Marsan, C., and Van Buren, J. M., Epileptiform activity in cortical and subcortical structures in the temporal lobe of man. In: *Temporal Lobe Epilepsy* (M. Baldwin, Ed.). Thomas, Springfield, Illinois, 1958: 78–100.

5. Andrioli, G., Angeleri, F., Bergonzi, F., Cantore, P., Ferroni, A., Gentilomo, A., Mingrino, S., Ricci, G. P., Rosadini, G., and Rossi, G. F., Inquadramento diagnostico dell'epilettico in neurochirurgia. *Minerva Neurochir.*, 1966, **10**: 49–144.

6. Angeleri, F., Il sonno notturno negli epilettici. In: *L'Epilessia* (E. Lugaresi and P. Pazzaglia, Eds.). Gaggi, Bologna, 1969: 181–204.

7. Angeleri, F., Ferro Milione, F., and Parigi, S., Electrical activity and reactivity of the rhinencephalic, pararhinencephalic and thalamic structures: Prolonged implantation of electrodes in man. *Electroenceph. clin. Neurophysiol.*, 1964, **16**: 100–129.

8. Bancaud, J., Rapport de l'exploration fonctionelle par voie stéréotaxique à la chirurgie de l'épilepsie. *Neurochirurgie*, 1959, **5**: 55–112.

9. Bancaud, J., Contribution de la stéréoelectroéncephalographie à l'étude physiopathologique et clinique des épilepsies. In: *L' Epilessia* (E. Lugaresi and P. Pazzaglia, Eds.). Gaggi, Bologna, 1967: 135–155.

10. Bancaud, J., and Talairach, J., *La stéréo-électroencéphalographie dan l'épilepsie*. Masson, Paris, 1965.

11. Bickford, R. G., The application of depth electrography in some varieties of epilepsy. *Electroenceph. clin. Neurophysiol.*, 1956, **8**: 526–527.

12. Bickford, R. G., Scope and limitation of frequency analysis. Computer techniques in EEG analysis. *Electroenceph. clin. Neurophysiol.*, 1961, **20**: 9–13.

13. Brazier, M. A. B., Depth recordings from the amygdaloid region in patients with temporal lobe epilepsy. *Electroenceph. clin. Neurophysiol.*, 1956, **8**: 532–533.

14. Brazier, M. A. B., An application of computer analysis to a problem in epilepsy. In: *Comparative and Cellular Pathophysiology of Epilepsy* (Z. Servit, Ed.). Excerpta Med. Found., Amsterdam, 1966: Int. Congr. Ser. No. 124: 112–125.

15. Brazier, M. A. B., Thiopental effects on subcortical mechanisms in temporal lobe epilepsy. *Anesthesiology*, 1967, **28**: 192–200.

16. Brazier, M. A. B., Electrical activity recorded simultaneously from the scalp and deep structures of the human brain. A computer study of their relationships. *J. Nerv. Ment. Dis.*, 1968, **147**: 31–39.

17. Brazier, M. A. B., Studies of the EEG activity of limbic structures in man. *Electroenceph. clin. Neurophysiol.*, 1968, **25**: 309–318.

18. Brazier, M. A. B., Modern advances in the use of depth electrodes. In: *The Surgical Control of Behavior* (A. Winter, Ed.). Thomas, Springfield, Illinois, 1971: 5–20.

19. Brazier, M. A. B., Schroeder, H., Chapman, W. P., Geyer, C., Farger, C., Poppen, J. L., Solomon, H. C., and Yakovlev, P. I., Electroencephalographic recordings from depth electrodes implanted in the amygdaloid region in man. *Electroenceph. clin. Neurophysiol.*, 1954, 6: 702.

20. Chatrian, G. E., and Chapman, W. P., Electrographic study of the amygdaloid region with implanted electrodes in patients with temporal lobe epilepsy. In: *Electrical Studies of the Unanesthetized Brain* (E. R. Ramey and D. S. O'Doherty, Eds.). Harper (Hoeber), New York, 1960: 351–368.

21. Cooper, R., Winter, A. L., Crow, H. G., and Walter, W. G., Comparison of subcortical, cortical and scalp activity using chronically indwelling electrodes in man. *Electroenceph. clin. Neurophysiol.*, 1965, 18: 217–228.

22. Corletto, F., Rosadini, G., and Rossi, G. F., Megimide intracarotideo per lo studio della soglia convulsiva emisferica. *Riv. Neurol.*, 1967, 37: 329–398.

23. Crandall, P. H., Walter, R. D., and Rand, R. W., Clinical applications of studies on stereotactically implanted electrodes in temporal lobe epilepsy. *J. Neurosurg.*, 1963, 20: 827–840.

24. Delgado, J. M. R., Permanent implantation of multilead electrodes in the brain. *Yale J. Biol. Med.*, 1952, 24: 351–358.

25. Delgado, J. M. R., and Hamlin, H., Direct recording of spontaneous and evoked seizures in epileptics. *Electroenceph. clin. Neurophysiol.*, 1958, 10: 463–486.

26. Delgado, J. M. R., Mark, V., Sweet, W., Ervin, F., Weiss, G., Bach-Y-Rita, G., and Hagiwara, R., Intracerebral radio-stimulation and recording in completely free patients. *J. Nerv. Ment. Dis.*, 1968, 147: 329–340.

27. Dodge, H. W., Jr., Hoiman, C. B., Sem-Jacobsen, C. W., Bickford, R. G., and Petersen, M. C., Technic of depth electrography. *Proc. Staff. Meet. Mayo Clin.*, 1953, 28: 147–155.

28. Dodge, H. W., Jr., Petersen, M. C., Sem-Jacobsen, C. W., Sayre, G. P., and Bickford, R. G., The paucity of demonstrable brain damage following intracerebral electrography: Report of the case. *Proc. Staff. Meet. Mayo Clin.*, 1955, 30: 215–221.

29. Ervin, F. R., Mark, V. H., and Sweet, W. H., Focal cerebral disease, temporal lobe epilepsy and violent behavior. *Trans. Am. Neurol. Assoc.*, 1969, 94: 253–256.

30. Ferrillo, F., Cavazza, B., Rosadini, G., and Sannita, W., Sull'impiego di una tecnica di "averaging" nello studio dei potenziali EEG epilettici nell'uomo. *Riv. Neurol.*, 1972, 42: 312–319.

31. Ferrillo, F., Gasparetto, B., Rosadini, G., and Siccardi, A., Applicazioni delle tecniche di "averaging" nello studio della forma di segnali elettrocerebrali spontanei e dei loro rapporti temporali in derivazioni multiple. *Riv. Neurol.*, 1971, 41: 373–383.

32. Ferro-Milone, F., Angeleri, F., and Parigi, S., L'attivita elettrica del lobo temporale ed il comportamento in rapporto a scariche postume archipalliali ed amigdaloidee. *Riv. Neurobiol.*, 1959, **5**: 477–507.

33. Fischer-Williams, M., and Cooper, R. A., Depth recording from the human brain in epilepsy. *Electroenceph. clin. Neurophysiol.*, 1963, **15**: 568–587.

34. Gastaut, H., Clinical and electroencephalographic classification of epileptic seizures. *Epilepsy*, 1970, **11**: 103–113.

35. Gersch, W., and Goddard, G. V., Epileptic focus location: Spectral analysis method. *Science*, 1970, **169**: 701–702.

36. Gibbs, F. A., Origin and spread of different types of seizure discharge. *Trans. Am. Neurol. Assoc.*, 1955, **80**: 15–17.

37. Goldberg, P., Samson Dolfus, D., and Gremy, G., Essai de reconnaissance automatique de figures paroxystiques en EEG. *Agressologie*, 1969, **10**: 565–569.

38. Hayne, R. A., Belinson, L., and Gibbs, F. A., Electrical activity of subcortical areas in epilepsy. *Electroenceph. clin. Neurophysiol.*, 1949, **1**: 437–445.

39. Heath, R. G., Common characteristics of epilepsy and schizophrenia; clinical observation and depth electrode studies. *Am. J. Psychiatry*, 1962, **118**: 1013–1026.

40. Ishikawa, O., Electroencephalographical study of human thalamus. *Folia Psychiatr. Neurol. Jap.*, 1957, **11**: 128–149.

41. Jung, R., Riechert, T., and Meyer-Michelheit, R. W., Uber intracerebrale Hirnpotentiales ableitungen bei hirnchirurgischen Eingriffen. *Dtsch. Z. Nervenheilkd.*, 1950, **162**: 52–60.

42. Kamp, A., Haayman, W. P., Schrijer, C. F. M., and Storm Van Leeuwen, W., La radiotélémetrie de l'EEG chez les malades avec électrodes implantées chroniques. *Rev. Electroenceph. clin. Neurophysiol.*, 1971, **1**: 287–294.

43. Kellaway, P., Depth recording in focal epilepsy. *Electroenceph. clin. Neurophysiol.*, 1956, **8**: 527–528.

44. Lichtenstein, R. S., Marshall, C., and Walker, A. E., Subcortical recording in temporal lobe epilepsy. *Arch. Neurol.*, 1959, **1**: 288–302.

45. Mark, V. H., Ervin, F. R., Sweet, W. H., and Delgado, J., Remote telemeter stimulation and recording from implanted temporal lobe electrodes. *Confin. Neurol.*, 1969, **31**: 86–93.

46. Meyers, R., Knott, J. R., Hayne, R. A., and Sweeney, D. B., The surgery of epilepsy. Limitations of the concept of the cortico-electrographic "spike" as an index of the epileptogenic focus. *J. Neurosurg.*, 1950, **7**: 337–346.

47. Niedermeyer, E., Lans, E. R., and Walker, A. E., Depth EEG findings in epileptics with generalized spike-wave complexes. *Arch. Neurol.*, 1969, **21**: 51–58.

48. Okuma, T., Shimazono, Y., Fukuda, T., and Narabayashi, H., Cortical and subcortical recordings in non-anesthetized and anesthetized periods in man. *Electroenceph. clin. Neurophysiol.*, 1954, **6**: 269–286.

49. Pagni, C. A., Riflessioni sull'importanza delle tecniche stereotassiche nella diagnosi e nella terapia dell'epilessia psicomotoria con focus EEG tem-

porale. In: *L' Epilessia* (E. Lugaresi and P. Pazzaglia, Eds.). Gaggi, Bologna, 1969: 157–163.

50. Passouant, P., Gros, C., Cadilhac, J., and Vlahovitch, B., Les post-décharges par stimulation électrique de la corne d'Ammon chez l'homme. *Rev. Neurol. (Paris)*, 1954, **90**: 265–274.

51. Penfield, W., and Jasper, H. H., *Epilepsy and Functional Anatomy of the Human Brain.* Little, Brown, Boston, 1954.

52. Perria, L., Rivano, C., Rosadini, G., and Rossi, G. F., The value of electro-diagnostic examinations in the assessment of cases of epilepsy for surgery. *Excerpta Med. Int. Congr. Ser.*, 1969, No. 193: 147.

53. Perria, L., Rosadini, G., Rossi, G. F., and Gentilomo, A., Neurosurgical aspects of epilepsy: Physiological sleep as a means for focalizing EEG epileptic discharges. *Acta Neurochir. (Wien)*, 1966, **14**: 1–9.

54. Perria, L., Rossi, G. F., Rosadini, G., Gentilomo, A., Giunta, F., Ottino, C. A., and Rivano, C., Valutazione epicritica di alcuni criteri diagnostici per l'indicazione operatoria nell'epilessia. *Minerva Neurochir.*, 1970, **14**: 173–178.

55. Pompeiano, O., Sleep mechanisms. In: *Basic Mechanisms of the Epilepsies* (H. H. Jasper, A. A. Ward, and A. Pope, Eds.). Churchill, London, and Little, Brown, Boston, 1969: 453–473.

56. Ramey, E. R., and O'Doherty, D. S. (Eds.), *Electrical Studies on the Unanesthetized Brain.* Harper (Hoeber), New York, 1960.

57. Rand, R. W., Crandall, P. H., and Walter, R. D., Chronic stereotactic implantation of depth electrodes for psychomotor epilepsy. *Acta Neurochir., (Wien)*, 1964, **11**: 609–630.

58. Ribstein, M., Exploration du cerveau humain par électrodes profondes. *Electroenceph. clin. Neurophysiol.*, 1960, Suppl. 16: 129 pp.

59. Rosadini, G., Gentilomo, A., Perria, L., and Rossi, G. F., Recherches sur les effets de l'injection intracarotidienne et intravertébral d'amytal sur les décharges convulsives EEG. *Neurochirurgie*, 1967, **13**: 537–546.

60. Rossi, G. F., La terapia chirurgica delle epilessie in rapporto alle indicazioni elettrodiagnostiche. In: *L'Epilessia* (E. Lugaresi and Pazzaglia, P., Eds.). Gaggi, Bologna, 1969: 253–269.

61. Rossi, G. F., Corletto, F., Gentilomo, A., and Rosadini, G., Essai d'interprétation sur une base neurophysiologique des mécanismes de production de décharges convulsives bilaterales et synchrones. *Neurochirurgie*, 1967, **13**: 547–556.

62. Rossi, G. F., Walter, R. D., and Crandall, P. H., Generalized spike and wave discharges and non-specific thalamic nuclei. *Arch. Neurol.*, 1968, **19**: 174–183.

63. Sheer, D. E. (Ed.), *Electrical Stimulation of the Brain.* Univ. of Texas Press, Austin, 1961.

64. Spiegel, E. A., and Wycis, H. T., Thalamic recordings in man with special reference to seizure discharges. *Electroenceph. clin. Neurophysiol.*, 1950, **2**: 23–27.

65. Stevens, J. R., Localization of epileptic focus by protracted monitoring of EEG by radio telemetry. *Epilepsia*, 1969, **10**: 420.

66. Takebayashi, H., Komai, N., and Imanura, H., Depth EEG analysis of the epilepsies. *Confin. Neurol.*, 1966, **27**: 144–148.

67. Talairach, J., and Bancaud, J., Lesion, "irritative" zone and epileptogenic lesion. *Confin. Neurol.*, 1966, **27**: 91–94.

68. Talairach, J., David, M., and Tournoux, P., *L'exploration chirurgicale stéréotaxique du lobe temporal dans l'épilepsie temporale.* Masson, Paris, 1958.

69. Torres, F., An averaging method for determination of temporal relationship between epileptogenic foci. *Electroenceph. clin. Neurophysiol.*, 1967, **22**: 270–272.

70. Van Buren, J. M., Some autonomic concomitants of ictal automatism. A study of temporal lobe attacks. *Brain*, 1958, **81**: 505–528.

71. Walker, A. E., and Marshall, C., The contribution of depth recording to clinical medicine. *Electroenceph. clin. Neurophysiol.*, 1964, **16**: 88–99.

72. Walker, A. E., and Ribstein, M., Chronic depth recording in focal and generalized epilepsy. An evaluation of the technique. *Arch. Neurol. Psychiatry*, 1957, **78**: 44–45.

73. Williams, D., A study of thalamic and cortical rhythms in petit mal. *Brain*, 1953, **76**: 50–69.

74. Wilson, W. P., and Nashold, B. S., Epileptic discharges occurring in the mesencephalon and thalamus. *Epilepsia*, 1968, **9**: 265–273.

75. Wycis, H. T., Lee, A. J., and Spiegel, E. A., Simultaneous records of thalamic and cortical potentials in schizophrenics and epileptics. *Confin. Neurol.*, 1949, **9**: 264–272.

DEVELOPMENTS IN DIRECT RECORDINGS FROM EPILEPTOGENIC REGIONS IN THE SURGICAL TREATMENT OF PARTIAL EPILEPSIES*

PAUL H. CRANDALL

Brain Research Institute, University of California, Los Angeles, California

The surgical treatment of focal or "partial" epilepsies imposes the need for an as accurate as possible localization. Enough successful results verified by long-term follow-ups have been achieved in temporal lobe epilepsy and with focal epileptic disorders of the cerebral convexities to validate the concept that removal of an epileptogenic cortex can be effective in the event that medical treatment fails. Jacksonian march seizures and visual seizures involving perception of patterned phosphenes can be localized largely by clinical criteria. The partial epilepsies also include focal motor/sensory seizures and secondary (etiology known) generalized seizures. Seizures of this type are more difficult to localize either by clinical criteria or by electroencephalography. It has been a common experience that more than one cortical epileptogenic area can give rise to similar seizure manifestations (2) and that these seizures frequently arise from foci inaccessible by means of electroencephalography and electrocorticography, for example, medial and inferior facies of the hemispheres or the limbic system. Equally successful results could be achieved in these groups if the preoperative diagnostic data were certain. The following method combines direct recordings from several suspected epileptogenic areas of the brain and recording during ambient conditions, especially during spontaneous seizures, to collect convincing electrographic data for purposes of surgical treatment.

Partial seizures represent an important fraction of the overall problem of epilepsy, especially in the medically uncontrolled group. It must always be considered that the partial epilepsies may be a symptom of any one of a variety of etiological conditions; the importance of the underlying cause may overshadow the epileptic condition. However, after a careful neurological evaluation has been performed, the majority of patients with chronic recurring seizures will not be found to have any other significant

* This research has been supported by Grant NS 02808 of the National Institute of Neurological Diseases and Stroke. The research was carried out at the Brain Research Institute, University of California, Los Angeles.

TABLE 1
AVERAGE ANNUAL INCIDENCE RATES PER 100,000 POPULATION
FOR EPILEPSY BY TYPE: FOUR POPULATION SURVEYS[a]

Survey	Primary grand mal	Petit mal alone	Secondary seizures[b]	Total seizures
Rochester [Kurland, 1959 (13)]	8	3	17	30[c]
Rochester (Hauser and co-workers, unpublished data)[c]	10	4	30	45[d]
Iceland [Gudmundsson, 1966 (9)]	19	1	13	33
Jutland [Kurtzke, 1968 (14),[d] Juul-Jensen, 1964 (12)]	17	4	15	36

[a] Reproduced by permission from *Epidemiology of Neurologic and Sense Organ Disorders*, Chapter 2, Convulsive Disorders, J. F. Kurtzke, L. T. Kurland, I. D. Goldberg, W. C. Nung, F. A. Reeder, Kurtzke *et al.* (11) Harvard University Press (15).
[b] Includes focal, psychomotor, and secondary (etiology known) generalized seizures.
[c] Includes 1 per 100,000 unclassified.
[d] Includes 2 per 100,000 unclassified.

disease (21). The prevalence of epilepsy among the adult population is about 0.4%. In Table 1 the results of four population surveys indicate that about one-half of epileptic patients are affected by secondary seizures, that is, partial epilepsies (15). Since the partial epilepsies tend to be more resistant to drugs and are more often associated with brain lesions, surgical treatment plays a special role. It is a challenge to physicians that, but for these seizures, many of these patients could be rehabilitated. A series of 27 consecutive patients with preoperative diagnoses of a drug-resistant form of partial epilepsy have been investigated with stereotaxically implanted depth electrodes and radiotelemetered recordings as a part of their surgical treatment at the UCLA Brain Research Institute. Our experience with this method in 16 patients having suspected psychomotor epilepsy has been reported previously (5). The subject of this preliminary report deals with the localization of origin of the focal sensorimotor seizures in 7 patients.

METHODS

Seven patients were referred for surgical treatment with a clinical description consistent with focal sensorimotor epilepsy, resistant to drugs, and who were adolescents or older. All patients underwent complete physical, neurological, and electroencephalographic examinations. Other tests included radioisotopic brain scanning, pneumoencephalography, and cerebral angiography. Patients with a diagnosis of possible brain tumor or arteriovenous malformation were excluded.

The clinical patterns accepted for depth electrode analysis included patients with seizure manifestations, such as adversive or contraversive head and eye movements; focal motor flection or extension or clonic movements;

unilateral, tonic facial movements; postural or torsion actions; unilateral, somatic inhibitory states (each with or without loss of consciousness and each with or without speech arrest). Some patients also had somatosensory symptoms, auditory or vertiginous components, autonomic or visceral manifestations, such as changes in respiration, sweating, urinary control, and mydriasis. One patient had epilepsia partialis continua. Such descriptors have not been especially localizing in our experience as there are at least four locations for seizure foci which may give these same manifestations. However, patients with Jacksonian march seizures, classic temporal lobe epilepsy, and others with visual-formed/unformed seizures are not included in this particular study. Most of our patients gave a history of experiencing generalized seizures as well, either in association with attacks of focal epilepsy or alone.

Five patients had abnormal neurological findings indicative of postictal paresis or congenital hemiparesis, such as asymmetrical reflexes or size of extremities. These signs were helpful for lateralization but not for localization purposes.

The electroencephalographic findings in all 7 patients were similar to either "secondary bilateral synchrony" or consisted of widespread electrographic abnormalities intermingled with focal frontal or temporal electroencephalogram (EEG) abnormality. Pneumoencephalograms in 3 patients showed large areas of cortical atrophy and various degrees of enlargement of one lateral ventricle and temporal horn. One patient had a parietal porencephalic cyst. Pneumoencephalograms in 3 patients were considered to be normal. One patient had a vestigial ascending frontal artery of the middle cerebral arterial complex (26), and 1 patient had a tiny meningeal angiomatosis, not recognized radiographically but found at the time of cortical resection.

The epileptogenic areas surveyed by depth electrode analysis for these types of seizures were the supplementary motor area (Ms II), the precentral motor cortex (Ms I), the cingulate gyrus, the limbic structures medial to the temporal lobe, and several thalamic nuclei. Not all of these areas were surveyed in each patient. In 5 patients the evidence for lateralization was sufficient that these epileptogenic zones were recorded in the abnormal hemisphere. In 2 patients the depth electrode placements were bilateral and symmetrical. The decision to record from these areas was guided by certain clinical features for each patient. During the seizures if the patient was fully conscious, then the depth electrodes were confined to supra-Sylvian sites, otherwise the deep temporal sites were included. Several thalamic nuclei were investigated in patients showing prominent generalization of discharges, but the findings were uninformative. We do not further recommend this step.

The stereotactic identification by coordinates of these regions was derived from the stereotactic atlases by Talairach and co-authors (27–29). The supplementary motor cortex was discovered by Penfield as a cortical area located largely on the medial aspect of the superior frontal gyrus anterior to the pre-central gyrus (18). Electrical excitation produced nontopographically organized responses such as vocalization, complex movements of the extremities and body (mostly contralateral), inhibition of voluntary activity, aphasia, eye movements, pupillary effects, cardiac acceleration, sensory responses, and arrest of breathing. He proposed the name *supplementary motor area* but also specified that it was a supplementary motor and sensory area. This is consistent with recent evidence that the Rolandic region consists of four distinct areas, each of which involves both sensory and motor function (31). Woolsey proposed that this be called *somatic motor-sensory area II* (Ms II). The abbreviations in parenthesis indicate, by capitals and lower case letters and by order, the relative dominance of sensory and motor features of the area. Talairach and colleagues have localized this cortical area stereotactically to the axis of the anterior–posterior cerebral commissures (AC-PC axis) (29). In relationship to a vertical at the anterior commissure, the vertical being at right angles to the AC-PC axis, the area Ms II is within 2 cm anterior to the vertical, 0.5–2.0 cm from the midline, and 1.0–3.0 cm deep to the inner surface of the cranial vault.

The image of the cingulate gyrus can be directly identified in stereotactic ventriculograms by air shadows in the pericallosal sulcus, the cingulate sulcus, and the calloso-marginal sulcus.

The limbic structures were located by coordinates measured from the VA-LT axes of the temporal horns and the midline of the third ventricle according to the stereotactic method of Talairach *et al.* (27). In lateral teleroentgenograms demonstrating the temporal horn, a line LT was drawn on the images of the most anterior tip of the temporal horn to another point 4.0 cm behind on the inferior edge of the lateral cleft of the temporal horn. VA is a line perpendicular to LT at the anterior point. The profiles of the hippocampus and the amygdala could be seen directly in the image of the temporal horn. The positions of the hippocampal gyrus were determined by coordinates taken from the atlas relative to LT-VA and the midline. The coordinates for thalamic nuclei were measured on a proportional grid determined by the anterior commissure–posterior commissure axis (AC-PC), the thalamic height and from the midline of the third ventricle (28).

Recordings were made from the precentral motor area (Ms I) by two epidural unipolar electrodes located at the F3-F4 motor point and T13-T14 Sylvian point of the 10-20 system of placements of the International Federation which has been adopted in many laboratories. Also other epidural electrodes—unipolar, stainless-steel nails insulated except for 1 mm of their tip were placed through the scalp and outer table of the skull in the frontal (F1-F2), anterior parietal (C5-C6), posterior parietal (P7-P8), posterior temporal (T17-T18) and anterior temporal (T11-T12) positions.

The stereotactic apparatus used in this series was the Todd-Wells system. Anteroposterior and lateral X-ray beams were aligned to intersect at the center of a fixed stereotactic hemisphere. The film–target distance was 14 ft. X-Ray images within 4.0 cm^2 of the center of the beam were not magnified by more than 3% so direct measurements were made from these films. The patient's cranium was fixed by transcutaneous pins in a base frame movable in any xyz axis in relation to the fixed stereotactic hemisphere. However, the sagittal and horizontal planes of the patient's head had to be correctly aligned with the similar planes of the stereotactic hemisphere. The internal anatomical landmarks of the brain were outlined in stereotactic ventriculograms after injection of filtered air and water-soluble positive contrast media. Since the operation was performed with the patient supine, these injections were made in the trigones of the lateral ventricles from a lateral direction. Sometimes the entire ventricular system was outlined by filtered air alone. In others, it was necessary to define the posterior commissure and posterior parts of the ventricles with positive contrast. No more than 5 cc of 60 Conray* diluted to a 1:3 mixture with saline was used as a total amount.

Plots were made on the X-ray films for the specific anatomical sites for the electrodes. Then the patient's head was moved to bring each anatomical zone into the focal point of the stereotactic hemisphere. Thus, each surgical target could be reached along any chosen radius of the hemisphere using this arc system. For the limbic sites the shortest approach was through the inferior temporal lobe by a horizontal approach. Thalamic sites were reached by an oblique paraventricular approach. The medial face of the hemisphere was approached from a vertical direction but not closer than 1.5 cm to the midline.

Hollow screws were fixed in place through twist drill holes in the calvarium (6, 19), and the dura mater was coagulated to open it. Bipolar, coaxial stainless-steel electrodes with blunt tips and flexible shafts were used in depth sites. The outside diameter was 0.5 mm. The inner wire was 8 mil in diameter and exposed for 0.5 mm. The other pole was a 0.5-mm wide band on the cylinder. Both electrode surfaces were separated by 0.5 mm. The electrodes were insulated with several layers of baked enamel.

The electrodes were advanced under X-ray control. When in the correct position each electrode was fixed and the electrode and hollow screw were sealed by the application of methylmethacrylate around the head of the screws. The leads from superficial electrodes were gathered into a plug which was later brought outside the head dressing.

One of the principal objectives following operation was to record the paroxysmal EEG activity during spontaneous seizures. This was achieved by continuous monitoring by remote radiotelemetry on the hospital ward.

---

* Conray-60, meglumine iothalamate U.S. Pharmacopeia 60%, Mallinckrodt Co.

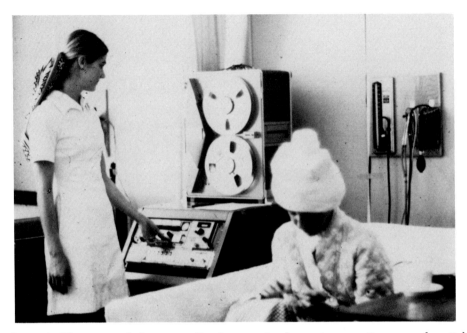

Figure 1. Electroencephalogram radiotelemetry is shown in operation on a hospital ward. The antenna is mounted on the wall behind the patient. The rectangular shape in the top of the patient's head dressing is a seven-channel pack. The continuous operation of the tape recorder allows unexpected seizures to be recorded.

The anticonvulsant medications were slowly withdrawn with the exception of diphenylhydantoin.

The EEG radiotelemetry system was designed and built by the UCLA Space Biology Laboratory and has been fully described in previous publications (1, 7). The patients wore a telemetry pack (Figure 1). The first packs recorded EEG data on five to seven channels and were worn in the head turban (size 6 × 4 × 2 in.) (Figure 1). At present we use a twelve-channel pack, which is larger and worn in a specially designed jacket. The battery life is about 30 hours. The range is sufficient for recording from a freely moving patient anywhere on the ward. The telemetry packs had an external multipin connector for the electrodes, and an on–off switch. All other adjustments were internal and were preset in the electronics laboratory. The telemetry pack was securely fastened, and all lead wires were taped down to prevent movements of cables.

After the telemetry unit was placed and turned on, the radio receiver was tuned to receive the transmitted signal, using an audio monitor to detect the characteristic sound of the summed FM subcarriers. All other settings on the equipment were preset prior to moving it to the ward. A tape was mounted on the recorder, the footage counter was zeroed, and the recorder was started. Besides periodically changing tapes, the only other requirement, once the system was in operation, was an occasional check on the receiver tuning. The nurse in charge of the equipment on the ward noted any occurrence, such as an epileptic seizure, on a form which also listed tape reel, track, time, and revolution counter reading. In addition the nurse wrote a description of the manifestations of each epileptic attack. Each morning the filled tapes and written forms were collected. The sections on the tapes that contained seizure events were recorded on a polygraph. This EEG record and the accompanying descriptions were available for interpretation. It was found desirable to collect information from at least three recordings of spontaneous seizures. Presently this technique requires the assistance of an electronic technician. It was well-received by nurses and easily fitted into their usual duties.

Results

The procedure of direct recording from suspected epileptogenic regions with EEG data obtained during spontaneous seizures was successful in localizing the earliest ictal discharges which progressively spread as the seizure developed in these patients. Later a localized excision of epileptogenic cortex was carried out in 6 of the 7 patients. In the unoperated patient, who had a parietal porencephalic cyst, the earliest ictal activity was observed in the homotopic parietal cortex. It was believed to be inadvisable for this patient to incur biparietal brain lesions, so an operation was not carried out.

In the remaining 6 patients, a small craniotomy was carried out under general anesthesia to explore the specific cortical area. Further electrocorticographic recordings were conducted in the operating room on the exposed cortical area to define the limits of the epileptogenic zone. Short acting barbiturates were administered to several patients to facilitate this recording. By the operations the following areas were removed: in 2 patients the inferior precentral motor cortex except the precentral gyrus (inferior Ms I); in 1 patient the superior precentral motor cortex except the precentral gyrus (superior Ms I); in 2 patients the supplementary motor cortex (Ms II) (1 of whom also had removal of anterior cingulate gyrus cortex); and in 1 patient an anterior temporal lobectomy at 6 cm from the temporal pole.

Postoperative observations have been carried out from 6 months to 3 years. In 4 patients the seizures have been fully controlled. In 1 patient the diagnosis proved to be a corpus callosum astrocytoma. His attacks were controlled for 9 months before recurrence of seizures as well as advancing contralateral hemiparesis became evident due to the tumor. One patient continued to have seizures which have been steadily decreasing in severity and frequency. All patients who had a preoperative history of generalized convulsions have had continued treatment with diphenylhydantoin in the postoperative period. In the 4 patients who are seizure free, other anticon-

vulsants were gradually eliminated. There were no additional neurological
deficits in these patients as an effect of the operations.

It has been found that interictal paroxysmal discharges recorded within
the epileptogenic zone are very frequent, most of which are not reflected
in simultaneous recordings from superficial leads. These interictal discharges are sporadic, unpredictable in occurrence, high in amplitude, and
vary considerably in wave form. Commonly there is a disorganized mixture
of spikes, sharp waves, and slow waves, generally termed a polyphasic type
of pattern. Also, of course, there is no clinical sign of their occurrence.

Ictal paroxysmal discharges in epileptogenic zones may begin in one site
or simultaneously in a few, closely adjacent sites. The interictal polyphasic
discharges in this region cease and are replaced by tightly organized, fast,
rhythmical wave form. Frequently this is either low voltage, fast activity,
or even "suppression" or flattening, apparently due to the rapidity of discharges. The initial rhythmical activity leads to a progressive slowing in
frequency and an increase in amplitude but still maintaining a highly organized form. As the wave pattern slows, it is replaced by a series of after-
discharges or high-amplitude spikes and slow waves. In the instance of
limbic system foci, the onset of the characteristic activity occurred in a
limited region for a variable period of time, and the clinical concomitants
did not appear until a wide propagation had occurred. The stepwise propagation is a specific feature of a focal type of epilepsy. There has been a
stereotyped repetition of the same patterns in the same regions during repeated seizures.

The findings during observed seizures may be best illustrated by examples from 4 patients. The following descriptions of seizures were each given
by either an experienced nurse or doctor who observed the attacks.

Case 1

This 18-year-old young man (R.C.) had a marked, spastic hemiparesis following a difficult birth due to uterine dystocia. He had had frequent seizures
since the age of 6. His seizures were often precipitated by sudden noises
or if he was tapped by someone unexpectedly. At that time he was unable
to speak, had a staring expression, and sometimes became limp with his
head slumped forward. On some occasions he had fallen down but he was
quite certain that he maintained consciousness throughout the attack.
These attacks could be as brief as 1 second or as long as 2 minutes. They
occurred as frequently as 5 to 6 per day, but the longest interval free of
attacks was 3 days. Numerous medications had been tried without benefit.

Neurological examinations revealed a hemiatrophy of the left side of the
body, decreased size of the right cranial vault, and a spastic left hemiparesis, most marked in the upper extremity. Mild decreased perception of sensory stimuli was noted. Electroencephalograms disclosed slow wave activity
over the central, parietal, and posterotemporal regions, sometimes accompanied by sharp waves. A pneumoencephalogram showed generalized atro-

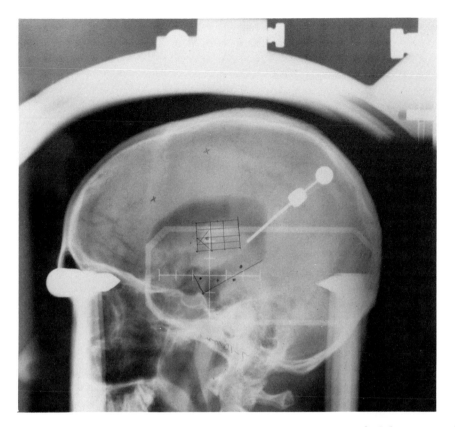

Figure 2. A stereotactic ventriculogram is shown with targets marked by means of a thalamic grid for the ventralis anterior nucleus, the VA-LT axis on a dilated temporal horn with, from front to back, amygdala, anterior pes hippocampus, mid-hippocampal gyrus, and posterior pes hippocampus. Above the ventricle are sites marked for the anterior cingulate gyrus and the posterior supplementary motor cortex. (Case 1.)

phy of the right hemisphere. A cerebral angiogram revealed a vestigial, ascending frontal artery of the right middle cerebral complex (30).

In May, 1971, depth electrodes were stereotaxically implanted in the right cerebral hemisphere in the anterior and mid-hippocampus, the mid-hippocampal gyrus, the thalamic nucleus ventralis anterior, the supplementary motor cortex, the anterior cingulate gyrus, and the posterior supplementary motor cortex (Figures 2 and 3).

Interictal depth EEG activity showed sharp waves followed by a slow wave intermittently in the right C4-P4 leads (Figure 4).

During the ictus there was the onset of rhythmical fast activity beginning in the right C4-P4 leads, spreading to the supplementary motor area of the same side, and finally involving the frontal and temporal skull leads on both sides, ending in generalized sharp and slow waves (Figure 5).

In October, 1971, a right frontal craniotomy disclosed a large cystic cavity in the Sylvian fissure below a wide area of cerebral malacia. The electrocorticogram showed an area of abnormal, large spikes over the shriveled

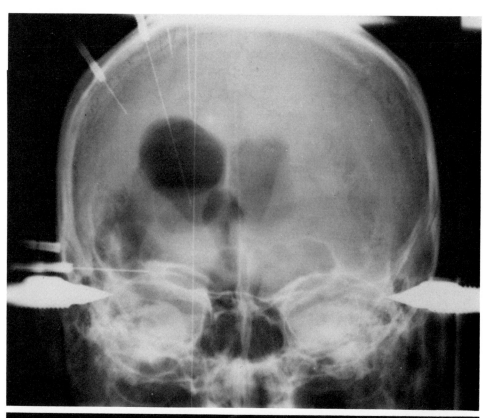
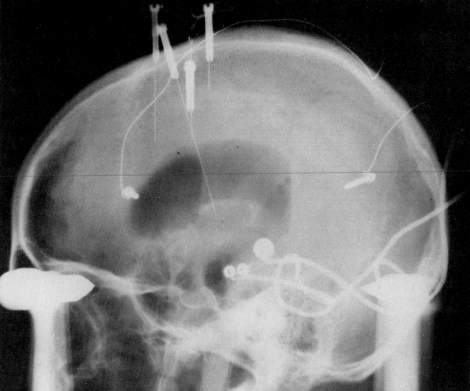

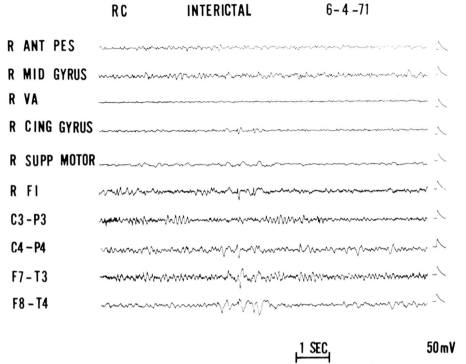

Figure 4. Interictal electroencephalogram activity recorded from indwelling electrodes—sharp waves followed by slow waves in several, superficial central areas with some homotopic effects as well. (Case 1.) R, right; ANT, anterior; VA, ventralis anterior nucleus; CING, cingulate gyrus; SUPP, supplementary; FI, precentral motor cortex; C3-P3, C4-P4, F7-T3, F8-T4; electrodes (international placement).

gyri of the frontal operculum. Three gyri were removed anterior to the precentral gyrus to a depth of 2 cm. Histological examination of the specimen revealed intense gliosis and atrophy.

Postoperatively the patient has been free of seizures. Many attempts to provoke seizures by startle have not elicited seizures. The functions of the left limbs remain as before. He continues to take 300 mg diphenylhydantoin daily.

Case 2

This 13-year-old girl (E.H.) was referred because of status epilepticus of focal type. Intermittent attacks of both generalized and focal seizures had occurred since age 7 at a frequency of 30 to 40 per month. Since 1969,

Figure 3. In the top picture, the ventricular system reveals widespread atrophy of the right cerebral hemisphere. Several indwelling electrodes have been placed in the anterior cingulate gyrus, supplementary and precentral motor cortices, thalamus, and one limbic site. In the bottom picture, two additional limbic sites and two calvarial electrodes have been placed. (Case 1.)

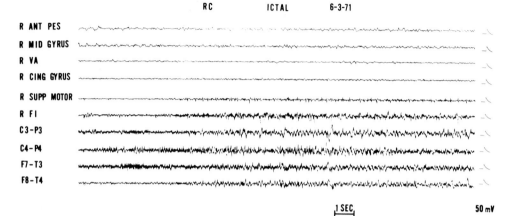

Figure 5. Ictal electroencephalogram activity recorded during the spontaneous seizure showed rhythmical, low-voltage fast activity beginning first in the C4-P4 leads, spreading to involve the right supplementary motor area and then to bilateral neocortical involvement. The patient remained conscious during the seizure. (Case 1.) R, right; ANT, anterior; VA, ventralis anterior nucleus; CING, cingulate gyrus; SUPP; supplementary; FI, precentral motor cortex; C3-P3, C4-P4, F7-T3, F8-T4, electrodes (international placement).

left-sided weakness and mild sensory loss was present, worse after seizures. Systematic trials of anticonvulsants failed to control the seizures.

During clinical seizures there was an involuntary, rigid extension of the left upper extremity and the patient complained of numbness in the left arm. Frequently she would grasp it with her right hand. Within a few seconds she became unconscious with dilated pupils, head and eyes turned to the right with clonic motions of the left upper extremity. The lower extremities were spread apart. Right facial twitching was also present in some seizures.

One EEG recorded at the scalp showed focal, right frontal slow waves and frequent right frontal sharp wave and spike wave complexes, Other EEG recordings showed focal spiking in the left central and temporal regions. A pneumoencephalogram revealed right periventricular atrophy manifested by rounding of the right superior lateral ventricle. Cerebral angiography was considered to be within normal limits.

Depth electrodes were placed in the right supplementary motor area, anterior cingulate gyrus, a thalamic nucleus (ventralis anterior), amygdala, anterior hippocampus and midportion of the hippocampal gyrus (November, 1971) (Figures 6 and 7). During the ictus, low-voltage fast rhythmical activity began first in the right hippocampal gyrus and hippocampus, culminating later in generalized discharges (Figures 8 and 9).

Right anterior temporal lobectomy was carried out in March, 1972. Some focal facial seizures without loss of consciousness occurred in the first week after operation. Otherwise she has remained seizure-free with improvement in the neurological status of the left limbs.

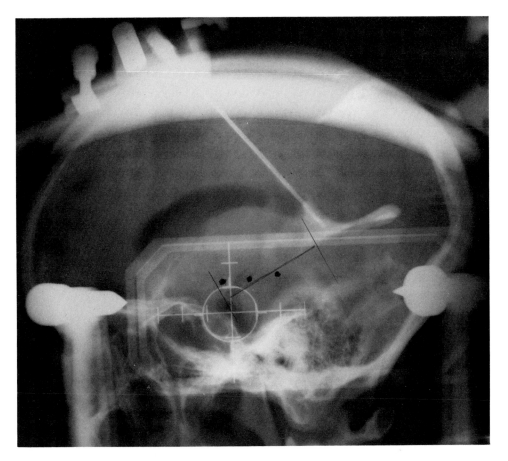

Figure 6. A stereotactic ventriculogram with combined gas and positive contrast with limbic sites marked for amygdala, anterior pes hippocampus, and mid-hippocampal gyrus. (Case 2.)

Case 3

This 17-year-old young man (P.F.) had focal seizures involving the right limbs since age 8 with a frequency of 6 to 12 per day. He has also experienced four generalized convulsions.

Each seizure was preceded by the onset of numbness in his right hand. At that point he generally tried to get to the floor or a chair because, shortly thereafter, his right upper limb was elevated and abducted in a stiff posture and his right leg became extended. During this time he could not move his head and he appeared to have clenched teeth. He could move his eyes in any direction and could speak during an attack. The initial rigidity was followed by clonic movements in the right limbs and abdomen, but not the face. Seizures lasted 30 to 50 seconds.

Numerous combinations of medications had been tried without success. In 1961 at another medical center, he had a craniotomy with multiple biop-

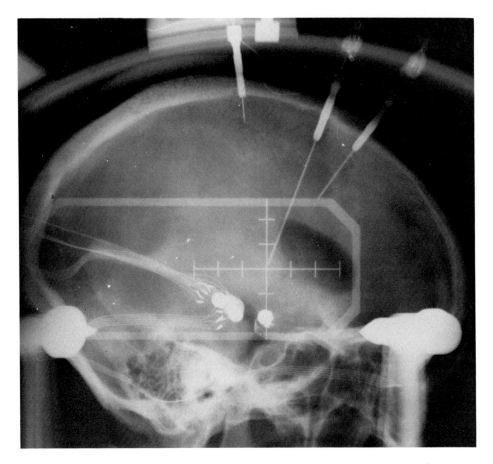

Figure 7. Indwelling electrodes have been placed in the right posterior supplementary motor area, anterior cingulate gyrus, thalamus, and three deep temporal lobe sites. (Case 2.)

sies revealing gliosis. In 1968 at a third center, he had a resection of part of the left parietal lobule without any significant change in his seizures. Several EEGs were slightly abnormal on the basis of intermittent focal left temporal and central slow waves which were apparent only during drowsiness and sleep. A pneumoencephalogram and arteriogram showed evidence of atrophy and loss of vasculature in the parietal area at the site of the previous operation.

In June, 1970, depth electrodes were placed in the left amygdala, left mid-hippocampal gyrus, left posterior hippocampal gyrus, and the midportion of the left hippocampus. Electrodes were also placed in the left pulvinar and left posterior ventrolateral nucleus of the thalamus. Calvarial electrodes were placed according to the 10-20 international system.

Recordings by EEG radiotelemetry during seizures showed the onset of fast rhythmical spiking in F3-F7 and C3-T3 leads (Figure 10). The

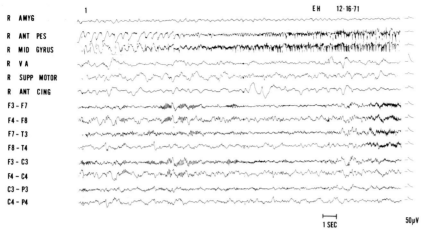

Figure 8. Ictal electroencephalogram activity clearly revealed the onset of low-voltage rhythmical, fast activity beginning in the right deep temporal sites during a seemingly left focal sensorimotor clinical seizure. (Case 2.) R, right; AMYG, anygdala; ANT, anterior; VA, ventralis anterior nucleus; SUPP, supplementary; CING, cingulate gyrus; F3-F7, F4-F8, . . . , electrodes (international placement).

changes were most marked in the left F3-F7 which quickly spread to the right C4-T4 lead. The termination was characterized by the appearance of bilateral slow waves in all leads (Figure 11).

In September, 1970, a left frontal craniotomy was made. Electrocorticograms revealed the major abnormalities were in the midportion of the middle and inferior frontal gyri located anterior to the precentral gyrus. A

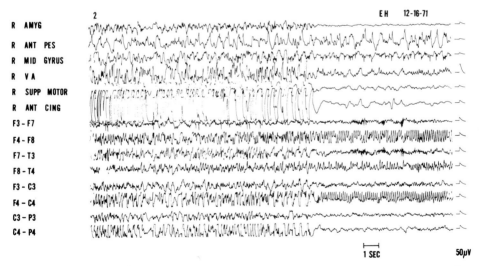

Figure 9. Depth electroencephalogram recording in the same patient as in Figure 8 after an interval of several seconds displayed generalization of the discharges. (Case 2.) R, right; AMYG, amygdala; ANT, anterior; VA, ventralis anterior nucleus; SUPP, supplementary; CING, cingulate gyrus; F3-F7, F4-F8, . . . , electrodes (international placement).

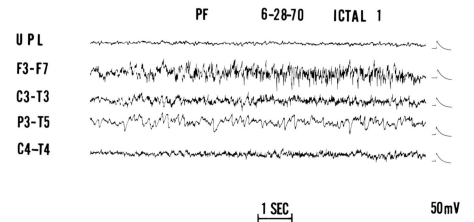

Figure 10. In this patient with focal motor activity in the right limbs with preservation of consciousness, the initial electroencephalogram ictal signal involved the right F3-F7 and C3-T3 sites. (Case 3.) UPL, n. posterior ventrolateral of the thalamus; F3-F7, C3-T3, P3-T5, C4-T4, electrodes (international placement).

block of tissue (3 × 4 cm and 2 cm in depth) was resected. Microscopic examinations showed an old cortical infarct.

Postoperatively the patient had hesitation of speech for a period of 3 weeks, which cleared completely. He has been completely free of further seizures. There is no neurological deficit. He continues to take diphenylhydantoin.

Case 4

A 22-year-old young man (G.McG) was referred with a diagnosis of psychomotor epilepsy and infrequent generalized seizures for 5 years. Ini-

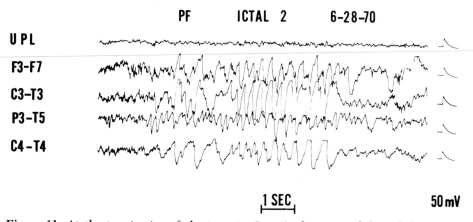

Figure 11. At the termination of the ictus in Case 3, there were bilateral slow waves in neocortical sites without abnormal activity in the left posterior ventrolateral nucleus of the thalamus. UPL, n. posterior ventrolateral of the thalamus; F3-F7, C3-T3, P3-T5, C4-T4, electrodes (international placement).

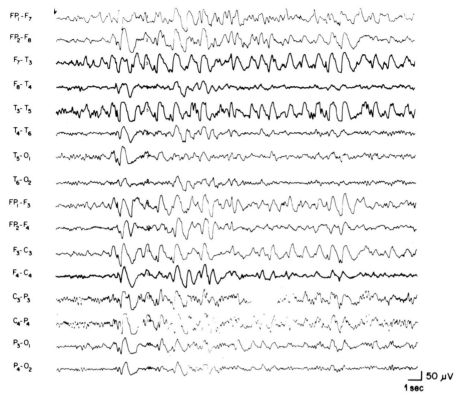

Figure 12. Scalp electroencephalogram recording in Case 4 showing generalized, high-amplitude slow waves with associated sharp waves in left frontal and temporal leads. FP₁-F₇, FP₂-F₈, . . . , electrodes (international placement).

tially seizures were controlled for 2 years by medications. The frequency of attacks was 3 to 4 daily despite many medications.

The clinical seizure began with the patient making a soft, whining sound; he became somewhat rigid with a tendency to fall backward; had smacking lip movements; was incontinent of urine and often pulled at his clothing. During the ictus he was not unconscious—he was able to indicate a response to some simple directions, although unable to speak. After the episode was over, he gradually regained his speech in the ensuing half-hour. The seizure usually lasted less than 2 minutes, and he remembered most of the events of the seizure. On other occasions the observers believed he briefly lost consciousness.

Physical, neurological, and radiographical studies were normal except for an equivocal depression of the roof of the anterior left lateral ventricle. Scalp EEGs demonstrated paroxysms of slow spike and slow wave activity, appearing at times focal from the right frontotemporal leads and at others, rather generalized (Figure 12). Other EEGs showed a bitemporal dysrhythmia maximal on the left especially in the left frontotemporal region.

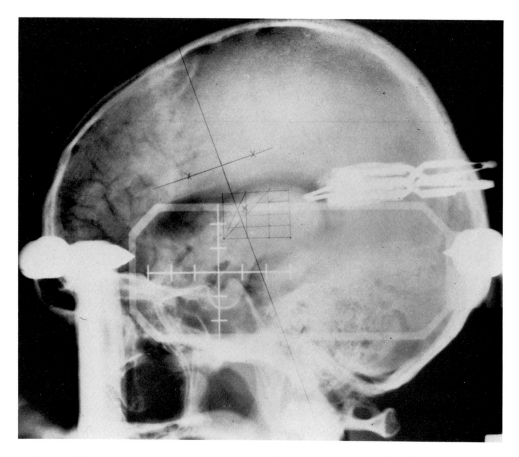

Figure 13. A stereotactic ventriculogram with gas showing the plots for the anterior and middle cingulate gyrus. (Case 4.)

Depth electrodes were placed stereotactically in bilateral, symmetrical positions. Plots were made based on the VA-LT axis for the basolateral amygdala, the anterior and posterior hippocampus, and the anterior and posterior hippocampal gyrus. Based on the AC-PC axis, the anterior nucleus of the thalamus was plotted. The anterior and middle parts of the cingulate gyrus were outlined by air-filled sulci (June, 1969) (Figures 13 and 14). Electrodes were placed in the cingulate gyrus because of the striking feature of urination (3). The clinical seizure was preceded by rhythmical, fast activity in the left anterior cingulate gyrus which spread to the left hippocampal formation (Figure 15).

A left frontal craniotomy was carried out in October, 1969. The parasagittal region of the frontal lobe was detached from the falx cerebri to allow electrocorticography of the medial and superior surfaces of the superior frontal lobe. Prominent EEG spikes were recorded from the cingulate gyrus and the superior frontal gyrus. In the course of the cortical resection, an

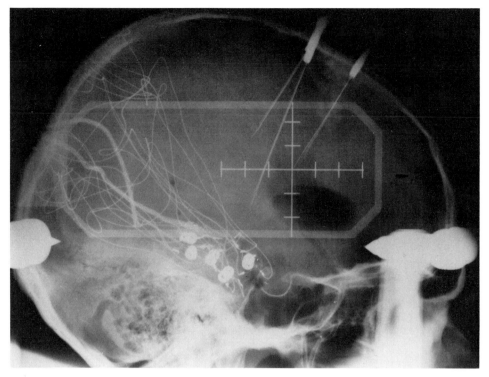

Figure 14. Stereotactically implanted electrodes placed symmetrically in the cingulate gyri, thalamus, and medial to the temporal lobe. (Case 4.)

astrocytoma was discovered which extended into the medial corpus callosum.

For 6 days after the operation the patient had dysphasia, which ultimately completely cleared. Postoperative radiation therapy was administered. Three weeks postoperatively he had a flurry of 10 seizures, then remained seizure-free for 9 months. Since then there has been the development of a progressive hemiparesis and recurrence of seizures with evidence of enlarging neoplasm. He has been receiving chemotherapy.

DISCUSSION

The problems connected with the identification of seizure foci are in lateralization and localization of characteristic activity. The usual preliminary material for a diagnostic analysis is derived from a history of the attacks and the recordings of interictal discharges by scalp electroencephalography. The difficulty in reaching a conclusion in the partial epilepsies, when relying solely on this type of material, is exemplified in one report by a group of French epileptologists (10). They collated their data from a large number of patients. In their syndromes of Bravais-Jacksonian paroxysms and "epilepsia partialis continua," four-fifths of the EEG foci involved

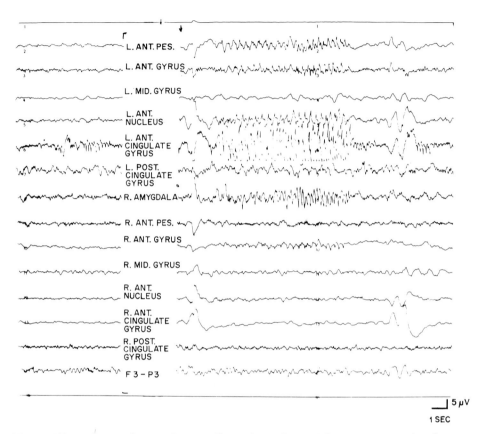

Figure 15. Ictal recording with indwelling electrodes and by means of radiotelemetry revealed the onset of focal, rhythmical discharges in the left cingulate gyrus which spread into the left hippocampal formation. (Case 4.) L, left; ANT., anterior; POST., posterior; R, right; F3-P3, electrodes (international placement).

the Rolandic region contralateral to the paroxysms. In contrast to this, in their group of adversive seizures, focal interictal discharges were rare and ictal discharges nearly always had a diffuse expression over one or both hemispheres, predominant on the side of the brain contralateral to the deviation. In patients having contraversive paroxysms the foci involved any region of the hemisphere, but especially the temporal region in half of the cases and the frontal region in nearly a quarter. Only a small number of patients had supplementary motor seizures but in one-half the EEG was almost normal and in the remainder EEG foci were divided between locations in the posterior frontal region, frontotemporal region, and in the temporal region. Therefore, the only high correlation was seen when the epileptic processes were superficial in the primary somatomotor cortices.

To derive better information there have been long-standing efforts by some investigators to photograph and electrographically record during ictal events. Simultaneous cinematographic recordings of the patient and of his EEG during seizures have been attempted since 1949 (11, 22, 23, 26).

These attempts were more successful in photographing the attacks than in electrographically recording during them. The electrographic changes during an ictus are probably the least well known and described of all the EEG changes. The occurrence of spontaneous seizures is relatively rare in routine EEG practice, and in the event it takes place, the presence of unexpected and uncontrollable artifacts rarely make an interpretation possible. A clinical electrographic analysis of Metrazol-induced attacks was undertaken by Ajmone Marsan and Ralston (2). With many precautions the numbers of usable records were increased. However, for certain types of attacks with vigorous motor actions, the likelihood of obtaining an artifact-free record was rather poor whether the seizure itself was spontaneous or induced. Also there was a continual question of separation of Metrazol-produced effects from the intrinsic epileptic activity. The photography of the ictus allowed good documentation and classification of the clinical features of the partial epilepsies. However, excluding seizures featured by automatism, aphasia, or ictal clonic movements, other clinical patterns of partial epilepsy could be found with focal EEG patterns in any one of five different regions.

Since the recent acquisition of miniature radio transmitters, it has been possible to record EEG in freely moving patients over hours or days (1, 24, 25). Since the transmitter moves with the patient's head and cable movements are eliminated, there are fewer artifacts. This makes it possible to record during many types of seizures which do not involve violent physical activity.

The two factors in the method presented here which permit the identification of seizure foci are (1) direct recording from deep cortical regions of the brain which are difficult of access and (2) continuous monitoring by radiotelemetry with ample time and under favorable conditions to examine interictal, preictal and ictal periods. These examples are not the first recordings of these events, but this method offers the possibility of regularly obtaining this information in patients for prospective surgical treatment. During stereotactic operations there have been rare, fortuitous recordings of ictal activities in the frontal supplementary motor, temporal, and para-rhinal cortices by Bancaud and co-workers (4). Focal ictal activity in the anterior cingulate gyrus leading to generalized epilepsy has been observed in chronic recordings by Mazars (16). Ictal activities during open craniotomies have been recorded by Penfield and Jasper (17). Also, in certain cases of generalized epilepsy, it has been shown that, when the scalp recording reveals generalized atypical spike-and-wave activity, the use of depth electrodes may reveal that the discharges emanate from discrete multifocal areas of frontal lobes (8). Examinations of these recordings from different regions, as well as comparing our previous cases of limbic system epilepsy, show strong similarities, which suggest that the ictal EEG signal is characteristic activity in its wave-form and propagation pattern when it occurs in several epileptogenic regions. Ultimately it leads to repetitive, high-amplitude spike discharges.

The method has the disadvantages that it interposes a surgical diagnostic operation into the patient's treatment and introduces possibilities of infection or bleeding. In our series of 60 patients examined with depth electrodes since 1960, we have had 1 instance of intracranial bleeding and 1 instance of transient meningitis. Balanced against these risks is that the improved preoperative data led to smaller craniotomies and cortical resections. In the past there have been other operations carried out for these seizure disorders, such as hemispherectomy or total frontal lobe resections, which involve much greater risks.

In conclusion, the preliminary results of recording the ictal EEG signal by surveying several possible epileptogenic zones by means of indwelling electrodes, and EEG radiotelemetry have been promising in instances of partial epilepsy which are drug-resistant. The follow-up period has been short. However, if temporal lobe epilepsy can be a guide, it is known that the ultimate result is present after 1 year in 90% of patients (20). These initial good results encourage us to study these difficult epileptic disorders further.

SUMMARY

Seven patients with partial epilepsy were studied by a method using stereotactically implanted electrodes and continuous monitoring by EEG radiotelemetry for several days to record the ictal EEG signal. The clinical patterns included adversive, contraversive, focal clonic, flection, extension, postural, somatic inhibitory, and focal status epilepticus seizures (with or without loss of consciousness and with or without speech arrest). The deep cortical areas surveyed by depth electrodes were the supplementary motor area, several limbic system sites such as cingulate gyrus, amygdala, hippocampus, hippocampal gyrus, and selected thalamic nuclei. The precentral motor cortex and other cerebral convexity regions were recorded from epidural calvarial electrodes placed in the international 10-20 EEG distribution. The ictal EEG signal was found to be valuable for purposes of localization. Clear recordings were obtained despite vigorous physical activity. The ictal wave form consisted of a cessation of interictal polyphasic waves of disorganized pattern which were replaced by focal, rhythmical, fast, low-amplitude, highly organized discharges or suppression. There followed a progressive slowing and increase in amplitude of waves as well as propagation into other regions. Focal sensorimotor manifestations of the type described appeared with seizure foci in any of the cortical regions studied. Four examples are submitted. The postoperative results after removal of these epileptogenic areas identified by this method have been promising in short-term follow-up (6 months to 3 years).

REFERENCES

1. Adey, W. R., Hanley, J., Kado, R. T., and Zweizig, J. R., A multichannel telemetry system for EEG recording. *Proc. Symp. Biomed. Eng., Marquette Univ.*, 1966, **1**: 36–39.

2. Ajmone Marsan, C., and Ralston, B. L., *The Epileptic Seizure.* Thomas, Springfield, Illinois, 1957.

3. Andrew, J., and Nathan, P. W., Lesions of the anterior frontal lobes and disturbances of micturition and defaecation. *Brain*, 1964, **87**: 233–262.

4. Bancaud, J., Talairach, J., Bonis, A., Schaub, C., Szikla, G., Morel, P., and Bordas-Ferer, M., *La stéréo-électroencéphalographie dans l' épilepsie.* Masson, Paris, 1965.

5. Crandall, P. H., and Walter, R. D., The ictal electroencephalographic signal identifying limbic system seizure foci. *Proc. Am. Assoc. Neurol. Surg.*, 1971, **1**: 1–9.

6. Crandall, P. H., Walter, R. D., and Rand, R. W., Clinical applications of studies on stereotactically implanted electrodes in temporal lobe epilepsy. *J. Neurosurg.*, 1963, **21**: 827–840.

7. Dymond, A. M., Zweizig, J. R., Crandall, P. H., and Hanley, J., Clinical applications of an EEG radio-telemetry system. *Biomed. Instrum.* **8**: 16–20.

8. Goldring, S., The role of prefrontal cortex in grand mal convulsion. *Arch. Neurol.*, 1972, **26**: 109–119.

9. Gudmundsson, G., Epilepsy in Iceland: A clinical and epidemiological investigation. *Acta Neurol. Scand.* 1966, 43 Suppl. 25: 1–124.

10. Hécaen, H., Gastaut, H., Bancaud, J., and Rebufat-Deschamps, M., Clinical and EEG aspects of the problem of cortical localization. In: *Cerebral Localization and Organization* (G. Schaltenbrand and C. N. Woolsey, Eds.). Univ. of Wisconsin Press, Madison, 1964: 67–88.

11. Hunter, J., and Jasper, H. H., A method of analysis of seizure pattern and electroencephalogram. *Electroencephalogr. Clin. Neurophysiol.*, 1949, **1**: 113–114.

12. Juul-Jensen, P., Epilepsy. A clinical and social analysis of 1020 adult patients with epileptic seizures. *Acta Neurol. Scand.*, 1964, **40**: Suppl. 5: 1–148.

13. Kurland, L. T., The incidence and prevalence of convulsive disorders in a small urban community. *Epilepsia*, 1959, **1**: 143–161.

14. Kurtzke, J. F., Some epidemiologic and clinical features of adult seizure disorders. *J. Chronic Dis.*, 1968, **21**: 143–156.

15. Kurtzke, J. F., Kurland, L. T., Goldberg, I. D., Nung, W. C., and Reeder, F. A., Convulsive disorders. In: *Epidemiology of Neurologic and Sense Organ Disorders* (L. T. Kurland, J. F. Kurtzke, and I. D. Goldberg, Eds.). Harvard Univ. Press, Cambridge, 1973: 15–40.

16. Mazars, G., Cingulate gyrus epileptogenic foci as an origin for generalized seizures. In: *The Physiopathogenesis of the Epilepsies* (H. Gastaut *et al.*, Eds.). Thomas, Springfield, Illinois, 1969: 186–189.

17. Penfield, W., and Jasper, H., *Epilepsy and the Functional Anatomy of the Human Brain.* Little, Brown, Boston, 1954.

18. Penfield, W., and Welch, K., The supplementary motor area of the cerebral cortex. *Arch. Neurol. Psychiatry*, 1951, **66**: 289–317.

19. Rand, R. W., Crandall, P. H., and Walter, R. D., Chronic stereotactic implantation of depth electrodes for psychomotor epilepsy. *Acta Neurochir. (Wien)*, 1964, **11**: 609–630.

20. Rasmussen, T., and Branch, C., Temporal lobe epilepsy: Indications for and results of surgical therapy. *Postgrad. Med.*, 1962, **31**: 9–14.

21. Rodin, E. A., *The Prognosis of Patients with Epilepsy*. Thomas, Springfield, Illinois, 1968.

22. Schwab, R. S., Some correlations of clinical and EEG patterns in short seizures. *Electroencephalogr. Clin. Neurophysiol.*, 1956, **8**: 148–149.

23. Schwab, R. S., Schwab, M. W., Withee, D., and Chock, Y. C., Synchronized moving picture of patient with his EEG. *Proc. Int. Congr. Electroenceph. clin. Neurophysiol.*, 3rd, 1953: 47.

24. Stevens, J. R., Kodama, H., Lonsbury, B., and Mills, L., Ultradian characteristics of spontaneous seizure discharges recorded by radiotelemetry in man. *Electroenceph. clin. Neurophysiol.*, 1971, **31**: 313–325.

25. Stevens, J. R., Lonsbury, B., Kodama, H., and Mills, L., Statistical characteristics of spontaneous seizure discharges recorded by radiotelemetry over 24 hour periods in man. *Electroenceph. clin. Neurophysiol.*, 1969, **27**: 691.

26. Stewart, L. F., Another simple method for the simultaneous cinematographic recording of the patient and his EEG during seizures. *Electroenceph. clin. Neurophysiol.*, 1956, **8**: 526–527.

27. Talairach, J., David, M., and Tournoux, P., *L'exploration chirurgicale stéréotaxique du lobe temporal dans l'épilepsie temporale*. Masson, Paris, 1958.

28. Talairach, J., David, M., Tournoux, P., Corredor, H., and Kvasina, T., *Atlas d'anatomie stéréotaxique*. Masson, Paris, 1957.

29. Talairach, J., Szikla, G., Tournoux, P., Prossalentis, A., Bordas-Ferrer, M., Covello, L., Jacob, M., and Mempel, E., *Atlas d'Anatomie stéréotaxique du télencéphale*. Masson, Paris, 1967.

30. Waddington, M. M., Angiographic changes in focal motor epilepsy. *Neurology (Minneap.)*, 1970, **20**: 879–888.

31. Woolsey, C. H., Organization of somatic sensory and motor areas of the cerebral cortex. In: *Biological and Biochemical Bases of Behavior* (H. F. Harlow and C. N. Woolsey, Eds.). Univ. of Wisconsin Press, Madison, 1965: 63–81.

HIPPOCAMPAL PATHOLOGY IN TEMPORAL LOBE EPILEPSY.
A GOLGI SURVEY

MADGE E. SCHEIBEL and **ARNOLD B. SCHEIBEL***

Brain Research Institute, University of California, Los Angeles, California

For more than a century, men have sought visible evidence of change in epileptogenic cortex which might provide clues to the cause of this enigmatic disease. Perhaps the earliest finding was the demonstration in 1825 by Bouchet and Cazauvieilh (6) of frequent changes in consistency, i.e. hardening or softening, in the hippocampus of epileptic patients. Approximately 20 years later, Bergmann (3) postulated a relationship between seizures and hippocampal asymmetry. Neither of these workers considered these changes to have etiological significance. In 1880, Sommer (42) and Pfleger (34) made somewhat more definitive contributions to the problem. The former reported that approximately one-third of the epileptic patients he had studied showed extensive loss of neurons in a circumscribed portion of Ammon's horn, an area now known as Sommer's sector (CA_1). The latter hypothesized that the sclerosis peculiar to the affected regions was due to repeated circulatory embarrassment provoked during the seizures themselves. This point of view that the lesions of temporal lobe epilepsy are secondary to the syndrome came to constitute one of two conceptual positions which, even today, polarize thinking in this area.

Gliosis gradually began to be recognized as a specific pathological substrate for virtually all cortical epileptic change, where change in appearance or consistency was recognizable at all. Alzheimer (1) and Chaslin (8) demonstrated neuron loss and associated glial overgrowth in the hippocampus and in the first layer of cerebral neocortex, respectively. Associated with the latter, at least during early portions of the life history of the disease process were unusually large concentrations of primitive bipolar cells in the molecular layer of cerebral cortex. Meanwhile, serious experimental histology by Monti (29) was establishing the fact that various types of nutritional insufficiency could produce changes in dendrites which included loss of dendritic spines, later described by Cajal (7), and the appear-

* *Acknowledgments:* This work was the supported by the U.S. Public Health Service Grant, NINDS 01063. We are indebted to Dr. Paul H. Crandall, Division of Neurosurgery, for supplying us with the human temporal lobe tissue upon which this study is based.

ance of nodular changes along the dendrites, changes which were, to some extent, reversible. At approximately the same time, De Moor (10) was using the Golgi methods, possibly for the first time, in the study of human epileptic cortex. The diffuse spine loss and moniliform deformity of virtually all of the dendrite shafts he examined pointed, by implication at least, to problems in blood supply or metabolic support.

In an important series of communication, Spielmayer (43–45) attempted to relate the neuronal loss and glial scarring which characterized sclerosis of Ammon's horn to peculiarities of the vascular bed supplying the region, especially the particularly vulnerable sector of Sommer. He postulated that angiospasm preceded, and possibly precipitated, the ictus, with the sclerosing lesion developing as a result of the ensuing ischemia. Recently Scholz (39–41) and Meyer and co-workers (28) have marshalled evidence in support of this position although the ultimate cause invoked by these authors, whether genetic or angiospastic, is never fully convincing.

The modern position that temporal lobe epilepsy stems from hippocampal sclerosis secondary to birth injury was apparently first suggested by Edinger (12). His concept of compression of ventromedial structures of the temporal lobe along the edge of the tentorium with herniation of the hippocampus was supported by Adolf Meyer (26). However, it was not till 30 years later that Earle and co-authors (11) supplied experimental evidence in support of this premise with their demonstration of the effects of severe lateral compression on the heads of stillborn infants. When lengths of rubber tubing were tied tightly around the heads of such infants and the entire specimen then frozen and sliced, the investigators were able to show clearly the herniation of uncus and hippocampus over the free edge of the tentorium. Removal of the tubing before freezing resulted in no visible displacement. It was concluded that herniation was reversible but that during the period of intense pressure and displacement, severe ischemia resulting in necrosis and eventual glial scarring might well develop. The relation to a difficult birth process received further support from a report by Nielsen and Courville (30) that 40% of all idiopathic epilepsies occurred in children from mothers bearing their first child.

Over the past two decades, a number of studies have added to the literature much descriptive pathology and a number of attempts to correlate the syndrome with the appearance of cortical tissue at postmortem examination or following partial resection of the temporal lobe. As an example, the reader is referred to a series of symposium presentations by Meyer (27), Scholz (41), Penfield (32), Norman (31), and Maspes and colleagues (25) on the pathological anatomy of the epilepsies presented at the 1954 Marseilles colloquium.

In the meantime, the development of laboratory techniques for generating experimental epileptic foci (23) has opened the way to studies of the development of the histopathological substrate, such as that of Westrum

and co-workers (50). At the same time, the extremely low seizuring threshold of normal hippocampus has become progressively more apparent over
three decades of neurophysiological experimentation (e.g., references 2, 21,
35). All of this work attests to the complex nature of ictal phenomena and
the unlikelihood of discovering a single, simple mechanism responsible for
all types of paroxysmal activity.

In the following sections we shall limit ourselves to descriptions of the
histological appearance of Ammon's horn removed from a number of patients with temporal lobe seizures and prepared for study under the light
microscope by means of the Golgi impregnation techniques.

The methods of Golgi cannot properly be considered within the roster
of routine neuropathological stains. Among the well-known drawbacks of
the method, the uncertainty of impregnation and the limited number of
neural elements that can be visualized are particularly trying when examining tissue specimens which are literally one-of-a-kind samples which can
neither be replaced nor duplicated. Clearly, for most diagnostic needs, more
reliable and broadly staining methods are preferable. Yet the capability
of the Golgi method to enable visualization of all pre- and postsynaptic
elements of the neural ensemble, including neuroglia, makes it a powerful
adjunctive technique in any neuropathological analysis. It, alone, can provide a panoramic view of cell bodies, axons, dendrites, and the specialized
structures, both pre- and postsynaptic, which line the soma-dendrite membrane. Although each of these items can also be studied at greater resolution with the electron microscope,[*] the Golgi method remains unique in
that its histopathological statement can be evaluated within the context
of the neural surround. One does not lose the forest for the trees as is
bound to happen in work performed exclusively at the level of electron
microscopy.

For this reason, we have not hesitated to apply the Golgi methods to
small blocks of human brain tissue removed during resections for temporal
lobe epilepsy. So long as part of the tissue is run up through routine stains
giving results that are predictable but limited, it has seemed reasonable
to us to venture the undeniable risk of partial or complete disappointment
in the hope of realizing the greater return of information that often follows.

Although we have tried a number of variations in staining technique,
we have realized the best results from a very simple modification of the
basic rapid Golgi method. Small blocks of tissue are removed from the
surgical field as quickly as possible into neutral 10% formalin solution.
After 2 to 4 hours, the blocks are cut down to a thickness of 3 to 4 mm
and immersed in a fresh mixture of osmic acid (1 gm) and potassium
dichromate (8 gm) in 300 ml of distilled water. After 4 to 7 days in the
dark, the tissue is removed from fixative, washed briefly in distilled water,

---

[*] See the chapter by Dr. Jann Brown in this volume.

and placed in the impregnating solution of 0.75 to 1% silver nitrate. After approximately 24 hours, the tissue is removed, placed on small cutting blocks, and encased in low melting point paraffin. Each paraffin–tissue block is then cut with a sliding microtome at 100 to 150 μm, and the sections are removed into absolute alcohol. Following clearing in oil of cloves and toluene, the sections are mounted and preserved under Permount or other synthetic resin. Despite the inevitable presence of myelin in these cortical specimens, the stained sections almost always have a sufficiently lucent background, i.e. the unstained surround, to enable either photography or drawing of the specimens. Other Golgi modifications which entirely avoid the use of osmic acid are also available. These methods often give a clearer, virtually colorless background which results in photographs of higher contrast. However, these entirely formalin-based methods are, in our hands at least, less reliable than the classic Golgi method and have accordingly been avoided in this study.

The interpretation of results in a study of this sort must be approached cautiously. Considerable variability marks the size and shape of dendrite domains and appearance of the soma-dendrite surface throughout the Ammon's horn. Furthermore, the range of patterns that may be considered to fall within normal limits in man is undoubtedly greater than in rodents, carnivores, or primates. Unfortunately, our access to normal control material is inadequate in man where the total amount of surgically removed temporal lobe tissue remains small and virtually limited to ictal syndromes. Relatively large amounts of tissue can be obtained from autopsy specimens, but it is rare to find a brain that has been perfused and/or removed sooner than 2–4 hours after death. This period of time is more than sufficient for the development of a number of gross morphological changes in Golgi-stained material removed from laboratory animals and must, therefore, be assumed to have similar effects in man.

Accordingly, we have used as controls, carefully prepared material from cats and a few rhesus monkeys. These have been compared and correlated with areas of human hippocampal-dentate tissue where essentially similar patterns have been found. Changes beyond these limits are then noted and considered as potentially or presumptively pathological in nature. Such changes include patchy or complete loss of dendrite spines, periodic swelling or nodulation ("string of beads" deformity) in dendrites, elongation or compression of dendrite domains, change—usually decrease—in the apparent density of dendrite branching, etc. More profound changes such as swelling or shrinkage of the cell body, fragmentation and loss of the dendrite tree, and obvious gliosis can be considered pathological with a higher confidence level.

We had hoped to establish correlations between the position, degree, and extent of hippocampal pathology and the nature and intensity of the clinical syndrome; however, the inevitably partial nature of Golgi staining makes this procedure an uncertain one. It is difficult to determine from study of Golgi sections alone whether or not one has seen all of the pathological areas and the full extent of pathology in any one area. Routine neurohistological and neuropathological methods must be consulted for further evidence here. For these reasons, the present study is limited to a qualitative description of neuronal and glial patterns in Ammon's horn that have been seen in 10 operated cases. Correlation of the nature and extent of the pathology with the severity of the clinical picture will be the subject of future studies.

Introductory Anatomical Comments

The fine structure of the hippocampus is well known from the Golgi studies of Cajal (7), Kölliker (22), and Lorente de Nó (24), among others, with important recent additions at the level of the electron microscope such as those of Hamlyn (19, 20) and Blackstad and his co-workers (4, 5). Utilizing the terminology of Lorente de Nó (24), there is fairly general agreement that the various subicular components of transitional temporal cortex merge insensibly with the three-layered zone of limbic archicortex. This structure, the classic Ammon's horn, can be divided into at least four major subdivisions: CA_1, CA_2, CA_3, and CA_4. Following Lorente de Nó, these can be assigned primarily on the basis of the morphology of the apical dendrites. In CA_1, the apical shaft originates from the soma as a single structure (Figure 1a). After a variable distance, this then divides into secondary and tertiary dendrites, forming the first stages of the apical dendrite bouquet. In CA_2 pyramids, the principal apical shaft is very short or nonexistent. The apical dendritic bouquet accordingly starts virtually at the neck of the soma (see Figure 2a). The CA_3 neurons are characterized, like those of CA_1, by the appreciable length of the single primary apical shaft prior to the development of the apical cluster, but with the addition of multiple short collateral dendrites which emerge from the primary shaft, often at right angles (Figure 1b). The pyramids of CA_4 are initially similar to those of CA_3 but as the hilus of the dentate fascia is progressively invaded, the cells become more polymorphic, finally coming to resemble in some cases the radiating dendrite-bearing elements found in the brain stem reticular core.

The granules of the dentate fascia are characterized by a spreading dendritic plexus emerging from one pole of the cell body, alone (Figure 10a–d), although we have found a number of examples where deep dendrites leave what is ordinarily the axonal pole and plunge into the underlying polymorph layer (Figure 11a and c). The dendrites of all of these elements appear covered with spines in the normal adult (see Figures 2c and 10e) and, with certain exceptions to be mentioned below, variations from this state will be considered abnormal.

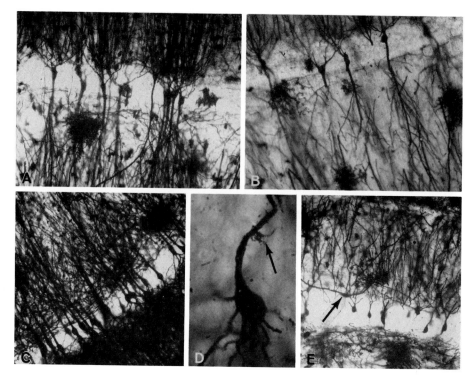

Figure 1. Neurons from hippocampus–dentate complex of adult cat. (a) Row of CA₁ hippocampal pyramids; (b) group of CA₃ hippocampal pyramids; (c) ensemble of CA₃ pyramids showing density of dendritic plexus; (d) CA₁ pyramid with mossy tuft on proximal portion of apical dendrite shaft; (e) row of dentate granule cells including several horizontal cells (arrow). Rapid Golgi variants. a, b, c, and e, magnification ×100; d magnification ×265.

Since the fine structure and connections of the hippocampus–dentate complex are known to most readers and are readily found in Cajal (7) and Lorente de Nó (24), further descriptions of normal structures are probably unnecessary. Ammon's horn contains a number of cell populations other than those mentioned above, notably short axoned components. Because our material has not included impregnations of significant numbers of these cells, we shall not consider them in this report.

PATHOLOGICAL CHANGES IN THE HIPPOCAMPUS

Spine Loss and Nodulation of Dendrites

The most obvious and frequent change to be seen in our series of resected hippocampi has been an apparent diminution or loss of dendritic spines and an increasing irregularity of dendrite silhouettes. Various stages of such changes can be seen in Figure 3. In our experience, patchy spine loss may occur anywhere along the apical or basilar dendrites. In the majority of

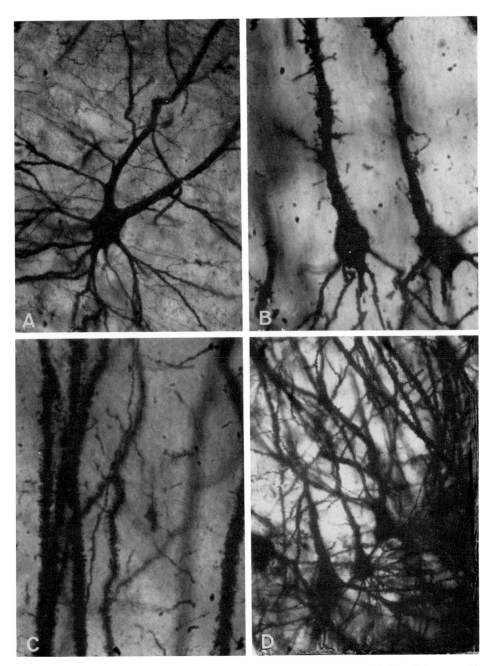

Figure 2. Apparently normal elements from human hippocampus. (a) The CA₂ pyramid showing richly branching basilar dendrites; (b) two CA₁ pyramids showing some pre- and postsynaptic detail. Several of the protruding structures probably represent terminating mossy fibers; (c) hippocampal dendrites showing clustering of spines; (d) ensemble of hippocampal pyramids at CA₁-CA₂ junction. Rapid Golgi variants. a and d, magnification ×225; b and c, magnification ×360.

cases, however, it appears to be accompanied by the development of series
of nodules or fusiform enlargements along the course of the dendrite. Since
this string-of-beads deformity seems usually initiated at the tips of basilar
(see Figures 3b, 4a, 9B) or apical (Figure 4b) branches, earliest evidences
of loss may occur here too. Although we are obviously unable to make
any statements about the rate at which the changes develop, our material
clearly indicates that both of these changes may be seen simultaneously

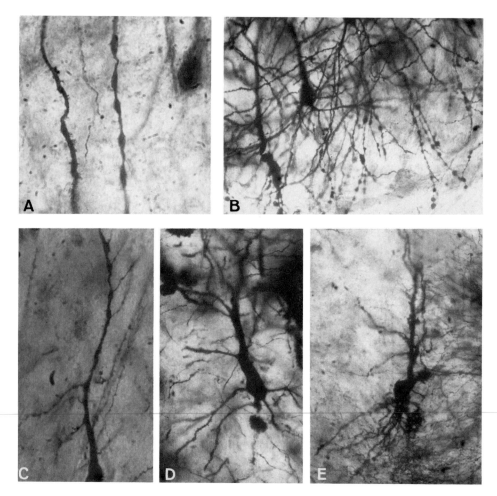

Figure 3. Several apparently pathological changes in neurons of the adult human hippocampal–dentate complex. (a) Two dendrites from the same hippocampal pyramid:
one shows early fusiform changes with residual patches of dendrite spines; the other
shows far advanced changes producing a typical string-of-beads deformity. (b) A
number of basilar dendrites of CA₃ pyramids show nodular changes with loss of spines.
(c) Apical shaft of CA₃ pyramid shows loss of spines and developing fusiform enlargements. (d) Large hippocampal CA₃ pyramid showing spine loss along dendrites and
swelling of proximal portion of apical dendrite. (e) Far advanced degenerative changes
in CA₃ pyramid with distortion and shrinkage of dendritic domain. Rapid Golgi variants.
a, magnification ×338; b, c, d, and e, magnification ×150.

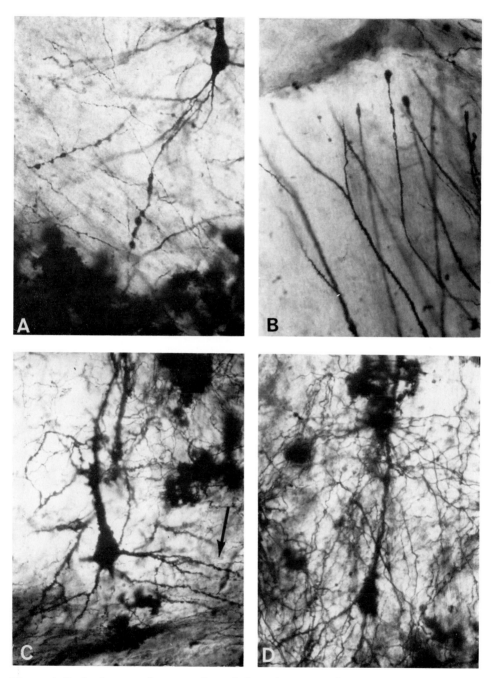

Figure 4. Early changes of apparently pathological nature in human hippocampal pyramids. (a) Nodular changes with loss of spines leading to string-of-beads deformity in basilar dendrites of CA₁ neuron. (b) Loss of spines and development of terminal nodules and knobs on the apical shafts of hippocampal CA₁ pyramids. (c) Large CA₁ pyramid showing development of early stage of string-of-beads deformity on part of the basilar dendrite system (arrow). (d) CA₁ pyramid showing diffuse architectural changes in a glial stroma rich in fibrillary astrocytic processes. This may represent a moderately scarred cortical focus. Rapid Golgi variants. a, c, and d, magnification ×225; b, magnification ×405.

in the same dendrite. For instance, in the dendrite on the left in Figure 3a, some evidence of nodulation can already be seen. Spines are still present although decreased in number; and where present, they appear to emerge from the convexity of each nodule or swelling. In the case of the shaft just to the right in the same photograph, the nodulation is far advanced, producing a clear-cut string-of-beads appearance, and no spines can be seen. In the case of the rather bizarrely distorted CA_2 pyramid in Figure 8, a number of dendrite branches show both spine patches and large nodular deformations, although seldom along the same length of dendrite. In the far advanced degenerative changes visible in the hippocampal pyramid in Figure 5c and d, the basilar dendrites are very short and curled, presenting a shrivelled appearance relieved only by several large nodules along their course. Although such nodules are seldom more than 2–5 μm in diameter, it seems clear that they can become appreciably larger, that is up to 6 to 8 μm as evidenced in Figure 8.

We have been particularly impressed by the erratic, patchy nature of these changes. We frequently find one or two cells showing such changes out of an ensemble which appears normal. Even more dramatic is the frequency with which a single dendrite will show these changes while all of the remaining shafts of the parent neuron appear unremarkable. In Figure 9B, approximately one-half of the basilar dendrites of a typical CA_1 pyramid show nodulation with loss of spines. Figure 9C shows that similar changes can be localized to the branches of a single apical shaft, and in many cases that we have seen, even greater selectivity can be demonstrated.

It would be of considerable importance to be able to evaluate properly the significance of such changes. Data from several laboratories have clearly shown that dendrite spines are lost following interruption of the presynaptic afferents terminating upon them (9, 14, 18, 48). This phenomenon has proven sufficiently consistent to form the basis for a powerful and sensitive hodological technique enabling precise localization of afferent axonal systems upon individual dendrites (15, 16, 46).

De Moor (10) was probably the first investigator to correlate neurohistological changes at the level of the individual neuron as visualized by the Golgi method with clinical (grand mal) epilepsy. He described a uniformly pathological state affecting all pyramidal cells (area not specified): "Ces neurones sont caracterisés par l'état moniliforme de tous les prolongements . . . de grosses nodosités . . . et tantôt absolument dépourvues de ces élèments [spines] (10)."*

In one of the few studies of experimental epilepsy to be controlled with Golgi Cox impregnation of the induced focus, Westrum and co-workers

---

* "These neurons are characterized by a moniliform state along their dendrites . . . large nodules . . . and virtually complete absence of these elements [spines]."

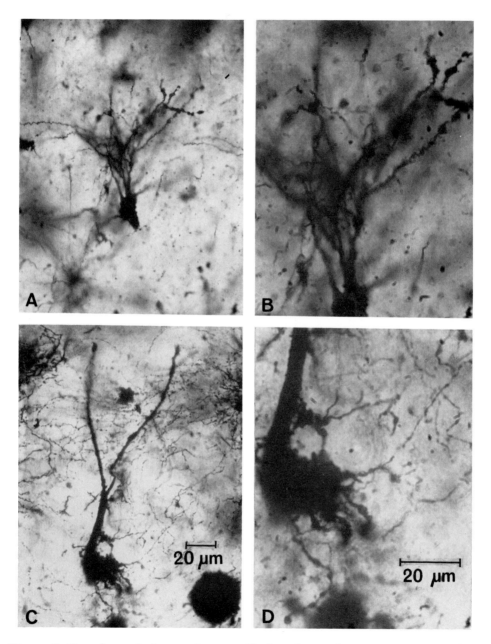

Figure 5. Far advanced changes in two cells from human hippocampus. (a and b) Small CA₂ pyramid showing marked shrinkage and distortion of apical dendrite system with loss of spines and terminal nodulation. (c and d). Degenerating pyramid from CA₁ showing loss of most of the apical dendrite system with extreme degree of shrivelling of basilar dendrites. Rapid Golgi variants. a and c, magnification ×170; b and d, magnification ×383.

(50) described the following changes in tissue subjacent to the zone of alumina cream destruction:

> There is neuronal depopulation involving predominantly the large neurons of the deeper layers and the small neurons of the superficial layers. The remaining neurons show marked alterations in dendritic structure . . . including . . . 1) reduction in branching, 2) bizarre angulations or distortions, 3) varicose-like swelling, 4) unexplained segments of poor impregnation, and 5) absence or severe reduction of spines or gemmules.

As will be seen presently, these authors have noted most of the changes in monkey neocortex that we have seen in human hippocampal tissue. In a group of unpublished studies (38) performed during the period 1953–1955, we noted spine loss, among other changes, in blocks of temporal lobe tissue from patients with characteristic uncinate fits. Although there is sufficient precedent for the finding, there is still no single satisfactory explanation as to mechanisms or significance. There is certainly no proof that in the clinical syndrome, spine loss represents the sequellae of deafferentation. If it did, the most attractive hypothesis would look to the loss as one of predominantly inhibitory elements to help explain the uncontrolled neuronal activity characteristic of the ictal episode. Deafferentation hypersensitivity would also have to be considered seriously in this context. Needless to say, both ideas have received careful consideration but the evidence for neither is, as yet, totally convincing.

However, spine loss is not an inevitable sign of pathological change. In the perinatal cortices of most mammals, the surfaces of pyramidal cells and dendrites are usually covered by large pleomorphic protospines. These disappear during the early postnatal period (1–3 weeks in the kitten) and are progressively replaced by spines of adult type (37). Similarly, in the case of ventral horn spinal motoneurons and in most neurons of the brain stem reticular core, nerve cells are covered with polymorphic protospines in the newborn state. These are gradually lost during the initial weeks of life. In the neurally mature or adult state, these neurons have smooth surfaces, virtually devoid of spinelike structures (38). In these cases, the loss must be considered a regular feature of the maturative process and without pathological significance (36).

Furthermore, there is some evidence to suggest that when spines are lost due to trauma or surgical intervention, they may, under certain circumstances, grow back. We have produced two types of deafferenting lesions in a short series of young rabbits, similar to the lesions described in earlier work in the visual system and corpus callosum (16, 17). Instead of sacrificing the animals after 30 days, we waited for a full year before terminating the experiment. In these cases, we were not able to find significant differences in spine counts between experimental tissue and normal controls. We have tentatively interpreted this as indicating that, under certain conditions, deafferented areas along dendrites may be reinervated, probably by fiber terminals other than the original afferent system. New spine populations may then develop in the place of the old (38). In a differently structured study, Valverde came to the conclusion that the recovery of dendrite spines for some apical dendrites in dark-reared mice, when finally exposed to light, may begin to occur as soon as 2 days after contact with light (47).

Spine growth, loss, and possible regrowth thereby assume an increasingly plastic, dynamic quality and must be considered among the normal activities of the nervous system. This need not eliminate part or all of this sequence as a sign of neuronal pathology. Careful study of control human and macaque hippocampus and dentate fascia stained with Golgi methods has seldom revealed obvious spine loss or dendritic distortions. We must assume that such changes are unusual in the normally functioning adult hippocampus and, therefore, in a very real sense, indices of pathology in the tissue we have examined. But it would also be prudent to consider spine loss, in its broadest context, as one of a relatively small group of changed states that a dendrite may show in a number of situations, normal or abnormal.

The nodular, moniliform or fusiform swelling along the dendrite represent a similar problem in evaluation. We have seen large numbers of archicortical neurons in varying stages of degeneration from the earliest loss of spines to the final stage of dendrite disintegration with swelling and shrivelling of the neuron soma (see Figure 9F). Invariably the periodic swellings develop early and stay late. Often, the final dendritic residue consists only of a few shrunken remnants of stalk and a couple of large nodules (Figures 5d and 9F).

On the other hand, many short axon (local circuit) cells, particularly in the neocortex are characteristically spineless (17, 33) and show regular swellings along their otherwise thin dendrites. Peters (33) has identified some of these zones under the electron microscope and finds that they contain many enlarged cisternae of the endoplasmic reticulum. It would, therefore, seem reasonable to assume that the string-of-beads deformity has a broader significance than simply as an index of pathology. It may represent a cell–dendrite system whose protein-synthesizing capacity is under challenge, whether it be for physiological or pathological causes.

With these provisos, our experience with surgically resected human material in comparison with control tissue persuades us that the appearance of nodules, periodic swelling, or the more generalized string-of-beads deformity in an adult hippocampal pyramid or dentate granule is a sensitive index of pathological processes in the cell.

Signs of More Extensive Pathology

Examination of Figures 5 through 9 reveals several other changes that characterize pathological cells in the human hippocampus. Irregular en-

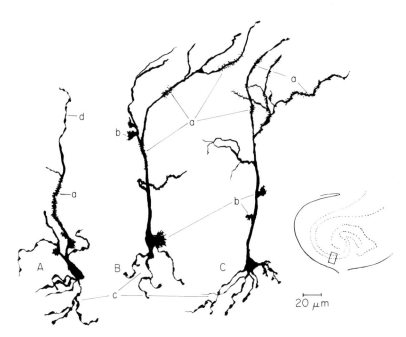

Figure 6. Drawing of three human hippocampal pyramids from CA₃ showing apparently far advanced states of pathological change. On each neuron there are patchy remaining areas of dendrite spines (a) and irregular leafy protrusions (b). There is marked distortion and angulation of basilar dendrites with typical string-of-beads deformities on all three cells. The apical shaft of cell A, in particular, shows similar changes at d. It appears obvious that all of these dendrite systems show marked shortening and loss of terminal branching when compared with a normal pyramid (see Figure 1a). Rapid Golgi variant.

largements occur haphazardly along the dendrite shafts (Figures 6b and 7b). They may resemble leafy excrescences, bulb or horn-shaped growths, or more simply, very marked and asymmetric dilatations of the dendrite stalk. The entire dendrite shaft, although shorn of spines, may appear swollen—sometimes over a length of several hundred micra. A good example of this deformation is seen in Figure 12 in two dentate granules.

Perhaps the most bizarre and obvious change that can occur to these cells rests in distortions of shape and size of the dendrite domain. Figures 6 to 8 show examples of this class of deformities. Because of the tightness in packing of the shafts, the changes are most obvious in the distal half of the apical shaft. The shorter basilar dendrites often show a more dramatic type of curling upon themselves (Figures 6A,B and 8A). These changes appear to lead directly to shrinkage and disintegration of the shafts (Figure 9D–F).

Ward (49) and Westrum and co-workers (50) have considered the problem of mechanical deformation of dendrites and its possible relationship to depolarization of the dendritic membrane. An intriguing analogy has

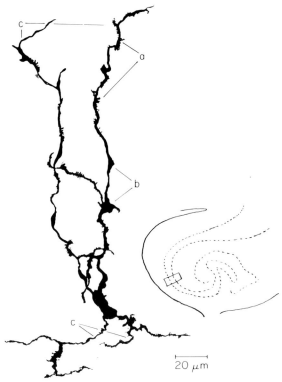

Figure 7. Drawing of human hippocampal CA$_2$ pyramid showing a number of dendritic changes which include partial loss of dendrite spines with patchy remnant areas (a); irregular enlargements along the course of the dendrite shafts (b); angular distortions of the shafts (c); loss of normal dendritic taper, etc. The tips of the apical dendrites and the entire basilar dendrite system show marked angular and directional distortions. Rapid Golgi variant.

been drawn between processes operating in the dendrites of sensory neurons in the crayfish ganglion and those possibly involved in dendrite tips of pathological cortical cells. The former are lodged in muscle masses where stress induced in them by changes in muscle length and tension depolarize the membrane and may induce propagated discharges (13). The dendrite tips are conceived as being placed under distortive stresses by an adjacent glial scar. The permanent, and sometimes progressive, nature of such a scar can be conceived as the focal pathological site which induces abnormal electrical activity in adjacent neurons. However, in the data reported by Westrum and co-workers (50), the number of distorted dendrite systems was very small and did not coincide geographically with sites of maximal paroxysmal activity. For this reason, they apparently discount tonic deformation of dendrite systems as a possible factor in epileptogenesis.

As we mentioned previously, our present data offer no conclusive insight into the numbers of neurons showing such changes at any one time, nor can we estimate the total number of cells that have disappeared completely

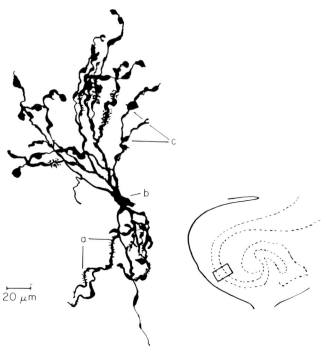

Figure 8. Drawing of human hippocampal CA₂ pyramid showing rather dramatic changes in the apical and basilar dendritic shafts. Although there are remaining patches of dendrite spines (a); the most obvious change is the large number of nodular and fusiform enlargements (c) contributing to a marked string-of-beads deformity. Some of these individual enlargements are 6–8 μm in diameter. The cell body (b) appears irregular in outline and may be showing early pyknotic changes. Rapid Golgi variant.

during the earlier history of the process. Such figures are of considerable interest but will have to be sought with the aid of techniques where quantitative results are reasonably reliable.

PATHOLOGY OF THE DENTATE GRANULES

In some respects, evaluation of pathological changes in the dentate fascia is beset with even more uncertainty than in the hippocampus. Despite the considerably smaller size of the dentate granules when compared to hippocampal pyramids, a greater range of sizes and shapes can be seen in their dendrite domains and shape and placement of cell bodies. Basic cell shape and domain architecture appear quite similar in a number of representative mammalian forms, such as in rat, cat, and man (Figure 10). However, in the human dentate tissue we have studied, a larger number of variant forms have been seen. Some of these are illustrated in Figures 11 through 14 and are summarized in Figure 15. The major change in dendrite domains which we have identified seems to involve an apparent compression of the dendrite stalks upon the axis of symmetry, leading to a

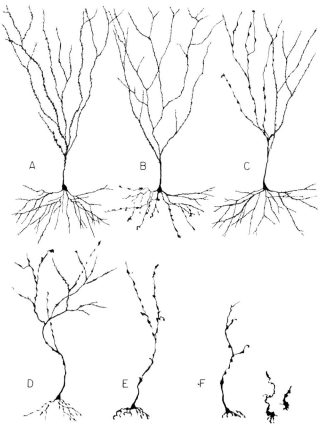

Figure 9. Drawing of human hippocampal pyramids from CA₁ area showing a series of changes of increasing severity leading to total cell destruction. Although all of these changes have been seen in many cells, it is not known that each cell in a pathological focus will follow this sequence of changes. (A) Apparently normal pyramid. (B) Loss of dendrite spines and development of nodulation (string-of-beads appearance) in approximately one-half of the basilar dendrites. All other dendrite branches appear normal. (C) Loss of dendrite spines and development of nodulation on approximately one-half of the branches of the apical shaft. The rest of the dendrite system seems normal. The changes in cells B and C represent alternatives. The same neuron would obviously be unlikely to go through both changes. (D) Some loss of branches and progressive distortion of the dendritic domain, patchy remaining areas of spines and extensive areas of dendrite showing string-of-beans patterns. (E and F) Apparently the terminal steps in cell death with progressive loss of dendrite substance, increasing irregularity of the remaining shaft segments, angular distortion or curling of the dendrite branches, and swelling and/or shrinkage of the cell body. Drawn from a number of sections stained by rapid Golgi variants.

kind of "closed parasol" appearance (Figures 11, 13, 15E). Since the dentate dendrite arbor is a true tridimensional structure, unlike the cerebellar Purkinje neuron, this effect cannot be attributed to the plane of section through the tissue block. A second domain variation is the "windblown look," illustrated in Figures 14 and 15F in which virtually all of the dendrites of an ensemble of cells, sometimes several hundred, appear sharply

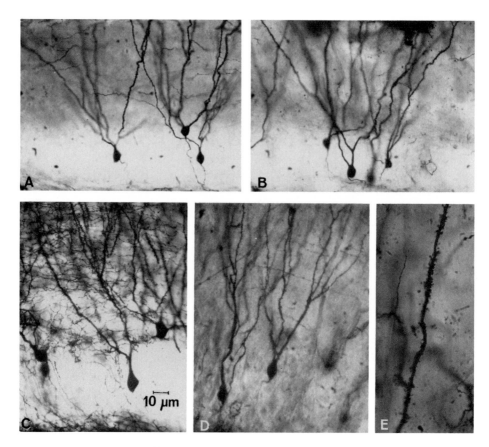

Figure 10. Dentate granule cells from several species. (a) Adult rat; (b) adult cat; (c and d) human dentate cells. Axons of the perforant pathway from entorhinal cortex can be seen passing among the dendrite shafts. Several dendrites in picture d show partial loss of spines and early nodular changes. (e) Apparently normal dendrite of dentate granule shows somewhat irregular distribution of spines. This is probably within normal limits. Rapid Golgi variants. a, b, c and d, Magnification ×165, e, magnification ×300.

deflected in a direction oblique or even parallel to the pial-glial surface of the dentate fascia toward which the shafts ordinarily extend.

A third variant, illustrated in Figures 11, 13, and 15Bb, is based in the atypical origin of one or more dendrites from the lower or axonal pole of the dentate granule. Such branches extend for varying distances into the subadjacent polymorph layer before turning laterally and then, often, superficially.

It cannot yet be stated unequivocally that all or indeed any of these domain variants invariably indicate dentate pathology. As already noted, it has been difficult thus far to develop an extensive experience in really well-preserved human control tissue. Careful study of Lorente de Nó's drawings of dentate material from monkeys (24) has not revealed any of

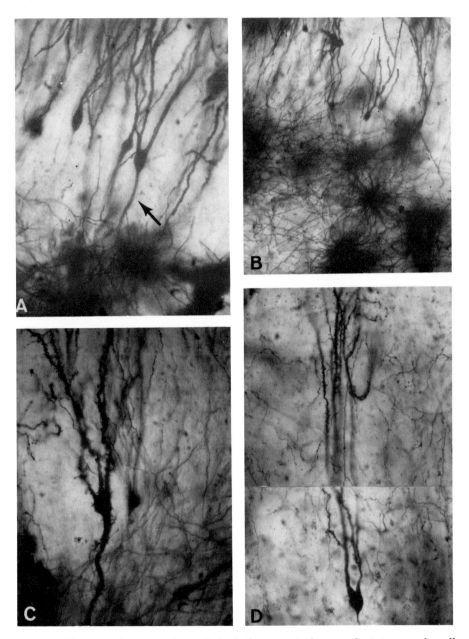

Figure 11. Changes of apparently pathological nature in human dentate granule cells. (a) Group of granules, some of which show the unusual dendrite developing from the lower (axonal) pole (arrow). (b) Intensive fibrillary astrocytosis deep to the granule layer. (c) Dentate granule with large lower pole dendrite and multiple excrescences along apical dendrites. (d) Dentate granule with unusuallly compressed dendrite domain (closed parasol pattern), and changes of dendrite surface including occasional nodular enlargements on several prominent shafts. Rapid Golgi variants. a, c, and d, Magnification ×215; b, magnification ×85.

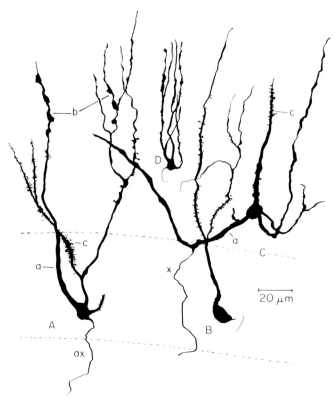

Figure 12. Drawing of group of presumed pathological dentate granules. The dendrite domains of A and B are apparently diminished in length and in number of shafts. Cell C is more horizontally oriented element, whereas cell D is an upward displaced dwarf cell. Among the features of pathological interest are swelling of individual dendrites (a); loss of spines and the development of nodular enlargements (b); and patchy areas where spines can still be seen (c). Rapid Golgi variant.

these variations, nor have our own limited analyses of macaque material. In view of the remarkable similarity of primate to human archicortex (24, 38), it seems at least reasonable to think that some of these changes are abnormal.

It would prove of considerable value if we could correlate these domain variations with some of the more generalized dendritic changes which have already been described as probably pathological in hippocampal pyramids. However, in our experience to this point, none of these variant patterns is consistently related to spine loss or dendritic nodulation. Of the three patterns, the closed parasol variant seems to be most frequently accompanied by loss of dendrite spines and development of the string-of-beads deformity. As indicated in Figures 11d, 13, and 15E the changes are more often partial than complete. The domain pattern variant based on origin of one or more dendrites from the axonal pole seems most usually accompanied by patchy or diffuse swelling of the dendrite shafts. Such changes

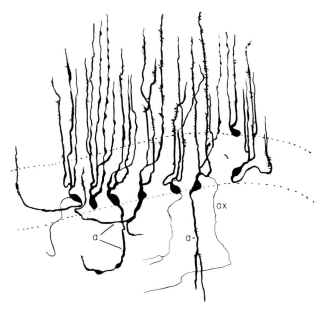

Figure 13. Drawing of cluster of human dentate granules showing unusual dendritic domain patterns and partial loss of dendrite spines. The unusually compressed dendrite patterns (closed parasol deformity) have been seen in a number of human tissue blocks removed at surgery, but not in blocks of animal dentate tissue used as controls. Several granules also show dendrites arising from the deep axonal (ax) pole of the cell (a). Rapid Golgi variant.

can be seen in Figure 11c and at a in Figure 13. Cells with dendrite systems showing the windblown look appear least likely to be associated with other anomalies of appearance. Further work is obviously necessary in deciding whether these apparent correlations help define the nature and pathological import of these variations in dendrite patterns.

As in the case of hippocampal pyramids, spine loss and nodular deformities are more frequently seen in patchy distribution than diffusely over the entire ensemble of dentate granules. Although Figure 15 is a composite built up from a number of preparations, it still provides a reasonably realistic interpretation of an individual specimen of dentate fascia removed at surgery. The dentate also resembles hippocampus proper in the idiosyncratic appearance of the individual dendrites on single granule cells. Figure 12 is instructive in this regard. Cell A shows almost normal spine distribution and density on the dendrite shaft (c). Shaft a in its proximal one-third is grossly swollen whereas more distally, it shows a series of nodular enlargements (b). The remaining dendrites are virtually spineless and show scattered regions of nodulation. Cell B is remarkable chiefly for a very simple dendrite arbor with patchy spine loss. Cell C shows upward displacement into the molecular layer and diffuse dendritic swelling. Cell D appears to be an even more displaced dwarf granule with a closed parasol domain pattern, dendritic nodulation, and almost complete loss of spines.

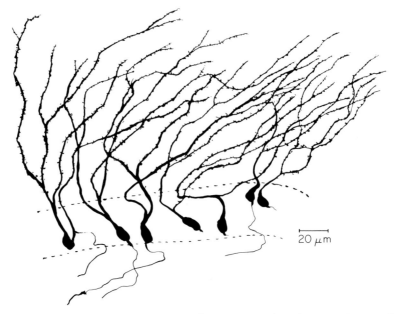

Figure 14. Drawing of cluster of human dentate granules showing the windblown appearance found in limited areas of some specimens. The distortion of dendrite patterns may be due to adjacent scar formation. Rapid Golgi variant.

NEUROGLIA

The nature and extent of neuroglial pathology is also uncertain from our Golgi studies so far, even though gliosis is the most consistently documented change in epileptic tissue. In the present material, as in an older series that we studied some years ago (38), it seems clear that certain areas of surgically excised Ammon's horn are densely infiltrated with fibrillary astrocytes. In many cases these astrocytes appear to bear enlargements along their individual stalks or at their terminals (Figure 16b). In the present series, we have noticed the most prominent gliosis in the zone of polymorph cells deep to the dentate fascia (Figure 11b) and in adjacent regions of CA₄; however, apparently abnormal numbers of fibrous astrocytes have been seen in the cortical laminae of each hippocampal zone. Reliable quantitative assessments of this glial component and of possible associated decrements in neuron density have yet to be made.

CONCLUSIONS

The Golgi methods can be used with considerable success in evaluating the appearance of cortical tissue removed from patients with temporal lobe epilepsy. Although the level of resolution provided by the light microscope is not likely to reveal evidence of those disturbances fundamental to the ictal process, it still provides opportunities for a unique overview of pathologically changed cells in their neuropil setting. The familiar, nonquantita-

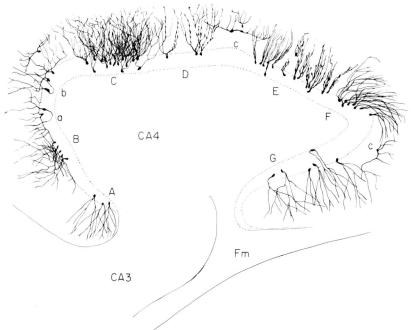

Figure 15. Composite drawing of the entire human dentate fascia showing the range of cell patterns found in surgically removed tissue. (A) Most usual appearance of dentate granules. (B) Granules with more extensive horizontal dendritic ramifications. Cells at Ba and Bb show atypical dendrite springing from the opposite (axonal) pole of the soma. This may be a normal or pathological variant. (C) Mass of normal granules showing density of dendritic plexus. (D) Several granules with string-of-beads changes in the dendrites. (E,F) Increasingly severe distortions of granules, some of whose dendrites show a windblown look. (G) Presumably normal granules with long and rather pleomorphic dendrite arbors. Cells c are granules with horizontal arbors, displaced from their normal site. Rapid Golgi variants.

tive aspects of Golgi impregnations limit us to a qualitative description of neuronal and glial elements. The variations that can be seen, especially loss of dendrite spines, dendritic nodulation, and the string-of-beads deformity, dendrite swelling, and variations in dendrite domain patterns will gain added meaning as our experience with the range of variation from normal human temporal lobe tissue is enhanced. These Golgi-revealed changes must also be correlated with routine histological and histopathological stains which provide reasonably quantitative estimates of gross histological change. Finally, a great deal can be expected by correlating results of Golgi and ultramicroscopic techniques in the mutual definition and documentation of patterns shown by each.

In the meantime, this initial study of hippocampal tissue from patients with temporal lobe epilepsy has served to emphasize the frequency with which minimal changes can be found in isolated neurons and even in portions of the dendrite systems of single nerve cells.

These localized zones of dendrite spine loss and nodule formation appear to represent the earliest phases of a sequence of increasingly severe

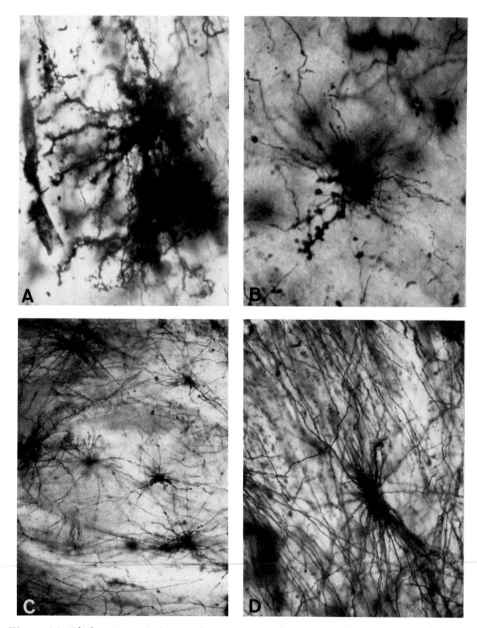

Figure 16. Glial patterns in human hippocampus–dentate complex. (a) Normal proto-plasmic astrocyte. (b) Small fibrous astrocyte showing abnormal nodules along several processes. (c) Field of fibrillary astrocytes in CA₁ area. (d) Dense fibrillary astrocyte zone. This may represent a glial scar. Rapid Golgi variants. a, b, and d, Magnification ×215; magnification c, ×85.

pathological change, culminating in cell death. Several interpretations are possible. The changes may represent immediate sequellae of the operative intervention itself or may be secondary to the implantation of recording electrodes 3 or 4 months previously and maintained *in situ* for 6 to 8 weeks.

The third and most intriguing possibility would relate these changes to the disease process itself. The concept of the epileptic syndrome as an ongoing process is, of course, not new (28, 39–41, 43–45) but has invariably been related to ischemic processes developing during recurrent ictal episodes. The nature and distribution of the early changes we have described appear too discrete to fit with this interpretation. At this point we can only suggest that, assuming the focal dendritic changes we have described are not surgical artifacts, these findings can be putatively assigned to some type of progressive pathological process, possibly of genetic-enzymic or slow virus nature. Although such a possibility is, at present, only speculation based on details of the Golgi picture, it obviously suggests new directions in epilepsy research as well as underlining the urgent need for the kinds of correlative studies already suggested.

REFERENCES

1. Alzheimer, A., Ein Beitrag zur pathologischen Anatomie der Epilepsie. *Monatsschr. Psychiatr. Neurol.*, 1898, **4**: 345–369.
2. Andy, O., and Akert, K., Seizure patterns induced by electrical stimulation of hippocampal formation in the cat. *J. Neuropathol. Exp. Neurol.*, 1955, **14**: 198.
3. Bergmann, G. H., *Allg. Z. Psychiatr.*, 1847, **4**: 361, quoted by W. Scholz, in *Pathology of the Nervous System* (J. Minckler, Ed.). McGraw-Hill, New York, 1972: 2635–2655.
4. Blackstad, T., and Flood, P., Ultrastructure of hippocampal axo-somatic synapses. *Nature (Lond.)*, 1963, **198**: 542–543.
5. Blackstad, T., and Kjaerheim, A., Special axo-dendritic synapses in the hippocampal cortex: Electron and light microscopic studies on the layer of mossy fibers. *J. Comp. Neurol.*, 1961, **117**: 133–159.
6. Bouchet and Cazauvieilh, *Arch. Gen. Med.*, 1825, **9**: 510, quoted by W. Scholz, in *Pathology of the Nervous System* (J. Mickler, Ed.). McGraw-Hill, New York, 1972: 2635–2655.
7. Cajal, S. Ramón y, *Histologie du système nerveux de l'homme et des vertébrés.* Maloine, Paris, 1909: Vol. 1.
8. Chaslin, P., Contribution à l'étude de la sclérose cérébrale. *Arch. Med. Exp. Anat. Pathol.*, 1891, **3**: 305–340.
9. Colonnier, M., Experimental degeneration in the cerebral cortex. *J. Anat.*, 1964, **98**: 47–53.
10. De Moor, J., La mécanisme et la signification de l'état moniliforme des neurones. *Ann. Soc. Sci. Med. Nat. Brux.*, 1898, **7**: 205–250.
11. Earle, K., Baldwin, M., and Penfield, W., Incisural sclerosis and temporal lobe seizures produced by hippocampal herniation at birth. *Arch. Neurol. Psychiatry*, 1953, **69**: 27–42.
12. Edinger, L., *Wien. Med. Wochenschr.*, 1917, **67**: 2020; quoted by W. Scholz, in: *Pathology of the Nervous System* (J. Minckler, Ed.). McGraw-Hill, New York, 1972: 2635–2655.

13. Eyzaguirre, C., and Kuffler, S., Processes of excitation in the dendrites and in the soma of single isolated sensory nerve cells of the lobster and crayfish. *J. Gen. Physiol.*, 1955, **39**: 87–119.

14. Globus, A., and Scheibel, A., Loss of dendrite spines as an index of pre-synaptic terminal patterns. *Nature (Lond.)*, 1966, **212**: 463–465.

15. Globus, A., and Scheibel, A., Synaptic loci on visual cortical neurons of the rabbit. The specific afferent radiation. *Exp. Neurol.*, 1967, **18**: 116–131.

16. Globus, A., and Scheibel, A., Synaptic loci on parietal cortical neurons. Terminations of corpus callosum fibers. *Science*, 1967, **156**: 1127–1129.

17. Globus, A., and Scheibel, A., Pattern and field in cortical structure: The rabbit. *J. Comp. Neurol.*, 1967, **131**: 155–172.

18. Gray, E., and Guillery, R., Synaptic morphology in the normal and degenerating nervous system. *Int. Rev. Cytol.*, 1966, **19**: 111–182.

19. Hamlyn, L. H., The fine structure of the mossy fibre endings in the hippocampus of the rabbit. *J. Anat. (Lond.)*, 1962, **96**: 112–120.

20. Hamlyn, L. H., An electron microscope study of pyramidal neurons in the Ammon's horn of the rabbit. *J. Anat. (Lond.)*, 1963, **97**: 189–201.

21. Kaada, B., Somatomotor, autonomic and electrocorticographic responses to electrical stimulation of rhinencephalic and other structures in primates, cat and dog. *Acta Physiol. Scand.*, 1951, **23**: Suppl. 83: 1–285.

22. Kölliker, A., *Handbuch der Gewebelehre des Menschen.* Engelman, Leipzig, 1889: 6th ed., Vol. 2.

23. Kopeloff, L., Barrera, S., and Kopeloff, N., Recurrent convulsive seizures in animals produced by immunologic and chemical means. *Am. J. Psychiatry*, 1942, **98**: 881–902.

24. Lorente de Nó, R., Studies on the structure of the cerebral cortex. II. Continuation of the study of the ammonic systems. *J. Psychol. Neurol., Lpz.*, 1934, **46**: 113–177.

25. Maspes, P., Grattarola, F. R., and Marossero, F., Etude anatomopathologique de 36 cas d'épilepsie temporale opérés. *Acta Neurol. Psychiat. Belg.*, 1956, **56**: 103–114.

26. Meyer, A., Quoted by D. Nieto and A. Escobar, in: *Pathology of the Nervous System* (J. Minckler, Ed.). McGraw-Hill, New York, 1972: 2627–2634.

27. Meyer, A., Lésions observées sur les pièces opératoires prélavées chez des épileptiques temporaux. *Acta Neurol. Psychiat. Belg.*, 1956, **56**: 21–42.

28. Meyer, A., Beck, E., and Shepherd, M., Unusually severe lesions in the brain following status epilepticus. *J. Neurol. Neurosurg. Psychiatry*, 1955, **18**: 24.

29. Monti, A., Sur les altérations du système nerveux dans l'inanition. *Arch. Ital. Biol.*, 1895, **24**: 347–360.

30. Nielsen, J., and Courville, C., Role of birth injury and asphyxia in idiopathic epilepsy. *Neurology (Minneap.)*, 1951, **1**: 48.

31. Norman, R. M., La sclérose lobaire dans l'épilepsie et l'encéphalopathie de la naissance. *Acta Neurol. Psychiat. Belg.*, 1956, **56**: 89–102.

32. Penfield, W., Epileptogenic lesions. *Acta Neurol. Psychiat. Belg.*, 1956, **56**: 75–88.

33. Peters, A., Stellate cells of the rat parietal cortex. *J. Comp. Neurol.*, 1971, **141:** 345–373.
34. Pfleger, L., Beobachtung über Schrumpfung und Sclerose des Ammonshornes bei Epilepsie. *Allg. Z. Psychiat.*, 1880, **36:** 359–365.
35. Renshaw, B., Forbes, A., and Morison, B., Activity of isocortex and hippocampus: Electrical studies with micro-electrodes. *J. Neurophysiol.*, 1940, **3:** 74–105.
36. Scheibel, M., Davies, T., and Scheibel, A., Unpublished data.
37. Scheibel, M., and Scheibel, A., Selected structural-functional correlations in postnatal brain. In: *Brain Development and Behavior* (M. B. Sterman, D. J. McGinty, and A. M. Adinolphi, Eds.). Academic Press, New York, 1971: 1–21.
38. Scheibel, M., and Scheibel, A., Unpublished studies.
39. Scholz, W., *Die Krampfschädigungen des Gehirns*. Springer-Verlag. Berlin and New York, 1951.
40. Scholz, W., Selective neuronal necrosis and its topistic patterns in hypoxemia and oligemia. *J. Neuropathol. Exp. Neurol.*, 1953, **12:** 249–261.
41. Scholz, W., Les lesions cérébrales recontrées chez les épileptiques; précisions sur la sclérose de la corne d'Ammon. *Acta Neurol. Psychiat. Belg.*, **56:** 43–60.
42. Sommer, W., Erkrankung des Ammonshorns als aetiologisches Moment der Epilepsie. Arch. Psychiatry, 1880, **10:** 631–675.
43. Spielmeyer, W., *Z. Neurol.*, 1920, **54:** 1; quoted by W. Scholz, in: *Pathology of the Nervous System* (J. Minckler, Ed.). McGraw-Hill, New York, 1972: 2635–2655.
44. Spielmeyer, W., Die Pathogenese des epileptichen Krampfes. *Ž. Gesamte Neurol. Psychiatr.*, 1927, **109:** 501–515.
45. Spielmeyer, W., The anatomic substratum of the convulsive state. *Arch. Neurol. Psychiatry*, 1930, **23:** 869–875.
46. Valverde, F., Apical dendritic spines of the visual cortex and light deprivation in the mouse. *Exp. Brain Res.*, 1967, **3:** 337–352.
47. Valverde, F., Rate and extent of recovery from dark rearing in the visual cortex of the mouse. *Brain Res.* 1971, **33:** 1–11.
48. Walberg, F., Role of normal dendrites in removal of degenerating terminal boutons. *Exp. Neurol.*, 1963, **8:** 112–124.
49. Ward, A., The epileptic neuron. *Epilepsia*, 1961, **2:** 70–80.
50. Westrum, L., White, L., and Ward, A., Morphology of the experimental epileptic focus. *J. Neurosurg.*, 1964, **21:** 1033–1046.

STRUCTURAL SUBSTRATES OF SEIZURE FOCI IN THE HUMAN TEMPORAL LOBE[*]

(A Combined Electrophysiological Optical Microscopic and Ultrastructural Study)

W. JANN BROWN

Brain Research Institute, University of California, Los Angeles, California

Attempts to uncover specific pathomorphological patterns in central nervous system tissues from patients with epilepsy have thus far failed. We have, however, come to understand that the limbic structures of the medial temporal lobes are somehow sensitive and are seemingly easy to activate into epileptic disorder. Moreover, it has become accepted that in this region there are sites of predilection for certain pathological conditions which are commonly associated with the variety of seizure patterns characterized by dreamy states and gross "feelings" related to the viscera and other sensory phenomena 9, 13, 14, 17–19, 27, 28, 31, 35, 43). One of the most common of these lesions is the sclerosis first described by Bouchet and Cazauvieilh as long ago as 1825, as a gross palpable hardness of the hippocampus (5). These changes in the hippocampus were subsequently thought to be the result of hypoxic brain damage induced by the repeated seizures (22, 37, 39) rather than the cause of the ictus. This view has been modified, based upon evidence advanced by Earle and co-workers (13) that the sclerosis may be the early lesion caused by compression of the uncus and more posterior segments of the hippocampal complex against the tentorium during molding of the infant's skull while being born. In the same vein, the studies of Lindenberg (26) relative to compression of long branches of the posterior cerebral artery against the tentorium in various types of brain swelling, thereby causing ischemic cell changes in parts of Sommer's sector, are rather convincing. Objectively, however, it must be remembered that similar lesions are also found in patients with no overt signs of epilepsy (11). The latter occurrence tends to weaken the causal relationship between this particular lesion and the clinical seizures. Corsellis (9) mooted this question by analyzing the structure of a number of brains from general

[*] *Acknowledgments:* This work was partially supported by U.S. Public Health Service Grant No. NS 02808, and HD 05615. The technical skill and interest at various stages of this investigation of M. A. Akers, M. Hall, H. Van Raan, S. Frommes, and M. Gianos is gratefully acknowledged. P. Blake's artistic craftsmanship is evident in diagrams. Special thanks are extended to Professor P. Crandall, Principal Investigator USPHS-NIH Grant No. 02808, whose surgical mastery has made available the tissues and clinical details on these patients.

and mental hospitals and found abnormalities of Ammon's horn in one or both sides in some patients, both with and without epilepsy. In the epileptic cases, however, the sclerotic Ammon's horn appeared to have a much older lesion than when such lesions were seen in brains injured by arteriosclerosis and other senile conditions. Such a study is of great usefulness but, unfortunately, the real basis for the seizures in such cases remains elusive.

From 1939–1955, Penfield and co-workers carried out numerous surgical procedures on the temporal lobe because of a variety of lesions believed to be causing seizures (29, 30, 34). These conditions varied from "simple" atrophy and cicatricial lesions to hemangioma calcificans, cholesteatoma, and other benign neoplasms. Electrocorticograms were utilized to demonstrate interictal discharges adjacent to lesions and to study neurophysiological features of the regions evoked by stimulation (24).

Twenty years ago, Gibbs persuaded Bailey to treat psychomotor seizures on the basis of the "low temporal" origin of scalp discharges even when gross temporal lesions were not evident (3). The resultant resections were made superficially in the temporal lobe cortex, but later were extended to include the limbic structures. The morphological substrate for this type of epilepsy was not really uncovered until Falconer (16) made "en bloc" resections of the offending lobes in which he included amygdala, hippocampus, hippocampal gyrus, and anterior temporal lobe. The entire panoply of microscopic alterations and lesions was then shown in significant locations within the limbic system. Falconer found hippocampal sclerosis in almost half his cases, glial hamartomata in 25%, and miscellaneous and/or no overt lesions in the remainder. Comparable figures have now been obtained from postmortem examinations of institutionalized patients known to have had preexisting epilepsy with temporal localization (27, 35). For some unexplained reason, glial hamartomata have been found only in surgically resected tissues. Our experience is similar. The hamartomatous category in the institutionalized series has been replaced by an increased incidence of developmental malformations.

Presently, there is no real agreement as to the morphological criteria which set apart from the normal an epileptogenic neuron; although Westrum and co-workers (47), employing the Golgi-Cox technique to study monkey cortex made seizure-sensitive with aluminum hydroxide, have observed decreased numbers of spines on dendrites and varicose swellings and abnormal angulations of dendrites. The significance of the loss or failure of development of spines on dendrites in such sensitive foci is also stressed by Scheibel and Scheibel (36). The neuroglia, commonly neglected in neuroanatomical studies, may well create mechanical distortion of the dendritic arborization of neurons in edges of cortical scars, as suggested by Ward (45, 46) or the number and position of astrocytes could alter electrical activity. To obtain a better estimate of the precise nature of some of these possibly aberrant anatomical complexities, we are endeavoring to map systematically the ultrastructural profile of the human hippocampus as each opportunity presents itself. The majority of the following 29 cases of temporal lobe epilepsy were studied by optical microscopy in combination with electrophysiological methods. The more recent cases in the series are being looked at more closely with ultrastructural techniques.

MATERIALS AND METHODS

Briefly, the depth macroelectrode is composed of a stainless-steel core 0.2 mm in diameter encased in Formvar insulation, except for a bared length of 0.5 mm. The insulated portion is 0.5 mm in length and is sloped over this length to an enveloping cuff which is 0.65 mm in diameter. These electrodes were emplaced by the stereotactic method using the atlas of Talairach and co-workers (42) as described by Crandall and colleagues (10).

Temporal lobes removed from selected patients were placed in 25 times their volumes of phosphate-buffered 10% formalin (pH 7.2) as soon after resection as possible. After several days of fixation, the entire lobe was smoothly sectioned across with long razor blades into blocks 0.75 cm in thickness. The sides and surfaces were oriented with India ink and embedded in paraffin. It was found that some portions of the edges of the hippocampus became lost with this type of blocking, and, therefore, in subsequent cases the entire lobe was embedded in paraplast after 12-hour periods in solutions of graded ethanol, and all pertinent segments of tissue were thereby preserved. The whole lobes were sectioned at 15 μm thickness, and every eighth group of sections was stained with H&E, cresyl violet, and Gomori iron stain. Weil myelin preparations were also done. Small iron deposits may be seen in the immediate vicinity of the electrode tips.*

In recently selected cases, an incision was made in the lateral aspect of the pertinent temporal lobe extending from the Sylvian fissure inferiorly, at a level 6 cm posterior to the temporal pole and anterior to the inferior anastomosing vein. This procedure ultimately gave access to the temporal horn of the lateral ventricle thereby baring the hippocampus (Figure 1). This approach preserved and maintained the blood supply from the posterior cerebral artery to the hippocampal formation. Slices were then taken transversely with a cold scalpel to the long axis of the hippocampal formation, for electron microscopy, Golgi impregnations, and tissue culture studies. The latter two investigations will be reported elsewhere. The material for electron microscopy was immediately immersed in 1.5% solution of redistilled norite-purified glutaraldehyde in 0.1 M Na cacodylate buffer, pH 7.2–7.4. From 1 to 2 mm thick slices were made across the longitudinal

---

* In a very early group the entire lobe was frozen and serially sectioned in the cold, but this proved to be awkward and difficult to interpret cytologically, and, hence, was abandoned in favor of the paraplast embedding.

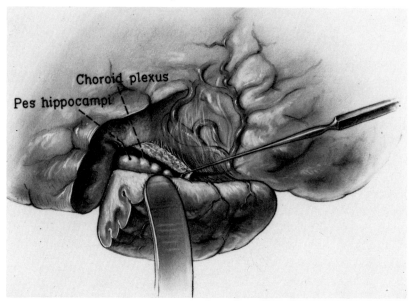

Figure 1. Diagrammatic essentials of temporal lobe resection procedure as carried out by Dr. Paul Crandall. At the point shown, although the superior, middle, and inferior gyri have been severed from the brain, the hippocampal formation has an intact blood supply derived from the posterior cerebral artery. The choroid plexus has been lifted forward with a nerve hook. Cold knife sections are then made transversely across the long axis of the hippocampus for electron microscopy, Golgi preparations, and tissue culture.

axis with cleaned razor blades. The tissue remained in fixative overnight at 4°C. Pertinent blocks from the alveus, subiculum, Sommer's sector, and other CA fields were then selected, oriented, and washed with fresh buffer, secondarily fixed in 1% OsO_4, and embedded in Epon 812 resin after dehydration in graded concentrations of methanol. The blocks were cut with glass knives for thick sectioning and the diamond knife for thin sections. Sections were mounted on pristine copper grids and stained with 4% aqueous uranyl acetate and lead citrate, according to the technique described by Venable and Coggeshall (44). Examinations of ultrastructure were carried out with the Siemens 1A microscope at 80 kV. The remainder of the temporal pole was fixed, as above, for light microscopic studies. Forty-four cases in all have been operated upon and examined. Five of these have had electron microscopy done on segments of the hippocampal gyrus.

CLINICAL OBSERVATIONS

Twenty-eight cases are included in this selected series and many of their important clinical details are catalogued in Tables 1–4. There are a number of other cases in the study, as is indicated above; but various aspects of their investigation in one way or another are incomplete. Hence, they have been deleted. Several case reports are given below in narrative detail. These detailed cases are included in the four tables. The first three were found to have typical types of hamartoma of the temporal lobe.

Case 6 (Table 1)

A 16-year-old girl had experienced attacks for 3 years described as starting with vocalizations such as "ah ah ah" and automatic behavior. Radiographic studies of the skull were unrevealing. Electroencephalographic changes were left-sided in the temporal region. Clinical seizures were recorded with depth electrodes and showed discharges originating in the left uncus and mid-hippocampal gyrus. A nodule which measured $7 \times 8 \times 20$ mm was found beneath the fusiform and inferior temporal gyri. The extent of the cystic fluid-filled compartments and solid portions of the resected lesion is indistinguishable (grossly) from an astrocytoma and is shown in Figures 2a–d and 3. She has been free of seizures since operation in 1962.

Case 55 (Table 1)

This patient had a precipitate birth but no obvious resultant injury. At age 7.5 years, he fell from a tree but was not rendered unconscious. Six months later, however, he began experiencing staring episodes during which he answered questions inappropriately and often elevated his arm overhead. Occasionally, a generalized seizure was experienced. Scalp electroencephalogram (EEG) showed generalized slowing and a right temporal lobe focus. Pneumoencephalogram and arteriogram appeared normal. Depth electrodes at age 18 showed abnormal interictal activity most prominent and frequent on the right side. During ictus, low-voltage fast activity was seen beginning in the right anterior hippocampus. Right anterior temporal lobectomy was done and a circumscribed mass found (see Figures 4a–d and 5). Withdrawal of suppressant drugs resulted in generalized seizures, but with restitution of Peganone and Mysoline he remains seizure-free.

Case 56 (Table 1)

A 12-year-old boy was treated for seizures in 1959, although they were first noted as staring spells at 8 months. Childhood seizures were characterized as having repetitive speech, immobility, lip-smacking, automatic clapping and rubbing movements, staring, rolling eyes, and facial pallor. During hospitalization several seizures were noted daily. He was a behavioral problem at school and was rated a low normal in intelligence. Roentgenograms of the skull revealed an irregular calcified mass at least 5×3 cm in size, near the floor of the right middle cranial fossa. The anterior wall of the middle fossa was thinned from pressure atrophy in an

TABLE 1

CLINICAL DETAILS OF CASES WITH HAMARTOMATA (17.2%)[a]

Case no.	Age at onset of seizure	Age at surgery (yr)	Handedness	Sex	Seizure character (incidence)	Locus of depth electrodes and complications (date)	Temporal lobectomy (date)	Pre/postoperative neurological defect	Pre/postoperative intelligence	Global result
56	8 mo	15	R	M	Repetitive speech, stares, lip smacking, hand clapping, eye rolling, pallor (150–240/mo)	No electrodes	R (8/59)	None/none	Low normal/better behavior	Excellent
2	23 yr	25	R	F	Chest sensation, ictal speech, automatism, chewing (20–30/mo; 0 grand mal/yr)	(12/61) R and L pes hippocampus; coagulation defect and 2-/cm hematoma	R (1/62)	None/L hemianopsia and L hemiparesis	Normal/normal	Excellent
6	12 yr	16	R	F	No aura, vocalization, automatic fumbling (60–90/mo; 5 grand mal/yr)	(4/62) L anterior hippocampal gyrus; transient visual field defect, coagulation defect[b]	L (11/62)	None/R. supraquadrantanopsia	Low normal/low normal	Good
38	14 yr	17	R	F	Stares, chewing, swallowing; sits upright (10–20/mo; 0 grand mal/yr)	(1/70) R temporal lobe	R (4/70)	Clumsy L hand/none	Normal/normal	Excellent
55	8 yr	19	R	M	Psychomotor, unilateral motor (8/12 mo; 2–3 grand mal/yr)	(10/71) R anterior hippocampal gyrus	R (12/71)	None/mild dysarthria. Resolving	Normal/improved school grades	Excellent

[a] R, right; L, left; M, male; F, female.
[b] Early focal coagulation was used as a marker.

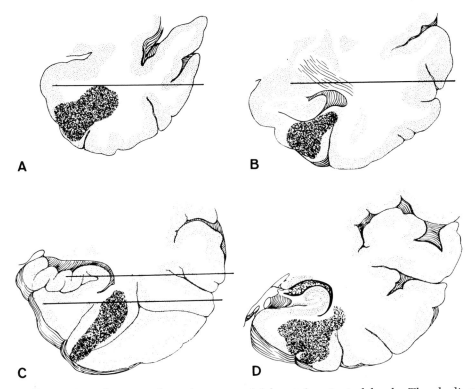

Figure 2. These diagrams show the temporal lobe at four typical levels. The shading reveals the extent of a hamartomatous lesion. (A) The nodule just behind the pole, extending to include portions of the superficial lamina of the cortex of the uncus medially and the inferior temporal gyrus laterally. The microelectrode depicted as a line, penetrates medially to the uncal cortex. (B) The shading includes the subependymal glial plate and cortex of the fusiform gyrus. The tip of the electrode at this level rests in the amygdaloid nucleus. (C) More posterior section revealing the lesion's relation to the edge of the ventricle, but lies deeper within the white matter of the lobe and more remote from the dentate gyrus. Two electrodes were in place at this level: the more superiorly placed terminates in the dentate gyrus, the inferior in the subiculum. (D) At this level, the lesion has again reached the cortical strip of the fusiform gyrus, beneath the subiculum and extends across the myelinated fibers emanating from and entering into the inferior and middle temporal gyri. (Case 6.)

anterior and inferior direction. The proximal right middle cerebral artery complex was elevated in angiograms. On pneumoencephalography, the right temporal horn was also slightly elevated and displaced posteriorly. Cerebrospinal fluid (CSF) protein content was within normal limits. Two EEGs during hospitalization, as well as several previous examinations, showed severe abnormalities with lateralized polyphasic spiking and slow waves over the central and temporal regions on the right, as well as some independent spiking from the left temporal region. The anterior 6 cm of the right temporal lobe was removed, and a calcified mass with an associated cyst containing 9 cm of yellowish fluid was found in the specimen.

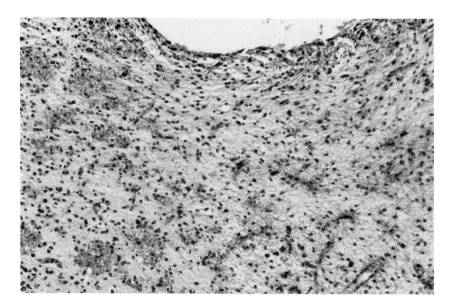

Figure 3. This microscopic field reveals the nature of the hamartoma outlined in Figure 2a–d. It is composed of fibrous astrocytes, enmeshed in a fibrillar matrix which contains numerous small vascular structures and cysts. The upper edge shows a portion of a large cyst. (Case 6.) H&E stains. Magnification ×335.

Further, the leptomeninges were chronically thickened and there appeared to be no lamination of the overlying cortex. Only a few of the larger pyramidal neurons were occasionally noted in the cortex and many appeared to be somewhat shrunken and distorted. Deeper in subcortex, masses of concentrically laminated calcific bodies were seen admixed with accumulations of vascular structures resembling both arteries and veins, and astrocytes (Figure 6). The diagnosis was hemangioma calcificans. Postoperatively, his seizures were almost completely abolished except for occasional warning symptoms. Dilantin and Mysoline were given, with a resultant improvement in behavior, and he was able to continue in school. One or two seizures occurred 10 years after surgery (1968) when he decreased his own medication. Several postoperative EEGs have shown right temporal slow waves. Spike discharges have been rare and are brought out only with hyperventilation.

Case 57 (Table 2)

This 24-year-old man was afflicted with tuberculous meningitis at age 4. He began to have automatisms with occasional warnings of "another world" at age 6. Some of these seizures were grand mal type, and several episodes of status epilepticus were encountered. The aggregate incidence of seizures was 30–40 per month. Medication mitigated grand mal seizures

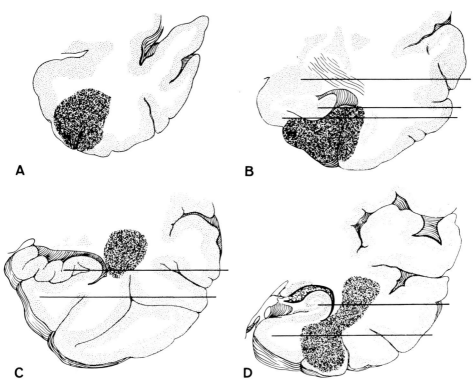

Figure 4. Camera lucida diagrams of several levels of temporal lobe with lesion shaded as in Figure 2A–D. The similarity of the hamartoma's outline and locus is probably coincidental. In diagram B, three electrodes are shown in place: the upper rests in the amygdala, the middle is placed in the anterior segment of the dentate gyrus, and the inferior electrode has crossed the lesion and ends in the anterior subicular cortex. There is some variation in diagram C in which the lesion has remained within the cortical strip just lateral to the collateral fissure of the hippocampal gyrus, then extends deep into the white matter to involve some fibers of the lateral portions of the anterior commissure. The upper electrode is in the main segment of the dentate gyrus; the inferior in the white matter just below the subiculum. (D) The lesion is now seen extending from the position shown in diagram C to subpial lamina of the inferior temporal gyrus. Two electrodes are in place: the upper tip terminates in the CA₄ region, the lower in the myelin below the subiculum. (Case 55.)

for 2 years prior to surgery. Neurological examination revealed a very mild ataxia and fine tremor with a CSF protein of 104 mg %. Scalp EEG disclosed diffuse slowing, a left midtemporal spike focus and left temporal slowing. Angiograms were normal. Depth electrodes were placed into mesial limbic structures; interictal recording showed frequent high-amplitude spikes on the left. Ictal responses were focal from left temporal sites. Observed fits were rather violent during which he pushed people around, head and eyes turned to the left, hypernea occurred, he picked at his clothing, moaned, crossed and uncrossed his legs, stared straight ahead, and experienced involuntary urination. A left anterior temporal lobectomy was

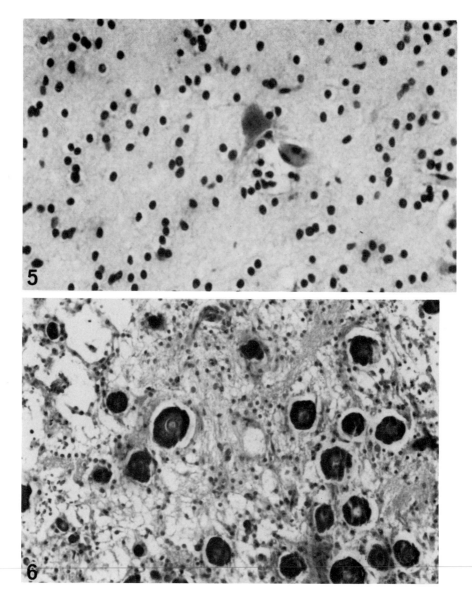

Figure 5. A typical microscopic field of the lesion delineated in Figure 4A–D. The cells are mostly oligodendrogliacytes admixed with occasional neurons. (Case 55.) H&E stains. Magnification ×335 in the original photograph.

Figure 6. Laminated masses of calcium are shown within a glial matrix with occasional small, primitive vascular channels. The calcospherites do not appear to have any special relationship to capillaries. The cells are fibrous astrocytes with a few oligodendrogliacytes. The nuclei are monotonously similar in size and shape. Temporal lobe. (Case 56.) H&E stains. Magnification ×490.

done and there have been no further seizures, but there is a residual right superior quadrantanopsia. Loss of neurons in the cornu ammonis with gliosis was found (see Figure 7 and ultrastructure Figures 14 and 16a–c).

Case 7 (Table 2)

At age 2 the patient suffered a fractured skull in a fall. There were no sequelae but at 5 years he began having seizures of multiple variety. Infrequently, the fits have been grand mal type and none have occurred in the past 2 years. The frequent seizures are of two types: the first is a brief loss of consciousness with staring and blinking, lasting a few seconds; the second involves a sudden loss of consciousness, sometimes preceded by a "strange feeling" with associated automatisms which may simply include hand movements, walking about, and sometimes mumbling. He has had from two to ten of these each month. He has had a limited response to drugs. Electroencephalogram records have shown focal spiking over the right temporal region with occasional slight spiking on the left. He has one twin brother in excellent health. At age 9, a diagnosis of lupus erythematosus was made with involvement of heart, lungs, and meninges. He has always been slow at school and has been depressed because his seizures have interfered with school and employment. Neurologically, he was estimated to have a dull–normal intellect, slightly thick and incoordinate speech, fine rhythmic nystagmus with lateral gaze in either direction, a suggestion of dysynergia in both upper extremities, and bilateral extensor plantar responses. Sleep and waking EEG records revealed sharp wave and spike discharges from the right anterior temporal region. Three awake and sleep EEGs with sphenoidal leads revealed prominent spike discharges from the right sphenoidal electrodes and from the right temporal scalp leads. The implanted depth electrode studies confirmed the right temporal localization. In 1962, a right temporal lobectomy was done. Gliosis and atrophy of the cornu ammonis was found (Figure 8a and b). Recovery was uneventful. A residual left homonymous hemianopsia was present 4 years later, but the patient is otherwise doing well. In 1970 he was found to be seizure free.

Case 58 (Table 2)

Grand mal seizures ushered in with numbness of the left hand and forearm and the tendency toward involuntary elevation of the arm began at age 7. The numbness usually spread to involve the whole left side of the body; the head turned to the left and there were clonic movements of the left foot. She did not lose consciousness. With the head turning, chewing motions were noted. On occasion, status epilepticus with clonic left seizures every 15–20 minutes were observed, as well as minor seizures with losses of consciousness. The seizures became mixed with adversive, generalized, or automatic features. Three years prior to operation (1969), weakness, Babinski sign, and decrease in sensation were noted on the left side. Scalp EEG (May, 1969) showed focal spiking in the left central and temporal region. Six months later the record appeared normal; but 1 year later

TABLE 2

CLINICAL DETAILS OF CASES WITH HIPPOCAMPAL SCLEROSIS (65.6%)ᵃ

Case no.	Age at onset of seizures (yr)	Age at surgery (yr)	Handedness	Sex	Seizure character (incidence)	Locus of depth electrodes and complications (date)	Temporal lobectomy (date)	Pre/postoperative neurological defect	Pre/postoperative intelligence	Global result
1	19 yr	25	R	M	Déjà vu, chewing, aggression, paranoia, hostility (10–12/mo; 1 grand mal/yr)	(8/61) Into right subiculum	R (9/61)	None/R hemianopsia and coagulation defectᵇ	Normal/normal	Excellent
4	25 yr	37	R	M	Organic dementia; epigastric sensation; automatism (20–30/mo; 0 grand mal/yr)	(2/62) L > R sub-iculum	L (4/62)	R hemiparesis/min or dysphagia, coagulation defectᵇ; R hemiparesis	Low/low	Poor
5	25 yr	47	R	M	Inadequate personality; epigastric cephalic sensations; automatisms (10–20/mo; 1 grand mal/yr)	(3/62) L anterior hippocampal gyrus	L (5/62)	None/mild dysphagia; coagulation defectᵇ	Low normal/low	Fair
7	5 yr	18	L	M	Suicidal schizophrenia, staring, psychic illusions, cephalic pressure, automatic fumbling (12–40/mo; 1 grand mal/yr)	(6/62) R posterior hippocampal gyrus	R (11/62)	None/L homonymous field cut	Low normal/low normal	Excellent
8	12 yr	33	L	M	Inadequate personality; illusion of floating; arrest stare (8–10/mo; 3–4 grand mal/yr)	(10/62) L amygdala	L (12/62)	None/recent memory loss and mild dysphagia	Low normal/low normal	Poor
9	15 yr	20	R	M	Epigastric aura, dreamy state, automatism, fumbling (15–60/mo; 0 grand mal/yr)	(4/63) R midpes	R (7/63)	None/L hemianopsia, slight tremor	Normal/normal	Excellent

Case	Duration	Age	Hand	Sex	Seizure description	Operation/location	Side (date)	Deficit (pre/post)	IQ (pre/post)	Outcome
11	1 yr	13	R	F	Fear, epigastric aura, automatism indeterminate; 1 grand mal/yr	(1/64) L hippocampal gyrus	L (3/64)	None/mild right hemiparesis, hemianopsia	Retarded/improved, but dependent	Excellent
13	1½	23	R	M	Epigastric aura, rushing thoughts, automatisms (10–50/mo; 2 grand mal/yr)	(3/64) R hippocampal gyrus	R (5/64)	None/none	Normal/normal	Excellent
15	3 mo	20	R	F	Vague aura, stare, chewing, (8/mo; 4–6 grand mal/yr)	(7/64) L anterior hippocampal gyrus	L (11/64)	None/paretic R upper extremity; dysphasia	Retarded/retarded	Poor
16	3 mo	20	R	M	Epigastric aura, lip smacking, stare (80–120/mo; 8–10 grand mal/yr)	(11/64) R amygdala, pes	R (3/65)	None/none	Low normal/improved	Excellent
17	15 yr	35	R	M	No aura, walking automatism fumbling (30–40/mo; 6 grand mal/yr)	(1/65) L amygdala, pes	L (6/65)	Memory loss/profound memory loss, right supraquadrantanopsia	Retarded/retarded	Poor
21	1 yr	27	R	M	Nausea, noisy, head and eyes to left; occasional automatism (8/mo; 2–4 grand mal/yr)	(5/66) R temporal lobe	R (7/66)	R peripheral VII palsy/same	Retarded/retarded	Excellent
26	18 yr	23	R	M	Turns pale, gulps, right hand elevated, head to right, automatisms (10–20/mo; 1 grand mal/yr)	(6/67) L hippocampal gyrus, pes	L (9/67)	None/R supraquadrantanopsia	Superior/superior	Excellent
31	5 yr	28	R	F	Aura, fullness in chest, stare, repetitive hand movements (6/mo; 0 grand mal/yr)	(5/68) R hippocampal gyrus	R (12/68)	None/L supraquadrantanopsia	Normal/normal	Excellent

TABLE 2 (Continued)

Case no.	Age at onset of seizures (yr)	Age at surgery (yr)	Handedness	Sex	Seizure character (incidence)	Locus of depth electrodes and complications (date)	Temporal lobectomy (date)	Pre/postoperative neurological defect	Pre/postoperative intelligence	Global result
47	10 yr	17	L	F	Visual aura, automatisms (12/mo; 2 grand mal/yr)	(2/71) R bilateral amygdala; anterior middle and posterior pes; hippocampal gyrus	R (5/71)	None/transient diplopia	Normal/normal	Excellent
48	7 yr	24	R	F	Aura of epigastric sensations, automatisms (3–13/mo; 3 grand mal/yr)	(3/71) R bilateral amygdala; anterior, middle, and posterior pes; 3 positions hippocampal gyrus	R (6/71)	None/none	Average/normal	Excellent
52	1 yr	33	R	M	Psychomotor cephalic aura, dysphagia, head to right) 3–4/mo; 0 grand mal/yr	(7/71) L Meningitis after electrode removal	L (10/71)	None/R supra quadrantanopsia	Average-dull normal/same	Excellent
57	6 yr	23	R	M	Psychomotor type (as many as 7/day; few grand mal/yr)	(11/71) Mesial limbic structure; subcortical foreign body reaction	L (2/72)	None/R supra quadrantanopsia	Normal/normal	Good (6 mo. postoperative)
58	7 yr	16	R	F	Confusion, nausea, emesis; auditory and visual phenomena (2–3/day; 1–2 grand mal/yr)	(11/71) R amygdala; anterior and middle pes; ventroanterior thalamus; anterior cingulate; supplementary motor	R (3/72)	None/dysdiadochokinesia	Low normal/low normal	No temporal lobe seizures; 1–2 nocturnal seizures (4 mo. postoperative)

[a] R, right; L, left; M, male, F, female.
[b] Early focal coagulation was used as a marker.

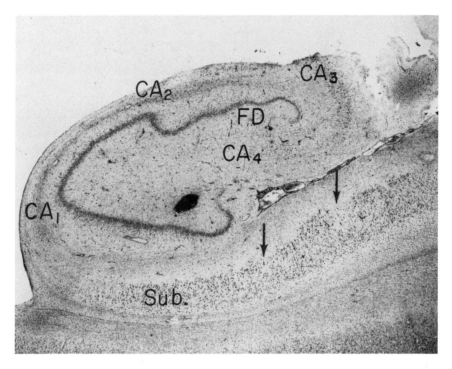

Figure 7. Cross section of the cornu ammonis showing the extent of injury present in the pyramidal cell layer. The neurons of section CA₁ are absent. Some of the neurons of area CA₃ just outside the hilus of the dentate fascia (FD) are present; however, CA₂ and CA₁ are almost completely devoid of any viable pyramidal cells. The cell loss extends into the presubiculum and edges of the subiculum (Sub). There are focal regions of cell loss (arrows) as the layer courses toward the entorhinal cortex. Not easily seen at this low magnification is the fine glial scarring present in the regions with absent neurons. The dark spot in the CA₄ portion of the tissue is due to iron deposited in the vicinity of the tip of an indwelling electrode. Segments of pyramidal cells and processes of the presubiculum and subiculum may be seen at higher power in Figures 14 and 16A–C. (Cases 57.) Gridley stain. Magnification ×10.

(March, 1970), focal right frontal slowing, frequent right frontal sharp wave and spike wave complexes were found in the right anterior temporal region. A pneumoencephalogram was done which revealed paraventricular atrophy manifested by rounding of the right superior lateral ventricle. Depth electrodes were placed in the right amygdala, anterior and mid pes, ventral anterior nucleus of the thalamus, supplementary motor, and anterior cingulate gyrus. The interictal record demonstrated frequent right temporal and generalized spiking. Ictal discharges clearly began in all leads. In March of 1972, right anterior temporal lobectomy was done. The specimen showed losses of neurons and increased numbers of astrocytes in portions of the posterior segments of the dentate gyrus. Further posteriorly transverse sections of the cornu ammonis and subiculum were removed and uti-

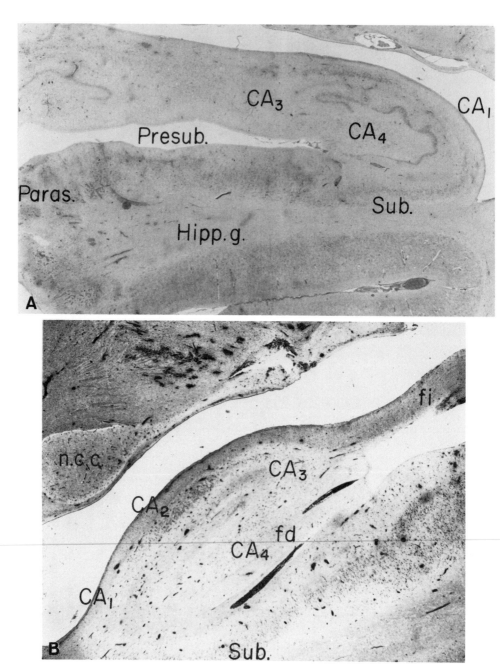

Figure 8. Profound cell loss is evident in all sectors of the cornu ammonis complex. In micrograph A, some of the granular cells of the fascia dentata are preserved. The loss of neurons and associated secondary gliosis, however, extends into the presubiculum (Presub.), subiculum (Sub.), parasubiculum (Paras.) and even more of the remainder of the hippocampal gyrus (Hipp. g.) cortex. Farther posteriorly, micrograph B reveals a few preserved neurons in sector CA₂, subiculum, and presubiculum. fd, Dentate fascia. (Case 7.) Nissl preparations. Magnification ×12.

lized for electron microscopy (see Figures 10 to 13). Additional similar sections were taken for Golgi-Cox preparations.

Light Microscopy

The majority of the cases in this series were studied primarily by light microscopic techniques. Hamartomata were found in the removed whole lobes in 5 of the cases (see Table 1). The pathological anatomy of these lesions varied in the individual cases but was not dissimilar to that described by Cavanagh (6, 7).

Figure 2a–d shows the geometric extent of an astrocytic hamartoma found in Case 6. The diagrams are stylized modifications of camera lucida drawings to show four transverse anatomical sections of a typical resected temporal lobe and here, in particular, Case 6. Straight lines may be seen extending across the drawings of Figure 2a–d at different levels to show positions of indwelling electrodes. The tips are located in regions from which recordings were taken prior to temporal lobe resection. The nature and extent of these abnormalities are unknown when emplacement is carried out; hence, the recording is usually somewhat remote from any interface between lesion and surround. The neurons of the uncal cortex (Figure 2a), the amygdala (Figure 2b), dentate gyrus (Figure 2c), and cornu ammonis (Figure 2d) showed only a minimal deviation from what might be designated as normal. The inferior temporal gyrus, however, revealed only a few neurons and those were caught up in the extensive, though low-grade, proliferation of astrocytes, glial fibrils, and slitlike vascular channels. The microscopic character of this mass may be observed in Figure 3. There is a striking similarity in the locus and extent of another example of this kind of disorder seen in Figure 4a–d, made of Case 55 (Table 1). Again, the cortices and nuclear groupings of the uncus, amygdala, dentate gyrus, and cornu ammonis were relatively normal. The inferior temporal gyrus (Figure 4a, b, and d) was extensively taken up by a hamartoma that involved a wide portion of the gyral cortex. One level in Figure 4c shows the lesion's relationship to the temporal horn of the lateral ventricle but no intimate contact with cortex. The lesion at this level, however, is in position to "intercept" traffic from the hippocampal complex. Only Figure 4b shows macroelectrodes closely adjacent to both lesion and normal-appearing cortex. Microscopically, this hamartoma was composed of numerous oligodendrogliacytes, scattered astrocytes, and a few clusters of neurons that had a rather normal appearance (Figure 5). There were no calcium deposits present.

Although the growth patterns of the lesions encountered in the two cases (Nos. 6 and 55) are rather indolent, the histological character of the tissue is nonetheless rather cellular. In comparison, the abnormal tissue taken from the temporal lobe in Case 56 is composed of only a few fibrous astrocytes, a great number of calcospherites, and fibrous-walled vascular channels (Figure 6). Indwelling electrodes were not utilized in the latter case because the lesion was so apparent from roentgenograms of the skull and the abnormal electrical activity was on the same side. The overall clinical result of lobectomy in the group of patients with hamartomata was very good (see Table 1).

Description of the spatial variations in neuron populations in sclerosis of the cornu ammonis in temporal lobe epilepsy has been adequately made by several investigators (9, 13, 14, 16, 19, 27, 28). Only two cases illustrated by light microscopy in this category are therefore shown here (Cases 57 and 7).

Some description of Case 57 is presented here in order to place subsequent ultrastructural studies in the more generally understood framework of light microscopy. The cornu ammonis and subiculum in this case are illustrated by Figure 7. The neurons of region CA_4 are absent, as are CA_1 and CA_2. There are a few neurons present in CA_3. The loss then extends into the subicular cortex. Ultrastructural studies (see below) were made in the region between the lower edge of CA_1 and the presubiculum. The linearly shaped glial scar, a consequence of the placement of an indwelling electrode, may also be seen in Figure 7. The scar lies deep to the hilus of the fascia dentata.

The findings in Case 7 (Table 2) are those of severe neuron loss of all CA sectors with only a thin residual of the fascia dentata. The severe involvement continues for some distance through the hippocampal cortex and includes the various subdivisions of the subiculum. The entire hippocampal gyrus appears scarred and contracted (Figure 8a). Figure 8b reveals the extensive change at yet another level. Here, however, there is some preservation of the cells of region CA_2, but the subiculum exhibits extensive replacement of neurons with astrocytes and gliosis. In some cases, the neuron loss seemed limited to one portion of the CA_1 sector; but most commonly, the loss and scarring was of much greater magnitude. For instance, in one case, neurons could not be found in any segment of the pyramidal layer.

We have found, as have others (27), that loss of neurons and scarring of the cornu ammonis may be accompanied by similar alterations of variable degree in other portions of the complex, that is, uncus, amygdaloid nucleus. The changes are often subtle in these more remote sectors, and a case pointing up the difficulty in interpretation of minor changes may be seen in Figure 9. The figure shows amygdaloid nucleus with small patches of missing neurons (Case 11). In addition, this patient had hippocampal sclerosis, but there was no continuity between the gliotic cornu ammonis and these small alterations of the amygdaloid nucleus. These losses may be the result of the same insult which was instrumental in the injury of the cornu ammonis or may be due to a completely unrelated episode of hypoxia. Slightly more than 65% of the cases in this series were

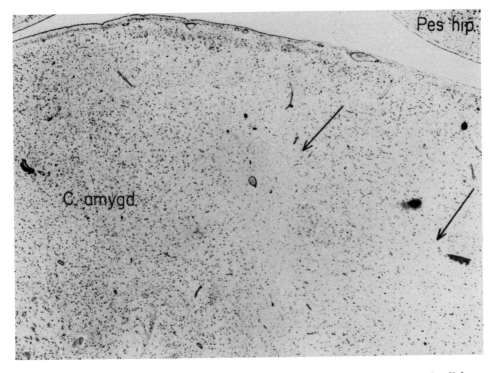

Figure 9. Section of the amygdaloid nucleus, showing a more subtle type of cell loss. At the foci indicated by arrows the neuron loss is most evident. Extending out in a wavelike fashion, however, there is a variable degree of neuron dropout and relative increase in astrocytic nuclei and fibers. Not shown is sclerosis of portions of the cornu ammonis, also seen in this case. amygd., amygdala; hip., hippocampus. (Case 11.) Gridley stain. Magnification ×12.

given the diagnosis of hippocampal sclerosis. The majority of the patients with this structural diagnosis responded very well clinically when the offending lobe was resected. Seventy-three percent did very well, whereas only 21% of these patients experienced a poor result (see Table 2).

Case 30 (Table 3) was found to have a malignant astrocytoma in the lobe resected in 1968. The general response to removal was excellent. Of great interest is the fact that the patient is still active and well.

The poorest clinical results were obtained in the cases in which lesions could not be found in the temporal lobes (Table 4). These tissues were serially sectioned and carefully examined so it is difficult to imagine that an abnormal structural focus might have been missed in such an examination.

ULTRASTRUCTURAL STUDIES

The pyramidal cells of the hippocampal cortex are normally in close parallel alignment. In the presubiculum and subicular cortex of Cases 57 and 58, however, numerous pyramidal cells are missing (see Figures 7 and

TABLE 3

CLINICAL DETAILS OF A CASE WITH A NEOPLASM (3.5%)[a]

Case no.	Age at onset of seizure	Age at surgery	Hand-edness	Sex	Seizure character (incidence)	Locus of depth electrodes and complications (date)	Temporal lobectomy	Pre/postoperative neurological defect	Pre/postoperative intelligence	Global result
30	10	17	R	M	Wandering automatisms, occasionally with left hand (120/mo; 0 grand mal/yr)	(3/68) Bilateral amygdala; and pes hippocampi	R (6/68)	None/L supra quadrantanopsia	Mild retardation/ mild retardation	Excellent

[a] R, right; L, left; M, male.
[b] Astrocytoma III.

TABLE 4

CLINICAL DETAILS OF CASES IN WHOM NO PATHOLOGY WAS FOUND (13.7%)[a]

Case no.	Age at onset of seizure	Age at surgery	Handedness	Sex	Seizure character (incidence)	Locus at depth electrodes and complications (date)	Temporal lobectomy	Pre/postoperative neurological defect	Pre/postoperative intelligence	Global result
10	22 yr	36	R	M	Déjà entendu, lip smacking, automatisms (50–60/mo; 1 grand mal/yr)	(11/63) L caudate nucleus[b]	L (3/64)	None/none	Normal/normal	Poor
18	6 yr	24	R	M	Focal motor (4–5/mo) no aura, walking automatism, lip smacking (15–30/mo; 1 grand mal/yr)	(2/65)[c]	R (5/65)	None/none	Low normal/low normal	Fair
44	21 yr	34	R	M	Focal motor (2–3 a day for 6 yr, automatisms, 1–10/day; 1 grand mal/yr)	(8/70)[d]	R (1/71)	Minimal L hemiparesis occult hydrocephalus/improved drainage	Average–dull/normal	Excellent
53	17 yr	25	R	F	Fear, visual and odor hallucinations, automatisms (40–50/mo; 0 grand mal/yr)	(7/71)[e]	R (10/71)	None/temporary L weakness and dyskinesia	Above normal/same	Fair

[a] R, right; L, left; M, male; F, female.
[b] Bilateral amygdala, uncus; anterior pes; posterior pes, anterior pes, anterior hippocampal gyrus; posterior hippocampal gyrus.
[c] Bilateral amygdala; pes; hippocampal gyrus.
[d] Bilateral amygdala, anterior middle, and posterior pes; 3 positions hippocampal gyrus.
[e] Bilateral amygdala, anterior middle, and posterior pes hippocampus.

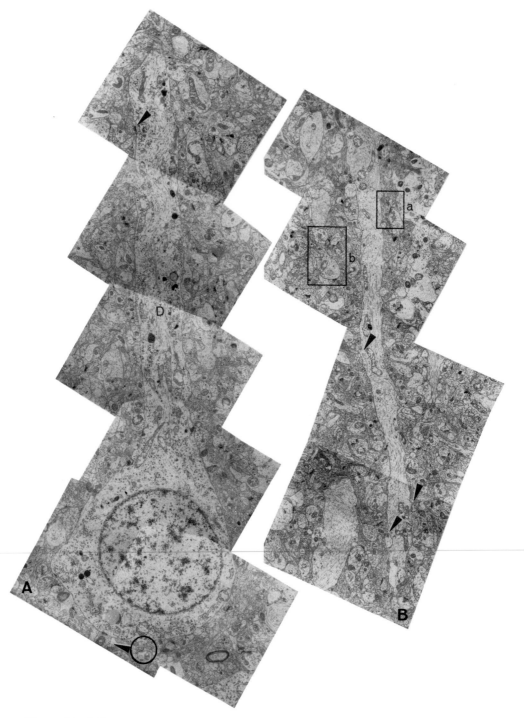

Figure 10. (A) Montage of electron micrograph of pyramidal neuron from the presubiculum. A thick apical dendrite (D) may be seen extending the neuron cytoplasm at one end. Both along the surface of the dendrite and on the neuron soma there are numerous Type I synapses, examples of which are marked (triangular wedge).

8a,b). The neuropil in this cortex is largely replaced by numerous astrocytes and bundles of glial fibrils. Viable pyramidal neurons from this segment of the disordered cortex of Case 58 are illustrated by Figures 10a,b and 11. The blocks from which these cells were taken were oriented parallel to the pyramidal cell apical dendrite. An attempt was made to study the cells in linear continuity. Only partial success is evident, and Figures 10a,b and 11 show the linear extent of such cells in montage. The neuron nucleus is large and occupies much of the flask-shaped cell body. The cytoplasm contains a rich array of lysosomes, rough endoplasmic reticulum, mitochondria, Golgi membranes, microtubules, and smooth vesicles. Spinous processes on these cells were rare, but did occur, and good examples of these are found in Figures 10a and 12. These somal spines are broad-based and straight-tipped and contain no special apparatus, although one or two coated vesicles are commonly found at the base (Figure 12). The boutons ending on these spines contain clear spherical vesicles and occasionally one is found with a dense-cored vesicle. Type I synapses may also be found directed against the soma, but in any one section these do not appear to be numerous. Slips of astrocytic glia are found discontinuously arranged about the neuron surface or along the apical dendrites. The plasmalemma of the cell is otherwise covered by many small dendrites.

In the crowded pyramidal layer, neuroneuronal contacts were apparent, but surface specializations were not found along these broad-based cell contacts. Serial sections of these surfaces were not done, however. Noteworthy, but not shown in figures were numerous alveolate indentations of the pyramidal cell surfaces.

The apical dendrite extends for some distance as a thick unbranched trunk directed toward the molecular layer and in this case (No. 58) toward the surface of the subicular cortex (at the edge of Rose's H_1 sector).

Spines are not found on the apical dendrite, although it must be recognized that the sampling thus far has been small. Microtubles are present within the body of the neuron, but this presence becomes strongly apparent only in the apical dendrite. The incidence of tubules increases in direct proportion to the distance from the cell body (Figure 10a and b). Moreover, as the tubules become more evident, as in Figure 10b, spines and

---

Two spines are found on the soma (one is encircled). (See also Figure 12.) None were found on the thick proximal segment of the apical dendrite. Nor are spines found on cross sections of dendrites at this level. (Case 58.) Ur and Pb stains. Magnification ×3525. (B) Montage of thinner distal segment of the apical dendrite prior to lateral branching. Note increased numbers of microtubules as compared with micrograph A. Along the slender trunk, there are numerous spines (triangular wedge). The complete longitudinal section of spine is located within rectangle a. Other spines are easily found projecting from cross-sectioned dendritic branches and are marked by rectangle b. These spines may be studied more closely in Figure 13A and B. Throughout the neuropil, there are many other spines and associated synapses which are attached to dendritic branchlets. (Case 58). Ur and Pb stains. Magnification ×2925.

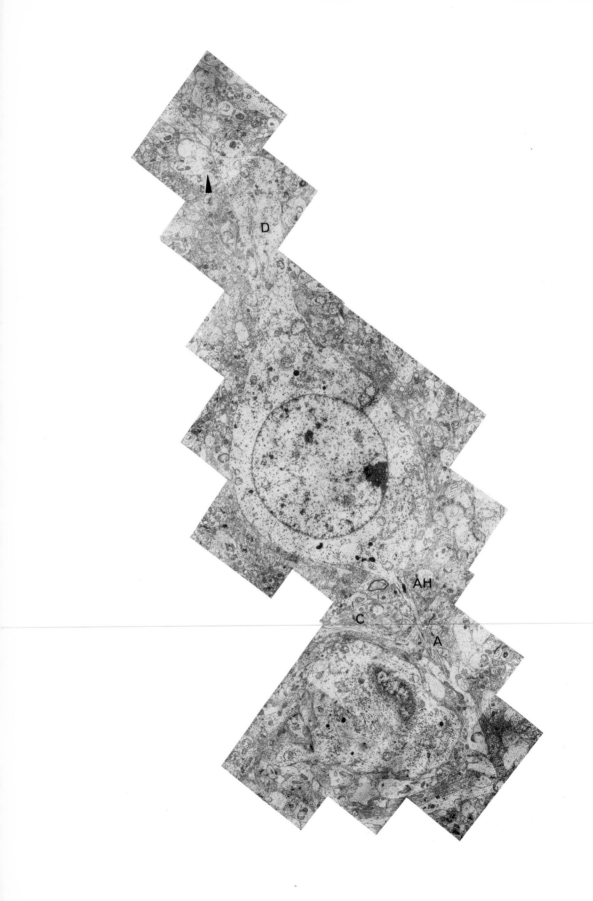

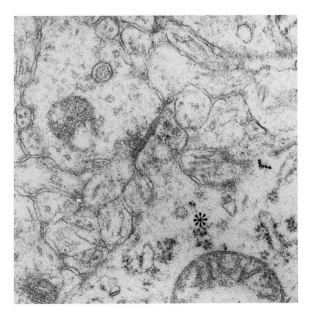

Figure 12. The peculiarly shaped somal spine appears here at greater magnification than that marked in Figure 10A. The appendage is short and blunt with a rather wide neck. One coated vesicle is evident at its base (°) in the neuron cytoplasm at the lower right of the illustration. The presynaptic bouton contains clear spherical vesicles adjacent to the synaptic bar. (Case 58.) Ur and Pb stain. Magnification ×32,800.

other types of synaptic specializations also become apparent. Cross and longitudinal sections of dendrites reveal lateral spinous extensions of dendritic substance. The tip of one type of spine commonly found in the stratum radiatum is blunt and slightly wider than its neck. The neck and proximal portion of this wedge-shaped spine contains an elaborate spine apparatus (Figures 10b and 13a,b). The presynaptic boutons on these spines feature numerous clear, variously sized spherical vesicles, many of which are crowded against a thick electron-dense bar.

The neuropil in this region is composed of myriads of spinous profiles, presynaptic boutons, dendrites, and astrocytes in closely packed array.

Figure 11. A pyramidal cell from the lower edge of CA₁ just before the presubiculum. This cell exhibits not only the initial portion of the apical dendrite (D) but also the axon hillock (AH) and the initial segment of the axon (A). The axon hillock and axon contain small fascicles of microtubules, two multivesicular bodies, but no apparent ribosomes or endoplasmic reticulum. A tangential segment of an additional large neuron may be seen at the lower level of the micrograph montage. There is a small axon (C) just above this unidentified cell which may represent some of a recurrent collateral from the larger neuron. Spines are evident on neither soma nor apical dendrite. An elongated but blunt spike is found projecting out from a cross section of a dendrite near the thick apical dendrite segment (triangular wedge). There are very few synapses on the body of the neuron, and none are found on either the axon hillock or axon. (Case 58). Ur and Pb stains. Magnification ×2850.

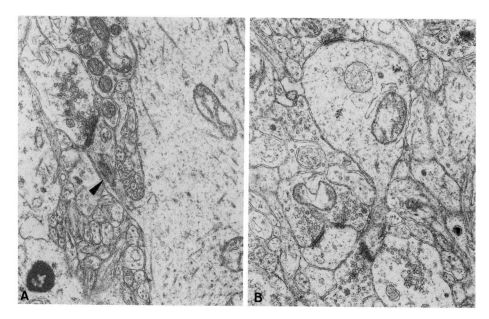

Figure 13. (A) An enlargement of the longitudinal section of a spine enclosed in rectangle a of Figure 10B. Note the wedge shape of the projection. The flat side is composed of the synaptic bar that abuts onto a broad surface of the presynaptic bouton which contains numerous variably sized spherical, clear vesicles and one dense-cored vesicle. Within the spine there is a large spine apparatus (triangular wedge), and a segment of a mitochondrion. The apparatus appears to be continuous with some smooth membranes which extend to the dendrite. The dendritic twigs between the spine and dendrite contain two to three microtubule profiles. (Case 58.) Ur and Pb stains. Magnification ×16,900. (B) A higher-power view of the transversely sectioned dendrite shown within rectangle b of Figure 10B. Projecting from the dendrite is a fairly complete wedge-shaped spine similar to that of Figure 13A, except the spine apparatus is rather indistinct. Also of interest at the top of the illustration is a Type I synapse on the opposite side of this same dendrite. (Case 58.) Ur and Pb stains. Magnification ×16,900.

Rarely are clearly defined unmyelinated or myelinated axons found in this layer.

More distally in the stratum lacunosum and lower reaches of the molecular layer, the synaptic input to the pyramidal cell dendrites becomes more varied and complex. On a short length of distal dendrite (see Figure 14) slim, more-or-less perpendicularly aligned spines with an extensive spine apparatus may be found opposed to each other. Adjacent to these are other short pointed spines with dense synaptic bars disposed within the fork made by spine and dendrite. Flattened synaptic vesicles were seldom found in any boutons examined.

In Figure 11 may be seen the neuron soma, thick apical dendrite, axon hillock, and initial axon segment. Microtubules in this axon segment are gathered in fascicles, irregularly disposed among multivesicular bodies, mitochondria, and lysosomes.

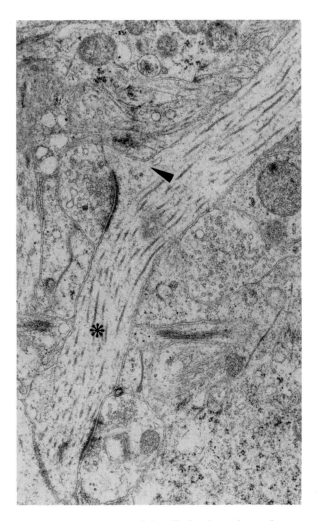

Figure 14. A short segment of pyramidal cell dendrite from the stratum lacunosum (also seen in lower reaches of the molecular layer). The synaptic connections are rich and various. Short conical spines (triangular wedge) synapse with boutons within a fork formed by dendrite and spine. Another form of spine is a narrow perpendicular projection, two of which are shown (°). These contain a large spine apparatus. Not shown on these two spines in apposition, are the presynaptic boutons that synapse on their tips and contain spherical vesicles. Finally, at the lower edge of the dendrites, there is a Type I synapse directly on the same dendrite. (Case 57.) Ur and Pb stains. Magnification ×19,000.

Abnormal Conformations

In each of the cases examined by electron microscopy, there was evidence of ongoing degenerative change in neurons, dendrites, synapses, and axons of various parts of the hippocampal cortex. In Cases 57 and 58, numerous postsynaptic elements of dendrites, including spines, appear as electron-dense profiles with all or most of the contained membranous components degenerated. Presynaptic boutons still exhibit vesicles crowded against

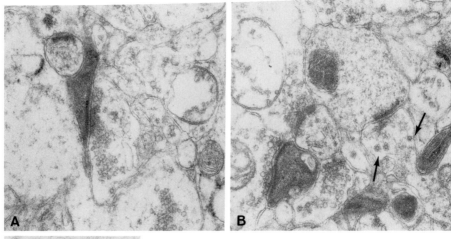

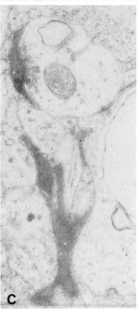

Figure 15. (A) A presynaptic bouton with numerous spherical clear vesicles clustered against the membrane opposite a contracted, electron-dense segment of a dendrite. There is a thick, very dark silhouette of a postsynaptic bar within the darkened receptor. Ur and Pb stains. Magnification ×25,600. (B) Micrograph shows several fragments of dendrite or spinous processes which are dark and contracted with a synaptic construct along one edge. Two segments show less advanced degenerative changes but have large autophagic vacuoles within the postsynaptic structures. In some presynaptic boutons, there are bodies (arrows) that closely resemble complex vesicles. Ur and Pb stains. Magnification ×25,600. (C) The upper portion shows a pre- and postsynaptic complex. The postsynaptic surface is dark and contracted. There are several other dark segments in the photograph which may be parts of the same degenerated neuron. Micrographs A–C are taken from the stratum lacunosum of Case 58. Ur and Pb stains. Magnification ×20,500 for micrograph C.

thick synaptic bars (see Figure 15a–c). The bars are visible as dark silhouettes partially obscured by the electron-dense postsynaptic surfaces. Some of these changes are more advanced than others with scattered autophagic vacuoles appearing amidst frayed and irregularly shaped dendrites. In many of the microregions showing these changes, there appears to be an unusual population of complex vesicles in presynaptic boutons (Figure 15a and b). These processes and altered cells were examined in tissue surfaces far removed from any regions adjacent to surgical incisions. Figure 15a–c are derived from the stratum lacunosum, molecular layer of the edges of the CA₁ sector and just beneath the molecular layer of the presubiculum. The pyramidal cell layer and apical dendrites are also being separately worked up using techniques that combine Golgi preparations and electron microscopy.

Further evidence of continuing neuronal disease may be seen in Figure 16a–c. These alterations in the normal conformation of axons were found in stratum oriens, alveus, and within and below the lower regions of the presubicular cortex. Altered myelinated axons were characterized by contained vacuoles (Figure 16a and c), absence of microtubules, and peeling away of myelin lamellae. In some regions where these changes were most advanced, thick fascicles of glial fibrils were found. It was not within the scope of this study to determine if the injured axons of the alveus were efferent or afferent.

DISCUSSION

That the patients in this series suffered with temporal lobe epilepsy was established by a descriptive history of the seizures and ancillary data obtained from both conventional electroencephalography and indwelling temporal lobe electrodes. Early in the study, electrodes were implanted depending on evidence of electrical abnormality on one side or the other as obtained from scalp electrodes. Presently it is deemed desirable to place indwelling electrodes bilaterally to establish the sidedness of the seizures. It often takes 4–6 weeks for a spontaneous seizure to be recorded and studied. Under such circumstances, the patient's drug regimen for seizure control, has had to be lightened in order that overt abnormal electrical patterns might be observed and lateralization established. The electrodes shown in Figures 2a–c and 4b–d were not drawn to scale, but their placement on the drawings is accurate and relative to existant lesions. Subsequent to adequate recording of both evoked and spontaneous activity, the electrodes were withdrawn and the tiny channels within the temporal lobe, bone, and scalp were allowed to heal. The opportunity to study healing in scalp and bony tissues has fortunately been lacking. The tissues of the temporal lobe, however, have usually shown a stringlike strand of densely packed astrocytes in the narrow electrode bed (see Figures 7 and 8a,b).

As with other case series of this type, we have not observed any differences in incidence of lesions in one sex or the other. Similarly, handedness is not a significant factor although it is of interest that more right-sided lobectomies have been done. Patients that were classed psychologically as being retarded prior to operation were improved only insofar as the seizure pattern might have contributed to their psychological deficit. Many patients were left with a superior quadrantanopsia or other degrees of visual loss relative to the severance of Meyer's loop. Two in the series suffered loss of recent memory and mild hemiparesis was found in 3. The rationale for many of the clinical details of this group of patients is considered in the chapters by R. D. Walter and by P. H. Crandall in this volume.

We were able, of course, to examine the temporal lobe on only one side

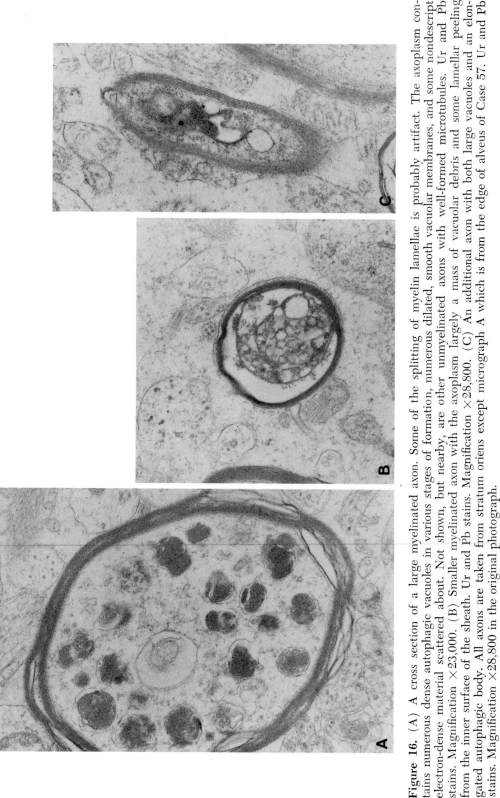

Figure 16. (A) A cross section of a large myelinated axon. Some of the splitting of myelin lamellae is probably artifact. The axoplasm contains numerous dense autophagic vacuoles in various stages of formation, numerous dilated, smooth vacuolar membranes, and some nondescript electron-dense material scattered about. Not shown, but nearby, are other unmyelinated axons with well-formed microtubules. Ur and Pb stains. Magnification ×23,000. (B) Smaller myelinated axon with the axoplasm largely a mass of vacuolar debris and some lamellar peeling from the inner surface of the sheath. Ur and Pb stains. Magnification ×28,800. (C) An additional axon with both large vacuoles and an elongated autophagic body. All axons are taken from stratum oriens except micrograph A which is from the edge of alveus of Case 57. Ur and Pb stains. Magnification ×28,800 in the original photograph.

and, since there have been no postmortems in the series,[*] one must either presume that the opposite side is normal or that there possibly may be abnormalities that are not contributing to any great extent to the abnormal electrical pattern obtained from scalp EEGs.

There is no real incongruity between this series of cases and those reported by Falconer (16) insofar as lesion substrates in epilepsy related to the temporal lobe are concerned. Hamartomata composed essentially of glia, both astrocytic and oligodendritic, reached the proportion of 25% of his cases, but slightly less than 18% in ours. The first three brief illustrative case reports (Nos. 6, 55, 56) are derived from data catalogued in Table 1, and each has a different histological variety of hamartoma. The third case (No. 56) features a rare epileptogenic lesion and merits some further comment. Hemangioma calcificans, in the context of temporal lobe epilepsy, has been reported (18, 20, 31). These masses have been found commonly in a periventricular subcortical location beneath the temporal horn or trigone. Other loci have been within or near the Sylvian fissure (31). Most have been apparent on standard roentgenograms of the skull; but, of course, are not characteristic enough to warrant histological diagnosis by this means.

Although these lesions are comprised of mixtures of abnormal hyalinized vessels and glia, angiograms do not reveal any unusual vascular makeup. Microgyria have been found associated with these masses in a father and his four children, pointing up a possible congenital nature (20). Similar calcifications, although in locations other than temporal lobe, have been observed with microencephaly (1, 25). The onset of fits associated with hamartomata generally has been above the age of 10 (28, 31). Seizures began in this case, however, at 3 months. This suggests that the situation of the stimulating nidus was especially favorable to excitation of mesial limbic structures, whereas others must grow and expand to reach such a point. At any rate, this is the only case (see Table 1) in the hamartoma group that had a history of seizures before 9 years.

In all reported series, including the present one, the site of predilection of the various degrees of neuronal loss and glial scarring found in most cases of psychomotor epilepsy, is the hippocampus (13, 14, 19, 28, 35). Hippocampal sclerosis was found in half of Falconer's cases (16) which is comparable to this present group although the latter is slightly higher (65.6%). The extent of cell loss and distribution varied. It included subtle lesions, in which only neurons of the CA_4 fields were absent except for an associated lesion in the amygdala (endfolium sclerosis as in Case 9, not illustrated). It also included more severe injury in which the neurons of

---

[*] There have been 3 deaths in the series; 1 patient died at the time of implantation, and 2 other patients who did not have temporal lobe resections subsequently died. In none of these instances have we had postmortem studies. Details of these 3 patients are not included in the tables.

the pyramidal layer were missing and a case in which the hippocampus is reduced to a dense glial scar (Figure 8a and b). In none of the cases was the loss confined to the CA$_1$ field or Sommer's sector (35, 38).

Three additional abbreviated case histories (Nos. 7, 57, and 58) of typical patients in the hippocampal sclerosis category (Table 2) have been included in this report because they serve to illustrate both the early age of onset of seizures with this lesion and the topical neuron loss. The latter varies from apparently complete neuron loss in Case 7 and loss of pyramidal cell layer and retention of dentate gyrus in Case 57 to restricted loss of CA$_4$ in Case 9 (only focal amygdaloid lesions are illustrated in Case 9). There is scattered loss of neurons but a similar pattern of preservation throughout the hippocampal gyrus of Case 58. Neuron losses in mesial sclerosis, in addition to EEG findings, clinical diagnosis, and study of hypoxic changes in the brain, as a whole, have been investigated in 55 autopsied cases by Margerison and Corsellis (27). They found other widely scattered hypoxic cerebral lesions in a great majority of a group of 55 brains, two-thirds of which had hippocampal sclerosis. Such variations may be present in our series, but there is little clinical evidence of it, and the generally good results precludes our immediate search for it.

In approximately 14% of our cases we could find no evidence of disease in the resected temporal lobes. It is of great interest that generally poor clinical results were achieved with this set of patients. Such an outcome could be due to a remote lesion effect as suggested by Falconer and co-authors (15). The EEG abnormalities in his patients seemed to originate in the anterior part of the temporal lobe, but small calcified glial neoplasms were found in the posterior portion of the middle temporal gyrus. The lesions were calcified; hence, local removal was done rather than complete anterior lobectomy. We did not find in this group any calcified lesion by roentgenogram, although there could be a small lesion posterior to the lobectomy resection line.

In retrospect, the patients without local disease in the cornu ammonis represented a unique opportunity from the ultrastructural point of view, since it may be possible to study "normal" neuronal patterns, dendritic arborization, branching, and spine types and numbers in the human hippocampal cortex.

The Scheibels (36) have cited Demoor (12) as probably the first investigator to use Golgi techniques to examine the cortex in human epilepsy. Demoor reported a uniform loss of spines from the pyramidal cells of a "cortex." Westrum and co-workers (47) have also reported a reduction in dendritic branching and spines in addition to dendritic varicosities—all occurred adjacent to epileptogenic foci experimentally induced with alumina cream injected into the monkey cortex. Similar findings have been reported by Scheibel and Scheibel (36) in human epileptogenic hippocampus (see also the chapter by the Scheibels in this volume). We have examined some of the pyramidal neurons of the CA₁ region and parts of the subicular cortex by ultrastructural techniques. The montage of pyramidal neurons shown in Figures 10a, b and 11 reveals the similarity of these neurons to those shown so well by electron microscopy in the rabbit by Hamlyn (23) and earlier with Golgi staining in various mammals by Cajal (32, 33).

The shafts of the apical dendrites examined were generally smooth, although distally in the stratum lacunosum, spines with an elaborate spine apparatus were encountered. Such spines had to be searched out, however. More remote, curved, finer dendritic processes often had a rather rich synaptic input with two kinds of spines, as well as nonspinous synapses. All the presynaptic sacs ending on spines and the dendritic shafts contained clear spherules with occasional dense cored vesicles. Flattened types of clear vesicles were not found in presynaptic sacs ending on dendrites or soma spines. Here, problems inherent in both sampling and immersion fixation must be appreciated. It is very possible that both factors might introduce errors, especially in regard to the existence of flattened vesicles in this cortex. It is tempting to speculate on the lack of inhibitory input their absence might infer, but with immersion fixation and lack of good normal human ultrastructural control, such speculations are dangerous. Varicosities seen in Golgi preparations were not encountered in toluidine blue-stained thick Epon sections. Hence, we have no data on the fine structure of these "nodulations."

The lack of spines on pyramidal cell dendrites may be the reflection of a plastic property by which spines respond negatively to a loss of presynaptic input (8); or the spines may not have developed from the outset in the newborn infant for similar reasons (21). This loss could result from either chronic injury stemming from the initial hypoxic insult eventuated in hippocampal sclerosis or from damage incident to the seizures. The possibility, then, of deafferentation as a cause of spine loss is real when one considers the contracted, darkly stained granular matrix of dendrites and associated synapses shown in Figure 15a, b and the evidence of ongoing axonal degeneration illustrated in Figure 16a–c. The dendritic and bouton degenerative changes here are similar to those described by Alksne and co-authors (2) in hippocampus of the rat after section of the ventral hippocampal commissure. Degeneration hypersensitivity possibly does influence the ictal substrate in these cortices.

To answer some of the problems that have arisen in the course of these studies, such as tracing the degenerating dendrites and axons, direct examinations of neurons shown to have deficient numbers of spines, and the meaning of the dendritic varicosities, we are exploring the possibilities offered by combinations of Golgi impregnation for survey and electron microscopy for fine detail in the manner of Stell (41) and Blackstad (4):

Summary

1. Twenty-nine patients with psychomotor epilepsy were investigated by the use of depth electrodes, treated by anterior temporal lobectomy, and evaluated by serial sections of the resected lobes.

2. In 65% of the lobes, hippocampal sclerosis was demonstrated; hamartomata were found in 18%; one malignant neoplasm was revealed, and no lesion was evident in 14%.

3. The majority (73%) of the patients with changes in the cornu ammonis and 100% of the cases with hamartomata responded very well to this surgical treatment. Less benefit could be demonstrated in most of the cases in whom pathological findings were either veiled or remote.

4. Electron microscopy was done on tissues from the most recently studied cases of hippocampal sclerosis. The apical dendrites of some pyramidal cells of the CA_1 sector and portions of the subicular cortex were found to have fewer spines than might be expected. Moreover, evidence of ongoing degeneration of boutons, spines, and axons in these cortices were obtained.

5. The current investigation being carried out on new cases utilizes supporting data obtained by closer collaboration with masters of other techniques such as Golgi impregnations and cytohistochemistry to aid in ultrastructural evaluation of whole neurons and glia which are shown to have evident abnormalities.

6. The possible meanings of these findings have been partially discussed.

REFERENCES

1. Alexander, L., and Woodhall, B., Calcified epileptogenic lesions as caused by incomplete interference with the blood supply of the diseased areas. *J. Neuropathol. Exp. Neurol.*, 1943, **2**: 1–33.

2. Alksne, J. F., Blackstad, T. W., Walberg, F., and White, L. E., Electron microscopy of axon degeneration: A valuable tool in experimental neuroanatomy. *Ergeb. Anat. Entwicklungsgesch.*, 1966, **39**: 1–31.

3. Bailey, P., and Gibbs, F. A., The surgical treatment of psychomotor epilepsy. *JAMA*, 1951, **145**: 365–370.

4. Blackstad, T. W., Mapping of experimental axon degeneration by electron microscopy of Golgi preparations. *Z. Zellforsch. Mikrosk. Anat.*, 1965, **67**: 819–834.

5. Bouchet and Cazauvieilh, De l'épilepsie considerée dans ses rapports avec l'aliénation mentale. *Arch. Gen. Med.*, 1825, **9**: 510–541.

6. Cavanagh, J. B., On certain small tumors encountered in the temporal lobe. *Brain*, 1958, **81**: 389–405.

7. Cavanagh, J. B., Falconer, M. A., and Meyer, A., Some pathogenic problems of temporal lobe epilepsy. In: *Temporal Lobe Epilepsy* (M. Baldwin and P. Bailey, Eds.). Thomas, Springfield, Illinois, 1958: 140–148.

8. Colonnier, M., Experimental degeneration in the cerebral cortex. *J. Anat.* 1964, **98**: 47–53.

9. Corsellis, J. A. N., The incidence of Ammon's horn sclerosis. *Brain*, 1957, **80**: 193–208.

10. Crandall, P. H., Walter, R. D., and Rand, R. W., Clinical applications of studies on stereotactically implanted electrodes in temporal-lobe epilepsy. *J. Neurosurg.*, 1963, **20**: 827–840.

11. Crome, L., A morphological critique of temporal lobectomy. *Lancet*, 1955, **1**: 882–884.

12. Demoor, J., La mécanisme et la signification de l'état moniliforme des neurones. *Ann. Soc. Sci. Med. Nat. Brux.*, 1898, **7**: 205–250.

13. Earle, K. M., Baldwin, M., and Penfield, W., Incisural sclerosis and temporal lobe seizures produced by hippocampal herniation at birth. *Arch. Neurol. Psychiatry*, 1953, **69**: 27–42.

14. Falconer, M. A., The significance of mesial temporal sclerosis (Ammon's horn sclerosis) in epilepsy. *Guys Hosp. Rep.*, 1968, **117**: 1–12.

15. Falconer, M. A., Driver, M. V., and Serafetinides, E. A. Temporal lobe epilepsy due to distant lesions: Two cases relieved by operation. *Brain*, 1962, **85**: 521–534.

16. Falconer, M. A., Hill, D., Meyer, A., Mitchell, W., and Pond, D. A., Treatment of temporal-lobe epilepsy by temporal lobectomy: A survey of findings and results. *Lancet*, 1955, **1**: 827–835.

17. Falconer, M. A., and Kennedy, W. A., Epilepsy due to small focal temporal lesions with bilateral independent spike-discharging foci. *J. Neurol. Neurosurg. Psychiatry*, 1961, **24**: 205–212.

18. Falconer, M. A., and Pond, D. A., Temporal lobe epilepsy with personality and behavior disorders caused by an unusual calcifying lesion. *J. Neurol. Neurosurg. Psychiatry*, 1953, **16**: 234–244.

19. Falconer, M. A., Serafetinides, E. A., and Corsellis, J. A. N., Etiology and pathogenesis of temporal lobe epilepsy. *Arch. Neurol.*, 1964, **10**: 233–248.

20. Geyelin, H. R., and Penfield, W., Cerebral calcification epilepsy. *Arch. Neurol. Psychiatry*, 1929, **21**: 1020–1043.

21. Globus, A., and Scheibel, A. B., Loss of dendrite spines as an index of presynaptic terminal patterns. *Nature (Lond.)*, 1966, **212**: 463–465.

22. Gowers, W. R., *Epilepsy and Other Chronic Convulsive Diseases: Their Causes, Symptoms and Treatment* (1881). American Academy of Neurology Reprint Series. Dover, New York, 1964: Vol. 1.

23. Hamlyn, L. H., An electron microscope study of pyramidal neurons in the Ammon's horn of the rabbit. *J. Anat.*, 1963; **97**: 189–201.

24. Jasper, H., Pertuisset, B., and Flanigin, H., EEG and cortical electrograms in patients with temporal lobe seizures. *Arch. Neurol. Psychiatry*, 1951, **65**: 272–290.

25. Jervis, G. A., Microcephaly with extensive calcium deposits and demyelination. *J. Neuropathol. Exp. Neurol.*, 1954, **13**: 318–329.

26. Lindenberg, R., Compression of brain arteries as pathogenetic factor for tissue necroses and their areas of predilection. *J. Neuropathol. Exp. Neurol.*, 1955, **14**: 223–235.

27. Margerison, J. H., and Corsellis, J. A. N., Epilepsy and the temporal lobes. *Brain*, 1966, **89**: 499–530.
28. Meyer, A., Falconer, M. A., and Beck, E., Pathological findings in temporal lobe epilepsy. *J. Neurol. Neurosurg. Psychiatry*, 1954, **17**: 276–285.
29. Penfield, W., and Flanigin, H., Surgical therapy of temporal lobe seizures. *Arch. Neurol. Psychiatry*, 1950, **64**: 491–500.
30. Penfield, W., and Paine, K., Results of surgical therapy for focal epileptic seizures. *Can. Med. Assoc. J.*, 1955, **73**: 515–531.
31. Penfield, W., and Ward, A., Calcifying epileptogenic lesions. *Arch. Neurol. Psychiatry*, 1948, **60**: 20–36.
32. Ramón y Cajal, S., *The Structure of Ammon's Horn*. Thomas, Springfield, Illinois, 1968.
33. Ramón y Cajal, S., *Histologie du systéme nerveux*. Consejo Superior De Investigaciones Cientificas, Madrid, 1955: Vol. II.
34. Rasmussen, T., and Jasper, H., Temporal lobe epilepsy: Indication for operation and surgical technique. In: *Temporal Lobe Epilepsy* (M. Baldwin and P. Bailey, Eds.). Thomas, Springfield, Illinois, 1958: 440–460.
35. Sano, K., and Malamud, N., Clinical significance of sclerosis of the cornu ammonis. *Arch. Neurol. Psychiatry*, 1953, **70**: 40–53.
36. Scheibel, M. E., and Scheibel, A. B., On the nature of dendritic spines— report of a workshop. *Commun. Behav. Biol.*, 1968, **1**: Pt. A: 231–265.
37. Scholz, W., The contribution of patho-anatomical research to the problem of epilepsy. *Epilepsia*, 1959, **1**: 36–55.
38. Sommer, W., Erkrankung des Ammonshorns als aetiologisches Moment der Epilepsie. *Arch. Psychiatr.*, 1880, **10**: 631–675.
39. Spielmeyer, W., Zur Pathogenese ortlich elektiver Gehirnveranderungen. *Z. Gesamte Neurol. Psychiat.*, 1925, **99**: 756–776.
40. Stauder, K. H., Epilepsie und Schlafenlappen. *Arch. Psychiatr.*, 1936, **104**: 181–212.
41. Stell, W. K., Correlation of retinal cytoarchitecture and ultrastructure in Golgi preparations. *Anat. Rec.*, 1965, **153**: 389–398.
42. Talairach, J., David, M., and Tournoux, P., *L'exploration chirurgicale stéreo-taxique du lobe temporale dans l'épilepsie temporale; Repérage antomique stéreotaxique et technique chirurgicale*. Masson, Paris, 1958.
43. Velasco, O. P., Contribuicao anatomo-clinica as atuais concepcoes sobre a epilepsia. *Arch. Neuropsiquiat.*, Sao Paulo, 1950, **8**: 301–334.
44. Venable, J. H., and Coggeshall, R. A., A simplified lead citrate stain for use in electron microscopy. *J. Cell Biol.*, 1965, **25**: 407–408.
45. Ward, A. A., The epileptic neurone. *Epilepsia*, 1961, **2**: 70–80.
46. Ward, A. A., Epilepsy. *Int. Rev. Neurobiol.*, 1961, **3**: 137–186.
47. Westrum, L. E., White, L. E., and Ward, A. A., Jr. Morphology of the experimental epileptic focus. *J. Neurosurg.*, 1964, **21**: 1033–1046.

AUTHOR INDEX

Numbers in parentheses are reference numbers and indicate that an author's work is referred to although his name is not cited in the text. Numbers in italics show the page on which the complete reference is listed.

M

MacCarty, C. S., 67(11), *93*
MacDonald, H. N. A., 67(11), *93*
McEwen, B. S., 200(32), *211*
McIntyre, D. C., 198(35), *211*
McLardy, T., 204(62), *212*
Maclean, P. D., 88(58), *96*, 196(59), 205(81), *212, 213*
McMurthy, J. G., 137(48), 146(48), *150*
Maekawa, K., 12(10a), 13, *24*
Magendie, F., 1, *9*
Magliocco, E. B., 174, *188*
Magnus, O., 69(47), *95*
Magoun, H. W., 80(7), 92(7), *93*, 121(32), *149*
Mailiani, A., 137(48), 146(48), *150*
Malamud, N., 339(35), 340(35), 369(35), 370(35), *374*
Mann, L. B., Jr., 174, *186*
Mano, T., 19(21a), *25*
Marchand, H., *230*
Marcus, E. M., 171(31), *186*
Marczynski, T., 229(59), *233*
Margerison, J. H., 100(15), *119*, 178, *187, 188*, 339(27), 340(27), 356(27), 370, *374*
Mark, V. H., 67(48), *95*, 261(26, 29, 45), 263(45), *282, 283*
Markham, C. H., 109(4), *118*
Marko, A., 123(29), *149*
Marossero, F., 19(2), *24*, 312(25), *336*
Marshall, C., 260(44), 261(71), *283, 285*
Marteret, H. G., 49, *63*
Martin, A. R., 145(30), *149*
Maso-Subirana, E., 52(49), *64*
Maspes, P., 312, *336*
Matthews, M. A., 143, *149*
Matthysse, S., 200(60), 205(61), *212*
Mattson, R. H., 226(47), *232, 233*
Maxwell, D. S., 32(7), *35*
Mazars, G., 307, *309*
Mazza, S., 220(18), 227(18), *231*
Mehler, W. R., 139, *148*, 204(71), *213*
Meier-Ewert, K., 219, 227, 228(38), *232*
Meldrum, B. S., 37(41), 48(41), 53(41), 61(41), *64*
Mempel, E., 289(29), 290(29), *310*
Menini, C., 39(12), 46(12), 47(48), 48(38, 42), 49(12), 53(38), 54(53), 58(35, 36, 42, 43), *62, 63, 64, 65*
Mergenhagen, D., 19(38), *26*
Merlis, S., 174, *186*
Merritt, H. H., 171(14), *185*
Mettler, F. A., 205(64), 208, *212*
Meyer, A., 100(16), *119*, 312, 335(28), *336*, 339(28), 340(16), 355(7), 356(16, 18), 369(16, 28), 372, 373, *374*

Meyer, M., 88(4, 5), *93*, 162(1), *167*
Meyer-Michelheit, R. W., 260(41), *283*
Meyers, R., 260(46), *283*
Meynert, T., 203(65), *212*
Mignone, R. J., 189(66), *212*
Miller, R. H., 67(22), *94*
Mills, L., 221(53), 223(53), 228(53), *233*, 307(24, 25), *310*
Milner, B., 116(19, 22), *119*
Milstein, V., 171(33, 54, 55), *186, 187*, 190(84), 200(84), 208(85), *213*
Mingrino, S., 260(5), 271(5), *281*
Mirsky, A. F., 171(34), 178(46), *179*, 180(36), 184(36), *186, 187*
Mitchell, W., 340(16), 356(16), 369(16), *373*
Miyazaki, K., 227(27), *231*
Moe, P. G., 173(37), *186*
Mombelli, A., 47(7), *62*
Moniava, E. S., 159, *170*
Monti, A., 311, *336*
Morel, P., 67(8, 9), 69(8), 74(8), 80(9), 88(8, 9), 91(8), 92(9), *93*, 99(3), *118*, 307(4), *309*
Morison, B., 313, *337*
Morita, H., 145(21), *149*
Morocutti, C., 21(39), *26*, 46, *64*
Morossero, M. D., 67(50), 80(50), 92(50), *96*
Morrell, F., 91(49), *95*, 198(67), *212*
Moruzzi, G., 121(32), *149*
Mountcastle, V. B., 139(33), *149*
Musella, L., 102, *119*
Musgrave, F. S., 17(44), *26*
Mutani, R., 220(6), 227(6), *230*

N

Nacimiento, A. C., 17(40), *26*
Nakajima, Y., 145(5), *148*
Nakamura, Y., 208(85), *213*
Naquet, R., 15(41), *26*, 37(27, 41, 45), 39(12), 46(12, 20), 47(48), 48(9, 40, 41), 49(9, 12, 13, 28), 52(9, 10), 53(9, 13, 34, 38, 41), 55(9), 56(27), 58(18, 35, 42, 43), 60(17, 39), 61(27, 41), *62, 63, 64*, 80(7), 92(7), *93*
Narabayashi, H., 260(48), *283*
Nashold, B. S., 261(74), *285*
Nathan, P. W., 304(3), *309*
Nauta, W. J. H., 88(84), *97*, 161, 162, *170*, 203, 204(68, 69, 70, 71, 91), 205, 208(44), *211, 212, 213, 214*
Neher, E., 19(37), *26*
Nelson, P. G., 146, *149*
Neuweiler, G., 19(38), *26*
Ng, L. K. Y., 201(15), *210*

SUBJECT INDEX